Recipes For life

Nourishing recipes from Australia's
favourite wellness influencers to feed
your body and soul

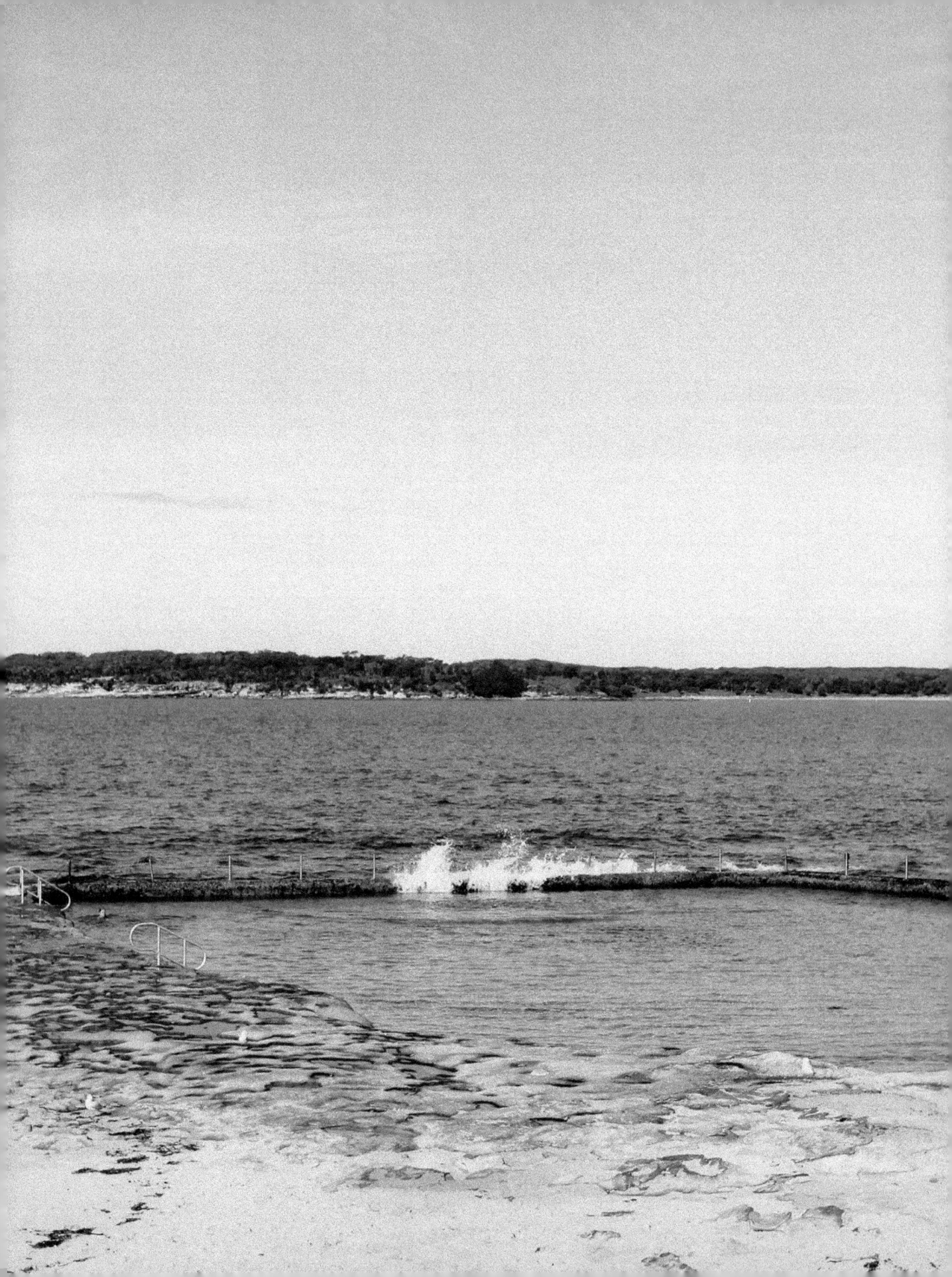

Contents

Introduction

In recent times, it seems that our relationship with food has become overly complicated, tied up in emotions, self-worth, body image and perfectionism. Due to the pressures of modern society, where self compassion is low and expectations are far too high, it has become all too easy to fall victim to diets that are overly restrictive, punitive and sometimes just whack.

We live in a world where we pick, poke and prod our bodies, wishing we could be better and look different. The latest diets are constantly pushed down our throats and make us believe they'll solve all our problems. The reality however, is that these diets serve to push us further into a cycle of self-criticism, guilt and shame.

Recipes for Life is a cookbook that aims to cut through the BS of this diet culture, helping you take back control of your relationship with food.

Here, you'll find a selection of simple, nourishing recipes contributed by some of Australia's favourite influencers in the health and wellness space. These contributors come from all walks of life. Some are registered dieticians, nutritionists and personal trainers, while others others use their social platform as a way to spread the message about body positivity and a balanced lifestyle. But one thing we all have in common is our passion for cooking delicious food and celebrating the joy that this brings to our lives.

Many of these women have had a challenging relationship with food and their bodies at some point in their lives, but have overcome this through support, education and, above all, learning to love food again. They now strive to promote a healthy, balanced lifestyle that replaces guilt and low self-worth with empowerment and self-compassion.

Within these pages you'll find recipes filled with nutritious ingredients that will fuel your body to be its best, without you having to overthink it. With each mouthful, you'll know you're getting a good dose of protein, fibre, vitamins, minerals and antioxidants that help your body do all the wonderful things it deserves to. While many of these recipes use more nutrient-dense alternatives, this by no means suggests that you're restricted to just eating this way.

For example, sometimes you'll see the use of cacao instead of chocolate, or quinoa pasta instead of wheat-based pasta. That's not because other foods are 'bad' or 'wrong'. If you want to eat pasta and chocolate, we're right there with you! We're simply using these alternative ingredients to help you get the best possible nutrition from your food.

Recipes for Life is a book about feeding your soul just as much as it is about feeding your body; sometimes that means having a smoothie bowl after a gym class and sometimes that means eating a piece of cake at your friend's birthday. It's called balance, and it's called life.

You'll also notice that we haven't included calorie counts or macronutrient breakdowns for these recipes, as we believe food is about so much more than the specific macronutrients it contains. It's about celebration, togetherness, fulfillment and, of course, deliciousness! Whether calorie counting is something you currently do, or whether you're trying to move away from that, Recipes for Life is a space where you can come to forget about the intricacies of food. It's a place to simply enjoy cooking delicious, healthful dishes that make you feel amazing inside and out.

So turn the pages and discover a life where food doesn't control or define you, but instead enriches you. These recipes will help you heal your relationship with food, teach you to stop being such a dick to yourself, and allow you to move around in this world proudly and unapologetically, perfectly you.

How to use this book

Recipes

Within these pages, you'll find our recipes divided into sections; breakfast, mains, snacks and desserts. But don't feel like this has to define the way you eat. If you want to have a breakfast tofu scramble at dinner, go for it! Breakfast for dinner is totally a thing. These dishes are here to help support you on your path to health, whatever that looks like.

Holistic Health

Throughout this book, you'll also find five chapters dedicated to Mindful Movement, Body Positivity, Self-Compassion and Work & Play. While a nourishing diet is indeed a very important part of a healthy life, it's only one small part of a much larger whole. These other five areas will help you achieve a completely holistic approach to your health, so that you can feel content and happy within yourself. There's no point in smashing it out at the gym and 'eating clean' if you're just going to hate on yourself when you look in the mirror, or beat yourself up at work.

Within each of these chapters you'll hear the story of some incredible Australian women who have faced challenges and hardships in each of these areas, which they have learned from and overcome. They are truly inspiring stories that we hope will embolden you to push through your own barriers of self-doubt, fear and judgement - whether that means becoming more accepting of your body, or finding a better work-life balance.

There will be practical tips and advice along the way that you can utilise in your everyday life to help you begin your own journey towards a similar place of holistic wellbeing.

We want to help you achieve the kind of internal peace that so many of us have found through focusing on these five areas of our lives, while combining them with a nutritious diet. It might feel like a lot of work at first, but we guarantee that once you begin to incorporate these elements into your routine, you'll wonder how you ever lived without them.

Tips & Tricks

Before you jump straight into cooking up a storm, take the time to have a look through some of the useful information we've created for you in the first few sections. You'll find helpful advice on everything from meal prep hacks and how to shop in season, to eating healthy on a budget.

We've also included all the important cooking-y stuff that you might need to know

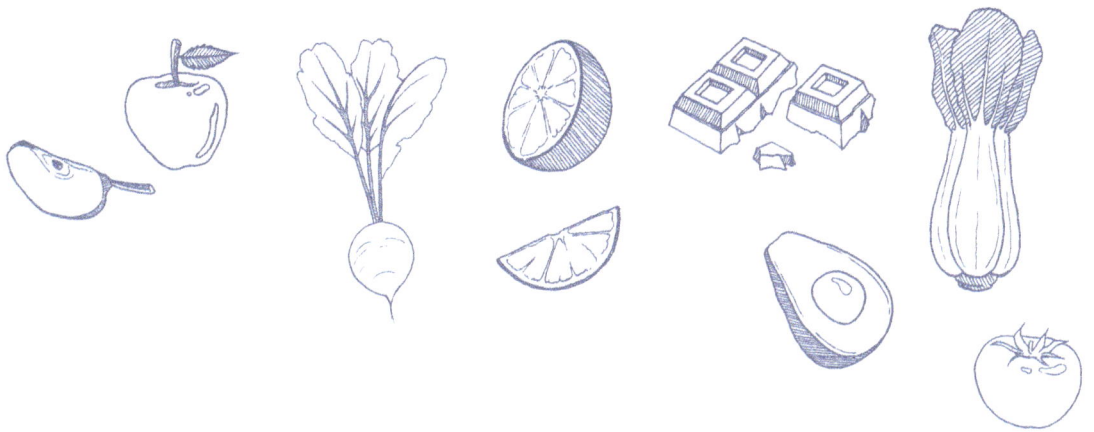

if you're needing to do anything like convert grams into ounce or celsius into fahrenheit - shout out to our American babes!

Eating Healthy on a Budget

It's the age old conundrum that plagues us all: do I buy that dress on The Iconic, or do I eat meals other than two-minute noodles this week?

Expensive health food products, such as protein powder, maca, bee pollen and acai, have become increasingly popular, leading people to believe they need to spend big to live healthily.

But we're here to tell you that you don't have to choose between healthy food and that dress!

While there's certainly a place for high-end ingredients like those mentioned above (you'll find them featured occasionally within this book), it by no means you need to eat them in order to achieve a diet that is full of all the nutrients your body requires to flourish.

When planning your meals, we want to help you get back to basics. Strip it all back and look beyond the branding, fancy packaging and hype. Fresh, whole foods are what will help your body thrive and that's some of the cheapest produce on supermarket shelves. The best examples of these foods are fresh fruits and vegetables, lean sources of protein, such as tinned or dry legumes, tofu, eggs and tinned tuna, and wholegrains like brown rice and oats. As long as you have some of these staples on hand, you can whip up a nutritious meal for only a couple of dollars per serve!

Here are a few of our favourite tips and tricks for eating healthily on a budget.

- **Shop in Season**

We're lucky to live in a place where most fruits and vegetables are available year round. You can get strawberries in winter, pumpkin in summer and asparagus in autumn - and we don't even think twice about it!

This may be convenient, but it isn't necessarily the most economical way to eat. When you buy produce that's out of season, it has had to travel further and will therefore lose some of its freshness, flavour and nutrients. The added effort involved in producing and transporting produce that isn't in season inevitably makes it more expensive too, so if you're trying to minimise your grocery spend, aim to purchase fruits and vegetables from that season.

Here are some common fruits and vegetables and when you can buy them in season. You'll notice that there's some crossover for certain produce, which means they might be seasonal a few times a year.

Summer (December - February)

Fruit

Apricots
Bananas
Blackberries
Blueberries
Cantaloupe
Cherries
Figs
Grapefruit
Grapes
Honeydew
Lychee
Mango
Nectarines
Passionfruit
Peach
Pineapples
Raspberries
Watermelon

Vegetables

Asparagus
Avocado
Beetroot
Cabbage
Capsicum
Carrot
Celery
Corn
Cucumber
Eggplant
Peas
Silverbeet
Tomato
Zucchini

Autumn (March - May)

Fruit

Avocado
Apples
Banana
Fig
Grapefruit
Grapes
Kiwi Fruit
Lemon
Lime
Manderine
Mango
Oranges
Papaya
Pears
Rockmelon
Strawberries

Vegetables

Artichoke
Asian greens (e.g. bok choy, choi sum)
Beetroot
Broccoli
Brussels sprouts
Cabbage
Capsicum
Carrot
Cauliflower
Celery
Cucumber
Eggplant
Fennel
Leek
Mushrooms
Parsnip
Peas
Pumpkin
Silverbeet
Spinach
Swede
Sweet potato
Zucchini

Winter (June - August)

Fruit

Apples
Cumquat
Grapefruit
Kiwi Fruit
Mandarins
Nashi
Pear
Persimmon
Quince
Tangelo

Vegetables

Asian greens (bok choy, choi sum)
Beetroot
Broccoli
Broccolini
Brussels sprouts
Cabbage
Cauliflower
Celeriac
Fennel
Kale
Leek
Mushroom
Onions
Parsnip
Potato Pumpkin
Silverbeet
Spinach
Swede
Sweet potato

- ## Buy in Bulk

Generally speaking, buying some of your staple pantry items in bulk is going to be cheaper, as you're eliminating the cost of additional packaging.

Avoid buying individually portioned groceries, instead choosing to purchase larger bags and then portioning out your own serves and putting them into tupperware. For example, instead of buying individual 30 gram servings of almonds, buy a larger packet from your supermarket or bulk food store and individually portion out serves at the start of your week for snacks.

You can then take these to school, uni or work, or keep them in your bag for an on-the-go snack.

Not only will you save money, but you'll also be decreasing your consumption of plastic packaging - yay for the earth!

- ## Embrace Tinned and Frozen Food

We're not talking about frozen party pies or tinned spam here. We're talking about the time-and-money-saving staples that allow you to whip up a quick, cheap meal when all you've got left in your fridge is a bottle of kombucha and a slimy cucumber.

Tinned pantry items, such as lentils, chickpeas, stock and tomatoes, aren't just convenient but also ridiculously cheap. Frozen fruits and vegetables are also very affordable and helpful to have on hand when you're in a rush. They often retain more nutrients than produce picked and left on the supermarket shelves for days, as they're frozen straight after being harvested.

Consider buying a couple of packets of frozen berries for smoothies and baked goods, and your favourite veggies to toss into stir fries, curries and soups.

Have some of these on hand and you can avoid a hefty UberEats bill when you get home late and you're tired and hangry!

- ## Make Home Brand your Bae

In most cases, when you're buying pantry staples - for example rice, tinned goods, grains and the like - you'll simply be paying more for the brand name. Shiny packaging, ambassadors and pretty websites all make it easy to get sucked into spending more money, but really what it all boils down to is marketing.

When you go to the supermarket, look at the items below eye-level, it's here that there'll often be similar items that are unbranded, or 'home brand'. Sure, your packet of brown rice might have an ugly yellow label and not own an Instagram account, but trust us, your wallet doesn't care about pretty packaging.

Be a #MealPrepQueen

The only thing better than tupperware, is tupperware filled with perfectly prepped, nutritious food stacked in your fridge. Truly, there's nothing more satisfying than knowing that after just a couple of hours spent cooking you've got heaps of healthy meals sorted for the week.

There's no denying that meal prep is where it's at. Not only will you save a tonne on UberEats, but you'll also avoid the last resort peanut butter toast for dinner after a long day at work.

If you're an aspiring meal prepper but haven't yet mastered the art, it's easy to think you can't achieve this level of organisation. Especially when you can hardly find the time to wash your socks regularly. If that's you, then read on and follow our tips below. Soon enough you'll be a true Meal Prep Queen.

What is Meal Prep?

'Meal Prep', or meal preparation, is the act of preparing some or all of your meals and snacks ahead of time. It's like having those pre-made frozen TV dinners... except made by you with way healthier, more delicious and unprocessed ingredients.

Before you start your meal preparation, it's important to evaluate how it will work for you. Don't be fooled into thinking that you need to prep every single meal for the whole week, just choose the meals you struggle with the most. Is it hard to cook a nutritious dinner because you get home late? Or perhaps you often find yourself racking up a hefty bill on Subway and sushi because you never bring your lunch to work It's important to choose a method that focuses on your goals and is suitable to your individual schedule and needs.

• Keep it Simple

Don't overwhelm yourself by trying to prep every single meal and snack for the week ahead. This will just overwhelm you. Instead, start off by preparing one meal that you know you struggle with and pick a recipe that you're familiar with to help ease you into the process.

Aim to keep ingredients, recipes and cooking methods as simple, cost effective and efficient as possible.

• Learn to Love Leftovers

Leftovers are a great way to reduce food waste and give yourself quick nutritious meals throughout the week. Many people associate meal prep with chicken, steamed broccoli and rice, but this doesn't have to be the case - the humble leftover makes the perfect meal prep!

All that matters is that the meals you prepare offer a wide range of nutrients and cover the important bases: lean protein, complex carbs and healthy fats. As a guide, aim to fill 50% your plate or container with colourful non-starchy veggies, 25% with a lean protein source and the final 25% with whole grains or Low GI carbohydrates.

For example, you can cook up a big batch of you favourite vegetable and tofu curry with quinoa on Sunday evening, then portion this into containers for lunch for the next three days. Alternatively, you can freeze the remaining portions so you can enjoy it for future dinners. No fuss, no stress and definitely more delicious than broc and boiled chicken.

• Plan & Shop Ahead

Planning your meals ahead of time will save you from having to run to the supermarket 476 times a week. To do this, simply choose the recipes you'll be preparing for the week ahead of your grocery shop, then write out a shopping list of all the ingredients you need to buy. Remember to do a quick inventory of what you already have, so you're not doubling up on ingredients.

• Snack Smart

If you often find yourself with your hand in your office's box of charity chocolates when the 3pm sugar craving kicks in, also factor snacks into your meal prep. Stock up on healthy snacks that will keep well in your desk at work, or that you can throw into your bag when you're on the go. Some great snack ideas include fresh fruit, a handful of mixed nuts, Greek yoghurt or even a small tin of tuna on crackers.

If you plan on making your own snacks (we highly recommend the bliss balls on page

167 and the Choc-Chip Cookie Dough Protein Balls on page 169, add the ingredients you need for these to your shopping list.

• Invest in Tupperware

You will need an assortment of tupperware containers to store your meals and snacks. Make sure these containers have airtight lids (trust us, you don't want salad dressing leaking into your bag!), are microwave-safe and BPA free to allow for quick reheating.

• (Food) Safety First

Meal prep is amazing. Unless it makes you sick. Follow our below advice to make sure you're meals keep you thriving, and not constantly diving to the bathroom.

Ensure that the maximum amount of lunches or dinners you prepare and plan on storing in the fridge is between 3-4 days. The general rule of thumb is three days for salads and seafood, and up to five days for cooked meats and vegetables, though it pays to err on the side of caution, particularly when preparing chicken. Generally, frozen meals can be kept in the freezer for between 3-6 months.

Reheat your food well. For safety, the recommended internal temperature you should reheat your food to is 75°C. If you're not reheating your food (for example, if you have a grilled chicken salad), just be sure you keep the item cooled and stored at the proper temperature of below 5°C.
Your refrigerator temperature should be set to 5°C or below, and your freezer should be at least -17°C or below.

If you are preparing several hot meals and plan on freezing them, you should allow the meals to cool down (nearly to room temperature) and then store them in the fridge or freezer within 1-2 hours of preparing.

If you plan on keeping meals frozen for a while, make sure you label them with the name of the meal and the date it was frozen. Thaw frozen foods or meals in your fridge overnight instead of on your countertop. For faster thawing, you can submerge foods in cold tap water, changing the water every 30 minutes.

The more times you cool and reheat a food, the higher the risk of food poisoning. That's bad. To avoid this, make sure you only reheat defrosted meals once.

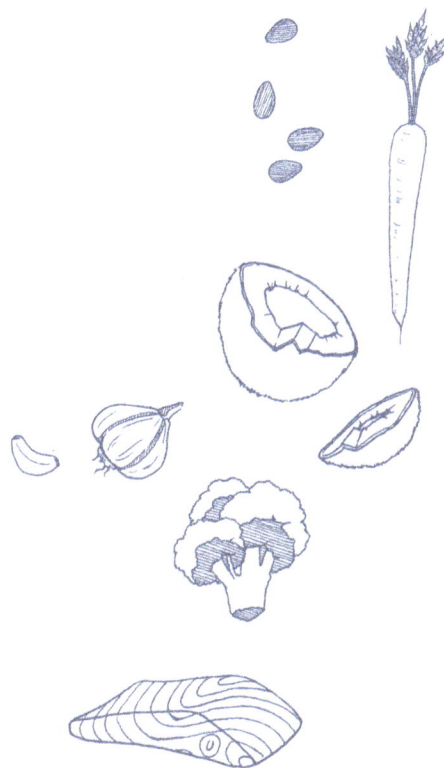

Common Ingredients

You'll find that throughout these recipes we've tried to use as many staple ingredients as possible to help make the process of cooking simple, healthy meals easier. For the most part, you should be able to find everything at your local supermarket and green grocers, and will likely have many of these ingredients already in your pantry or fridge.

We wanted to include this helpful list of common ingredients used within Recipes for Life and their nutritional benefits, just in case you're not familiar with all of them. It'll also give you a bit more information about some of the wonderful nutritional benefits of some of your staples that you may never have even known about.

Acai Berries:

Heralded for their high levels of antioxidants, acai berries grow on acai palm trees in the rainforests of Central and South America. In the Western World, they can typically be found as a frozen fruit puree, powder or pressed juice.

Almonds:

Almonds are rich in healthy fats, fiber, protein, magnesium and vitamin E, and have been said to lower blood sugar levels, reduced blood pressure and lower cholesterol levels. They're a great on-the-go snack and can be sprinkled on muesli, salads or used as a spread in almond butter form.

Aloe Vera Gel:

This is an optional ingredient used in Tarni Deutsher's green smoothie bowl. While best known for treating skin injuries, it is also thought to be helpful for digestion.

Arborio Rice:

Arborio rice is an Italian short-grain, starchy rice that's most traditionally used for cooking risotto, however it also works well for paella and rice pudding. It's starch content and short, round shape gives it a luxuriously creamy texture that makes it perfect for risotto.

Avocado:

The avocado is a unique fruit, being mostly made up of heart-healthy monounsaturated fats rather than carbohydrates. They're loaded with fibre and contain a wide variety of nutrients, including 20 different vitamins and minerals.

Bananas:

You may have heard some people talk about bananas not being good for you - these people clearly want to eliminate all that is joyous from the world.

Bananas are one of the best fruit sources of vitamin B6, with one medium banana containing around one quarter of your daily needs. Vitamin B6 is important for the production of red blood cells and metabolising carbohydrates and fats. Furthermore, they are rich in manganese, fibre and vitamin C.

Ignore the haters and enjoy your god damn bananas.

Black Beans:

Delicious in tacos and stews, these little beans are fibre powerhouses, making them an amazing choice for your digestion. They also contain protein and iron, making them a great meat-alternative for those following a plant-based diet.

Black Rice:

Also known as "forbidden rice", black rice is the rice with the highest level of antioxidants. The outermost layer of this rice contains one of the highest levels of the antioxidant anthocyanin found in any known food and is thought to help in the prevention of cardiovascular disease, improve brain function and reduce inflammation. It also looks really pretty when thrown into a mix with brown or red rice!

Brown Rice:

Brown rice is an unrefined and unpolished whole grain that retains its nutrient-dense bran and germ layer. While most of the recipes in this book will use brown rice instead of white rice, this by no means white rice is "bad" or off-limits. We simply love the slightly chewy texture and nutty flavour of brown rice.

Buckwheat:

Despite its name, buckwheat is in fact a seed and contains no wheat, making it an ideal alternative for those sensitive to gluten. This ancient grain is a fantastic source of amino acids, vitamins and minerals that can assist in lowering blood pressure.

You can cook buckwheat "groats" just like rice or quinoa in boiling water, or else keep them raw for granola and baked goods. Buckwheat flour is also often used as an alternative for gluten-free baking.

Bee Pollen:

This is a bit of a bougie ingredient that came onto the scene a few years ago when #healthspo became a thing. Don't feel that this is something you need to eat for optimal health, but if you have a little cash to splash and want to jazz up your meals with these pretty balls of golden pollen, then go for it!

Bee pollen is a mixture of flower pollen, nectar, enzymes, honey and wax, and is known for its anti-inflammatory and antibacterial properties.

Berries:

While all berries will have a slightly different nutrient make-up, they're all fantastic sources of fibre, vitamin C and antioxidants. Try adding a handful of blueberries, raspberries or strawberries into your breakfast for a low-sugar alternative to dried fruit.

Beetroot:

While we love so many vegetables, beetroot is one that definitely gets a special mention, due to its exceptional nutritional value.

Beets are an excellent source of folic acid and a very good source of fibre, manganese and potassium. And don't ignore the green tops either, they're rich in calcium, iron and vitamin A. Use them just as you would spinach.

Chlorophyll:

Chlorophyll is a pigment that gives plants their green color and can be found in the form of drops, pills, or capsules. People have used chlorophyll as a health supplement for many years, with a variety of medical studies suggesting that it may be helpful for skin conditions. However the evidence isn't conclusive, so don't feel like you need to go out of your way to buy it!

Cacao:

Not to be confused with cocoa powder (that's the drinking chocolate!), raw cacao is chocolate in its most natural form. Often touted as a superfood, this powder is rich in magnesium, which plays a vital role in energy production and relaxing your muscles. It may also increase the body's production of serotonin and dopamine, both of which are known mood enhancers.

Cacao is delicious when used in smoothies and smoothie bowls, or used as a chocolate alternative in baking. You can find it in health food stores and most supermarkets in powder form.

Cacao Nibs:

Cacao nibs are essentially the unground version of cacao powder. These crunchy little nibs are made from the cacao bean after it's been roasted, had the husk removed and been slightly crushed. With all the benefits of cacao powder, these chocolate-y chunks are also delicious.

Cashews:

Eaten whole, ground into a meal or turned into a butter or milk, we can't get enough of cashews. They're rich in copper, which aids in skin and hair health (yes please!), calcium for bone strength and are a good source of branched chain amino acids.

Chia Seeds:

These little seeds may not look like much, but what they lack in size they more than make up for in fibre! This is an incredibly important nutrient for maintaining good gut health. They also contain all nine amino acids making them a complete source of protein, so make a great addition to a vegan or vegetarian diet. They contain plenty of heart-healthy omega 3 fatty acids, vitamins and minerals, so sprinkle these nutrient powerhouses over smoothie bowls, mix into salads or use in your baking.

Chickpeas:

Another legume powerhouse, chickpeas contain a significant amount of fibre and are great for gut and digestive health. In tinned form they're also incredibly easy to keep in your cupboard and whip out to throw into curries, salads and stews for an added dose of protein.

Chickpea Flour:

Also known as besan flour, this flour is made from dried and ground up chickpeas. It's a fantastic gluten-free alternative for baking, especially in savoury dishes such as Chloe Munro's crepes on page 37, and contains more protein than typical wheat flour.

Cinnamon:

As well as being a delicious addition to porridge and baked goods, cinnamon has been prized for its medicinal properties for thousands of years. In a study that compared the antioxidant levels of 26 spices, cinnamon came out on top, and has also been linked to reducing inflammation.

Dates:

Dates are Mother Nature's perfect sweet treat and are an amazing natural sweetener for smoothies and raw desserts. Packed with fibre, they're the perfect snack when you need an energy boost.

Eggs:

Eggs are an inexpensive, high quality source of protein. They're a rich source of selenium, vitamin D, B12 and minerals such as zinc, iron and copper. They also make Sunday brunching particularly delicious!

Make sure you buy organic free-range eggs!

Extra Virgin Olive Oil:

Olive Oil is rich in healthy monounsaturated fats and has strong anti-inflammatory properties.

Flaxseeds:

Also known as linseeds, flaxseeds are high in omega-3 and fibre, which can help stabilise your blood sugar and make you feel fuller for longer. You can use flaxseed meal (finely ground flaxseed) in your baking to add an extra nutritional boost to your muffins, cakes and slices.

Goji Berries:

This shrivelled red berry has risen to 'superfood' fame in recent years, but has been used in traditional Chinese medicine for more than 2,000 years.

Sweet and a little tart, they contain 11 essential amino acids and are extremely high in vitamin C and selenium. Gojis taste great in granola, sprinkled on smoothie bowls or used in baked goods.

Greek Yogurt:

A great source of protein and calcium, perhaps what we love most about Greek yogurt is its level of probiotics. These are healthy bacteria that typically live in your intestines and promote a healthy balance of good bacteria in the gut.

When choosing your yogurt, make sure you opt for a brand that is unflavoured, low in added sugar and preservatives.

Hemp Seeds:

These earthy-flavoured seeds are a complete source of protein containing all 9 essential amino acids and a good dose of omega-3 fatty acids. For this reason they're an excellent addition to a plant-based diet. Try sprinkling them into smoothies, on salads and using them in baking.

Kefir:

Traditionally made using cow's milk or goat's milk, Kefir is a fermented drink that is made by adding kefir grains (colonies of yeast and lactic acid bacteria) to milk. High in nutrients and probiotics, it's very beneficial for gut health, and has a high calcium content which is good for your bones.

Lentils:

Keeping a tin of lentils in your cupboard is a quick and easy way to include a good source of protein and fibre in your meals. Throw them into soups, curries, salads or create a delicious lentil bolognese.

Liquid Smoke:

This one might sound a little strange, but bear with us, because once you use it in your cooking you'll understand why you need it in your life. Usually found in specialty grocers and food stores, liquid smoke adds an authentic smoky flavour to dishes.

Maca Powder:

Maca is a Peruvian plant grown in the Andes mountains and is related to broccoli and kale. When the plant is ground up, it forms a powder that is great source of several important vitamins and minerals, including vitamin C and iron. Maca is often used in smoothies and baking.

Manuka Honey:

Manuka honey is a special type of honey that's native to New Zealand. It has incredible antibacterial, antiviral and anti-inflammatory properties that set it apart from your regular, run-of-the-mill sticky stuff.

It's also been said to aid in soothing a sore throat. Simply add ½ a tablespoon to a glass of warm water along with a little grated ginger and stir. This also tastes delicious!

Mushrooms:

Mushrooms are packed with nutritional value, being a great source of fiber and protein, which makes them awesome for those on a plant-based diet.

Mushrooms are also often described as having a 'meaty' flavour and texture, making them a favourite for vegan alternatives such as burger patties and bolognaise.

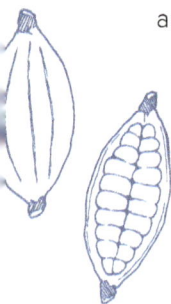

Oats:

Oats are the poster child for cheap, healthy food and, as you'll see from our wide range of oat recipes, they're a personal favourite of ours. Oats are a wonderful source of low-GI carbohydrates and fibre in the morning and are loaded with important vitamins, minerals and antioxidant plant compounds.

Quick oats are typically used in porridge, where as rolled oats are more frequently found in muesli and granola. Oat flour can also be used in baking as a substitute to wheat flour. It tends to be more moist, making it a good choice for cookies and quick breads.

Papaya:

Tropical and sweet, the papaya is loaded with vitamin C and antioxidants that can reduce inflammation and fight disease. Try out Sally O'Neil's incredible baked papaya recipe on page 40 and we guarantee you'll be a convert.

Pitaya Powder:

Otherwise known as dragon fruit, pitaya is a fruit grown in tropical regions of South America and South East Asia. In its powdered form, this bright pink superfood can easily be added to smoothie bowls, desserts, juices and sauces for a fantastic dose of fiber, vitamin C, antioxidants and essential fatty acids.

Plus, it makes everything pink - yay!

Protein Powder:

While protein powder isn't necessary to meet your protein requirements, it can help if you struggle to eat enough protein, or are trying to build muscle. Also, in flavours like salted caramel, chocolate and vanilla, it also just tastes damn good!

Before buying, look at the ingredients and make sure it's not packed with preservatives or 'fillers'. Get recommendations about flavours from friends and try out a few before committing to a big purchase. Protein powder can be quite expensive and there's nothing worse than buying a bulk order of one you're not happy with.

Pumpkin:

Roast it, bake it, steam it or blend it. Whichever way you use it, pumpkin is an incredibly versatile vegetable and is also usually very cheap - bonus! Furthermore, it's packed with Vitamin A, which is important for your vision and the immune system.

Pumpkin Seeds:

Delicious sprinkled over porridge or toasted and tossed through salads, pumpkin seeds (also known as pepitas) contain tryptophan, which increases serotonin and can promote better sleep quality. They're also packed with B vitamins and minerals, such as iron, zinc and magnesium which supports a healthy immune system and helps to regulate blood glucose levels.

Quinoa:

Not to be mistaken for a grain, quinoa is actually a seed, making it a great gluten-free alternative. It's also a great choice for those following a plant-based diet, as it contains higher levels of protein in comparison to many other carbohydrate sources and is one of the few plant foods that contains sufficient amounts of all nine essential amino acids.

Reishi Mushrooms:

When a superfood is referred to as the

"magic mushroom", you know something special is going on. Reishi mushrooms began trending in 2018, though have been used in the East for their health benefits for hundreds of years.

Today, they're grown commercially and sold in various forms, including in teas, capsules and powders. These mushies are said to stimulate the immune system and liver function, producing an anti-inflammatory effect in the body.

Spirulina Powder:

Spirulina is a type of cyanobacteria, which is a family of single-celled microbes that are often referred to as blue-green algae...

Thank you for coming to our Ted Talk.

But seriously, usually found in tablet or powder form, this green stuff has a high protein and vitamin content. Research also suggests that spirulina has antioxidant and inflammation-fighting properties, as well as the ability to help regulate the immune system.

Sunflower Seeds:

Rich in protein and heart-healthy fats, sunflower seeds also contain vitamin E, which is known for its anti-inflammatory properties and improving skin and hair health.

Sweet Potato:

While the potato debate (are you team sweet potato or white potato?) still rages, there's no denying the humble sweet potato definitely reigns supreme in the health department.

Containing both soluble and insoluble fibre, sweet potatoes are great for promoting a healthy gut and also contain an impressive range of vitamins and antioxidants.

Tahini:

A paste made from ground up sesame seeds, tahini contains more protein than milk and most nuts. It's also a rich source of B vitamins that boosts energy and brain function, vitamin E, which is protective against heart disease and important minerals such as magnesium, iron and calcium.

Tofu:

This cheap, flavour-sponge is heralded as one of the best sources of vegan protein. Also known as bean curd, tofu is made by curdling fresh soya milk and pressing it into a solid block before cooling it.

Tofu is a good source of protein and contains all nine essential amino acids. It's also a valuable plant source of iron and calcium, as well as zinc and selenium.

Walnuts:

Would you believe us if we told you that for the past 50 years, a group of scientists have gathered in California for the sole purpose of discussing the health benefits of the walnut. It's literally a convention for walnuts...

But given its high omega-3 and antioxidant content, we feel like it deserves its own party, and we're so here for it.

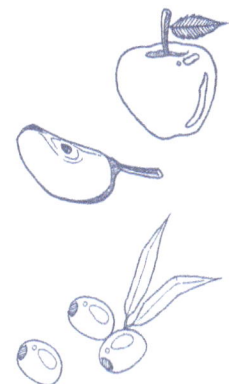

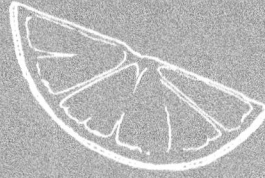

Breakfast

Whether it's fluffy pancakes, a warming bowl of porridge or a veg-packed omelette, breakfast is easily our most loved meal of the day. And it should be yours too!

By giving your body a balance of protein, complex carbohydrates and healthy fats, a filling nutrient-dense breakfast sets you up for your day, both physically and mentally.

These recipes were chosen not just because they give you the energy you need to be a total boss lady, but also because they taste amazing. So amazing that they'll make you excited to get out of bed in the morning. Yes, we promise it's possible.

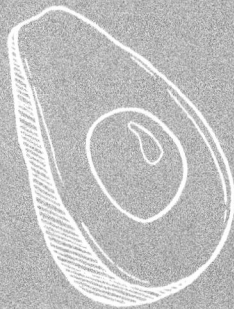

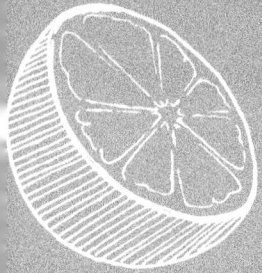

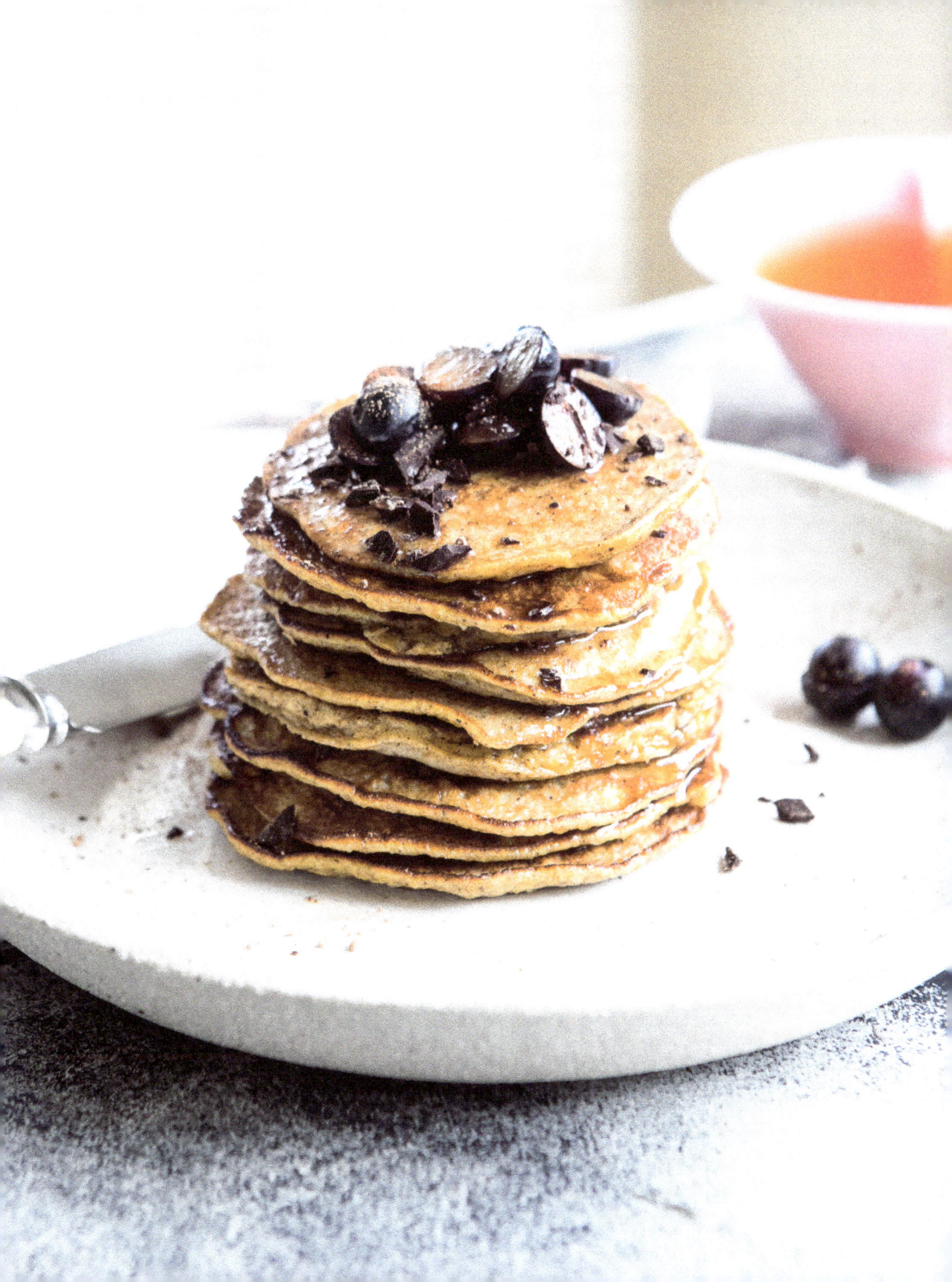

Vegan Matcha & Banana Porridge

Sarah Holloway @spoonful_of_sarah

Entrepreneur, founder of Matcha Maiden and all round Boss Lady Sarah Holloway admits to being a breakfast fiend. And when she's not at her favourite local enjoying her morning meal, she can be found whipping up this porridge at home.

It showcases matcha powder, one of Sarah's favourite ingredients. Made from ground up Japanese green tea leaves, matcha contains 137 times the number of antioxidants of a regular cup of brewed green tea. This magical cup of goodness is said to help improve energy, focus, skin and the metabolism.

Beyond it's nutritional benefits however, the matcha truly makes this porridge something special, lending it an earthy flavour that works perfectly against the sticky caramelised banana. You could say it's a matcha made in heaven.

Vegan, dairy-free, refined sugar-free

Ingredients

For the porridge

½ cup rolled oats

1 heaped teaspoon matcha_ maiden matcha powder

½ teaspoon spirulina

1 cup of almond milk (or plant-based milk of choice)

1 banana, sliced lengthways (1 half mashed for porridge, 1 half reserved for caramelisation)

Granola, almond butter, rice malt syrup or honey, to serve

For the caramalised banana

Remaining half of sliced banana

Ground cinnamon

Rice malt syrup

Method

For the porridge, place the oats, matcha and spirulina together in a saucepan over a medium heat and stir to combine.

Add the milk and mashed banana to the saucepan and bring to the boil. Let simmer for 4 to 5 minutes, stirring regularly until the oats are cooked or reach your desired consistency.

Cook your caramalised banana (recipe below).

Pour porridge into a bowl, top with caramelised banana and toppings!

Caramelised banana

Place the remaining half of the banana on a non-stick fry pan set over a medium heat.

Drizzle rice malt syrup and sprinkle cinnamon on the banana. Once the banana begins to brown on one side, flip it and cook for a further few minutes on the other side. Once golden and caramelised, take off heat and serve on top of porridge.

Serves 1

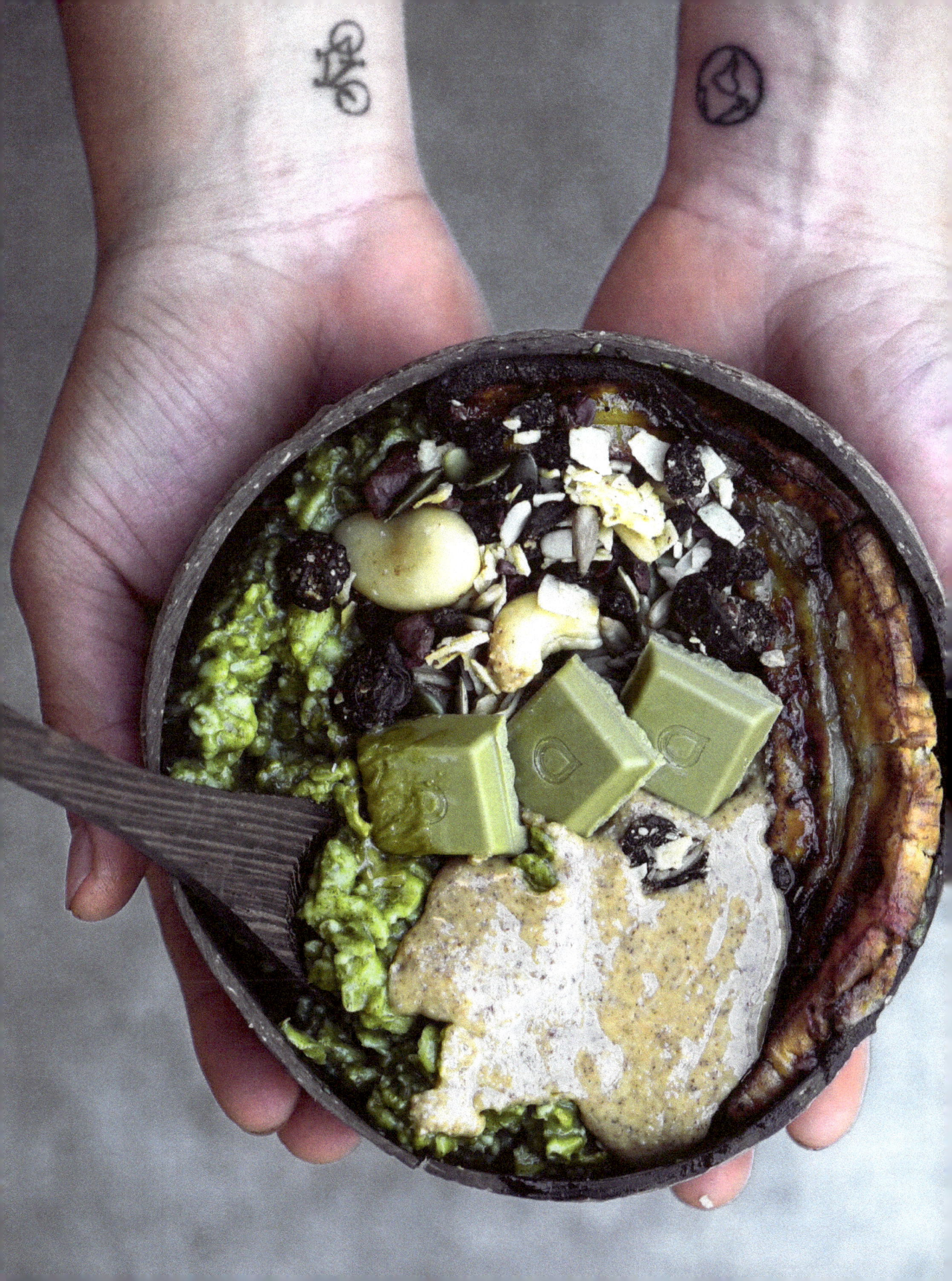

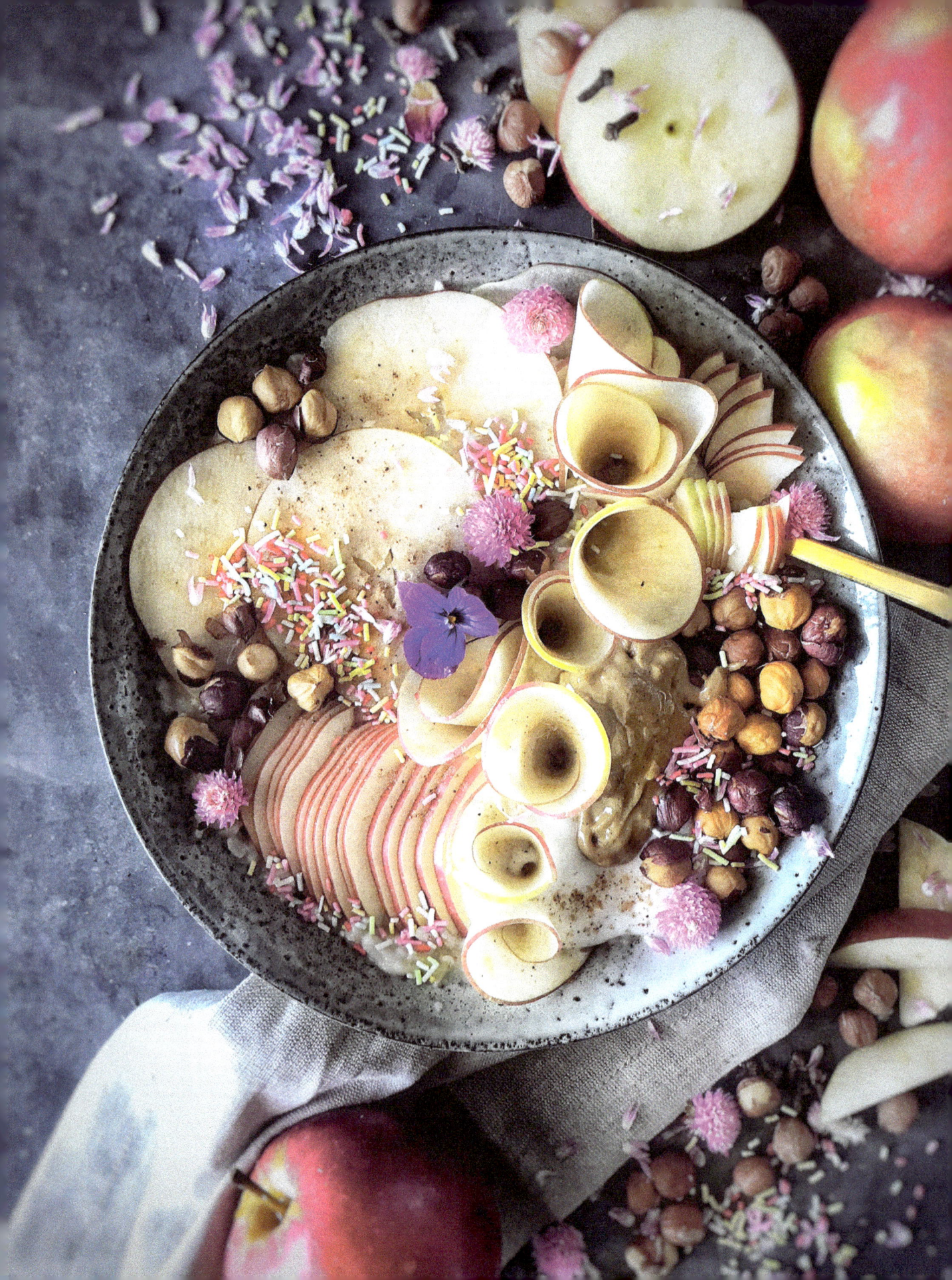

Apple Pie Oatmeal

Ami Shoesmith @the_sunkissed_kitchen

While a warming bowl of oats might be comforting for most of us on a winter morning, it's especially so for vegan food stylist Ami Shoesmith, who has a freezing cold shower every morning. But we're not suggesting you need to do that to enjoy this cosy bowl of goodness!

Filled with cinnamon and nutmeg, these spices will make you feel as though you're being hugged from the inside out - freezing shower or not.

Vegan, dairy-free, refined sugar-free,

Ingredients

For the oats

1 cup rolled oats

3 cups water

1 apple, grated

1/2 teaspoon cinnamon

1/4 cup sultanas

Pinch of nutmeg

Pinch of ginger

Pinch of ground cloves

To serve

1 large apple, thinly sliced

2 tablespoons coconut yoghurt

2 tablespoons hazelnut butter

Cinnamon

Fresh roasted hazelnuts

Edible flowers (optional)

Natural sprinkles (optional, but so pretty!)

Method

To make the oatmeal, place all the ingredients for the oats into a saucepan and warm over a low heat until it begins to boil.

Simmer until thick and creamy, around 4-5 minutes, or until cooked to your liking.

Pour the oatmeal into two bowls and top with the sliced apples, coconut yoghurt, and nut butter. Sprinkle with cinnamon and edible flowers and sprinkles, if using.

Serves 2

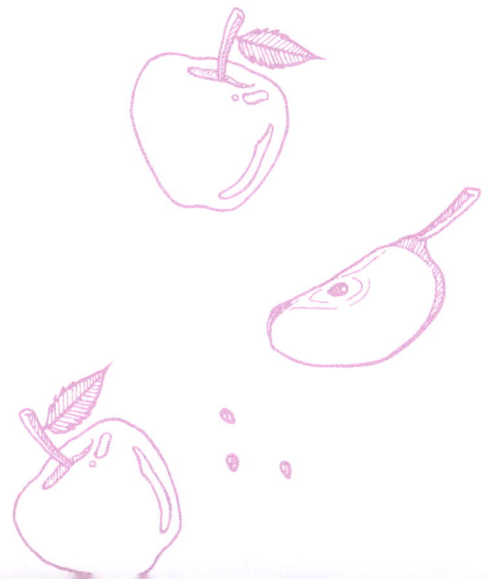

Chia Buckwheat Porridge with Berry Compote

Gabrielle O'Dea @nourishtheday

Growing up in Adelaide Hills sparked dietician Gabrielle O'Dea's love of food and fresh produce. From a young age, she could be found helping her mum make jams and preserves from the fresh fruit they collected in their garden.

This inspired the creation of the sweet and delicious berry compote that accompanies this warming, creamy porridge, though Gabby says you can also enjoy this hearty breakfast topped with chopped nuts, seeds, fresh fruit or nut butters.

'This is the perfect breakfast to cook up for yourself and loved ones on a cold winter morning,' says Gabby. 'The buckwheat gives it a really nice soft texture and adds a bit of diversity to my breakfasts, rather than always using oats. This is an old favourite with a twist.'

Vegan, gluten-free, dairy-free

Ingredients

For the porridge

1 cup buckwheat groats

1 1/2 cups soy milk or milk of choice

1 cup water

1 tablespoon chia seeds

1 teaspoon vanilla paste or vanilla extract

1-2 tablespoons coconut sugar or stevia (to taste)

Pinch of cinnamon (optional)

Extra milk, fresh fruit, hulled tahini or nut butter, extra coconut sugar, to serve

For the quick raspberry compote

1 cup raspberries, fresh or frozen

1 tablespoon maple syrup

Method

To make the porridge, place the buckwheat groats in a medium saucepan with the soy milk and water. Bring to the boil over a high heat. Once boiling turn down to a simmer (watch out, it can get foamy and overflow if too high).

Simmer for 15 minutes, or until the buckwheat is tender. It should be only just be starting to get a bit mushier.

Turn off the heat, add the chia seeds, vanilla, coconut sugar and cinnamon, if using. Add an extra splash of milk if needed here, but the buckwheat and chia will continue to soak up the liquid.

While the porridge is cooking, start on the compote. Place the berries in a small saucepan and heat gently over the stove, using a fork to gently smash them up a bit. Add the maple syrup to taste. You could also do this step in the microwave if you wish!

Once your porridge is cooked, divide into two bowls and top with raspberry compote, a dollop of tahini or nut butter and any fruit you fancy. Add a splash of extra soy milk if desired.

Serves 2 hungry people

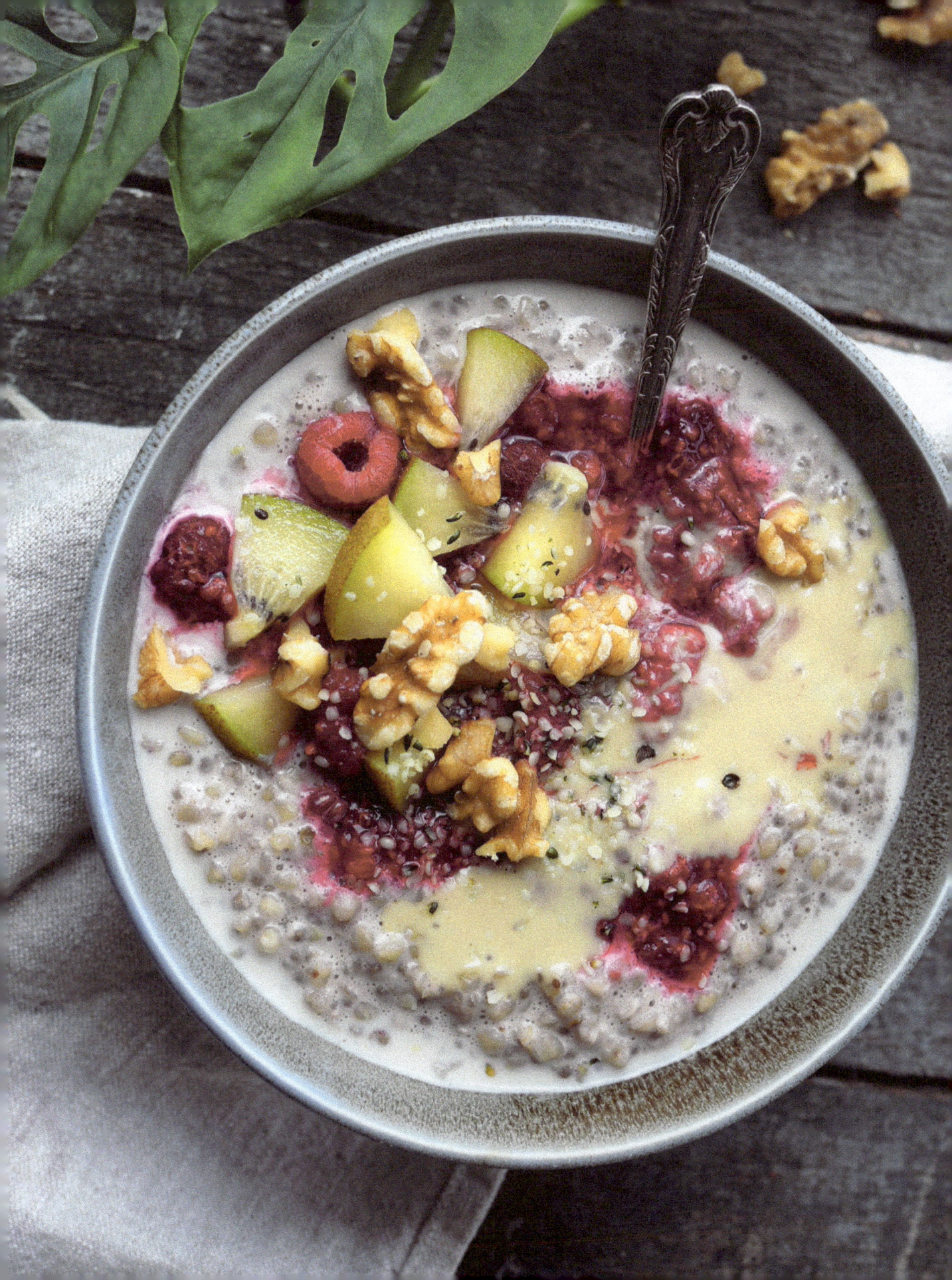

Chunky Monkey Rawnola

Michelle Chen @run2food

Filled with hearty oats and nutrient-dense walnuts, it's hard to believe this recipe was inspired by Ben and Jerry's. When Sydney food blogger Michelle Chen attended a free cone day from the ice cream magnate, she found inspiration for this wholefood vegan recipe from the flavours on display.

'This flavour just looked so fun, so I had to recreate it,' she laughs. 'I love textural things, so the chewy oats with the crunchy walnuts makes this really satisfying. I made a baked version of this dish which people loved, but as I was making another batch I tried it raw and it was so good that I decided to leave it uncooked.'

Vegan, gluten-free alternative, dairy-free, refined sugar-free,

Ingredients

Dry ingredients

3/4 cup oats (sub for quinoa or rice flakes for a gluten-free alternative)

1 scoop vegan vanilla protein powder

Handful of walnuts

25 grams (1 oz) dark chocolate, chopped

Wet ingredients

1 large ripe banana

2 tablespoons natural peanut butter

Optional: maple syrup or other liquid sweetener to taste

**Some almond milk may be if required, depending on the size of your banana and brand of protein powder.

Method

Combine all the dry ingredients in a bowl and mix thoroughly.

Blend the wet ingredients in a blender to create a nutty 'banana milk'. Pour the wet mixture into the dry and stir until well combined and all the liquid is absorbed.

Tip into a bowl and eat!

Serves 1

This rawnola should be consumed soon after being made, as it contains raw banana. But at least you can eat a lot in one go - yay!

Tropical Berry & Chia Oats

Tarni Deutsher @healthywholefood

There are some mornings when a simple smoothie or smoothie bowl topped with fresh fruit will be enough to satisfy you. And then there are mornings when, inexplicably, you're so ravenous you feel like you could eat a small village. This oaty bowl created by Melbourne food blogger and dietician-in-training Tarni Deutsher is for such munchy mornings.

While fresh and fruity, the oats make this dish wonderfully substantial, giving you fuel to power through your morning. Serve them straight out of the fridge in summer for a refreshing breakfast, or else warm them up for something more cosy on cold winter mornings.

Vegan, dairy-free, refined sugar-free

Ingredients

3/4 cup oats

1/2 cup coconut milk

3/4 cup water

2 teaspoons desiccated coconut

1 teaspoon chia seeds

1/2 teaspoon cinnamon

1 teaspoon honey or maple syrup

Toppings: Passionfruit, berries of choice

goji berries

Method

In a saucepan set over a medium heat, add all the porridge ingredients and stir for five minutes until thick and creamy.

If you want to have a few thawed, melted berries dotted throughout your porridge, stir them through the oats for the final minute of cooking. If not, just leave them to top at the end.

Pour your porridge into a bowl and top with fresh passionfruit, goji berries and more berries!

Serves 1

If you want to make this the night before, put all the base ingredients into a container and stir thoroughly. You can add the toppings either the night before or the next morning. You may also need to add some extra liquid as the oats and chia seeds soak up a lot of it during the night.

Breakfast Chia Pudding

Kat Nguyen-Thai @katnt

To say that Melbourne food blogger Kat Nguyen-Thai loves breakfast is an understatement. She loves it so much in fact, that she admits to going to bed each night excited about the prospect of waking up to eat her first meal.

'I'm the type of person who could eat breakfast at any time of the day,' she laughs. 'It's a meal I could never skip because I'm most hungry in the morning and it gives me energy for my busy days.'

This chia pudding is the perfect example of how Kat loves to cook and eat: simple, delicious, plant-based recipes that nourish her body from the inside out.

Chia seeds are naturally packed with protein, fibre and Omega 3, which makes this quick breakfast deceptively satisfying. Simply make it the night before, and in the morning grab it out of the fridge, add your favourite toppings and you're good to go.

Vegan, gluten-free, dairy-free, refined sugar-free

Ingredients

For the chia pudding

3 tablespoons chia seeds

1 cup water

3 tablespoons coconut yoghurt

Toppings

Caramalised buckinis

Roughly chopped nuts (hazelnuts, pistachios and macadamias are Kat's favourite)

Sliced banana

Hemp seeds

Fresh berries (optional)

Method

In a glass container, add the chia seeds and water. Stir to combine and store in the fridge overnight.

In the morning, remove the chia pudding from the fridge and stir through the coconut yoghurt until well combined and white in colour.

Divide the chia pudding into two bowls. Top with the carmalised buckinis, nuts, hemp seeds, banana and berries and serve.

Serves 2

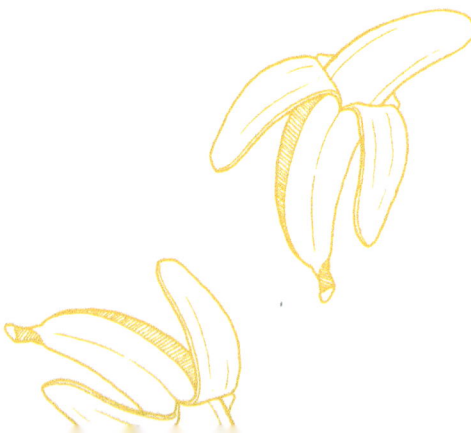

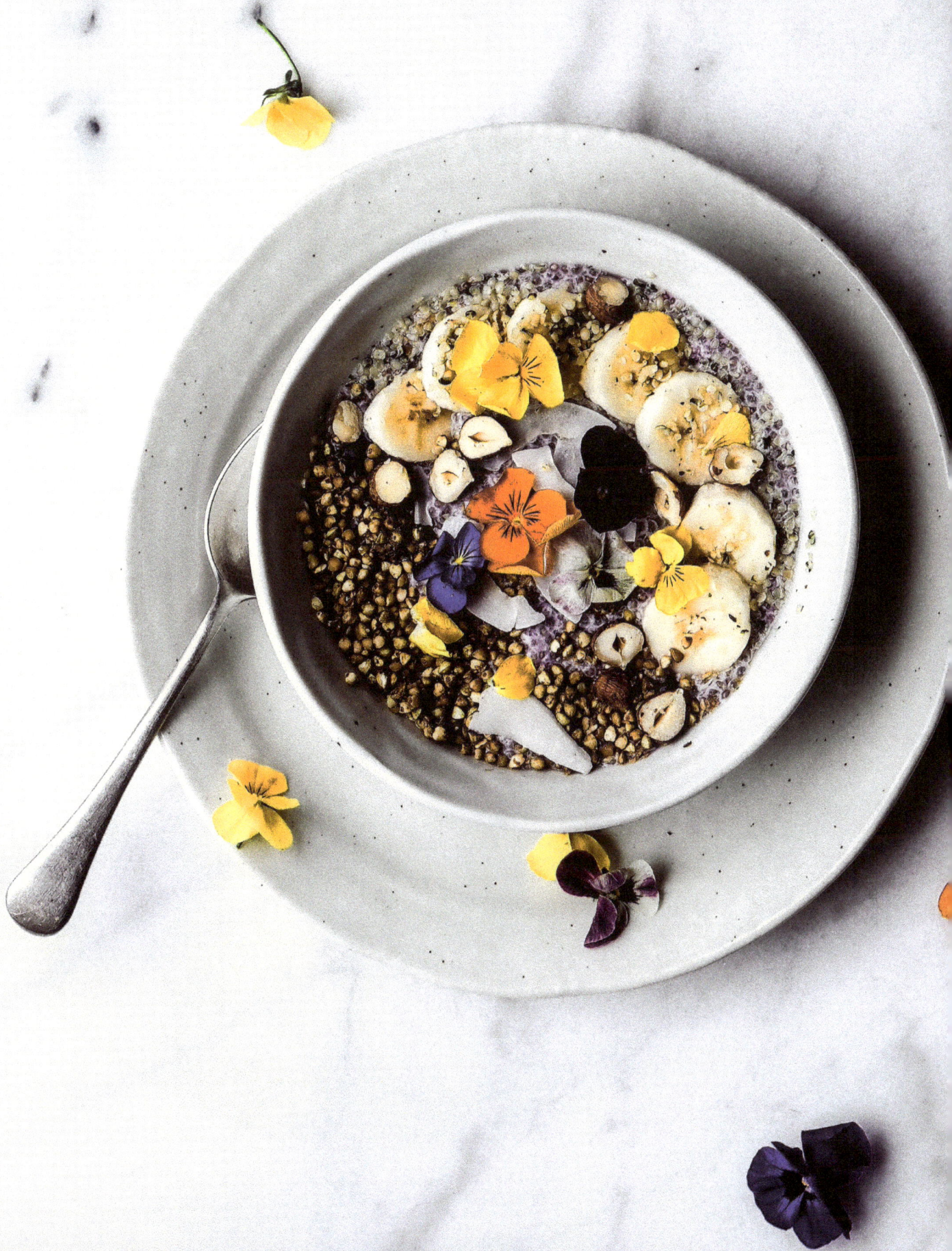

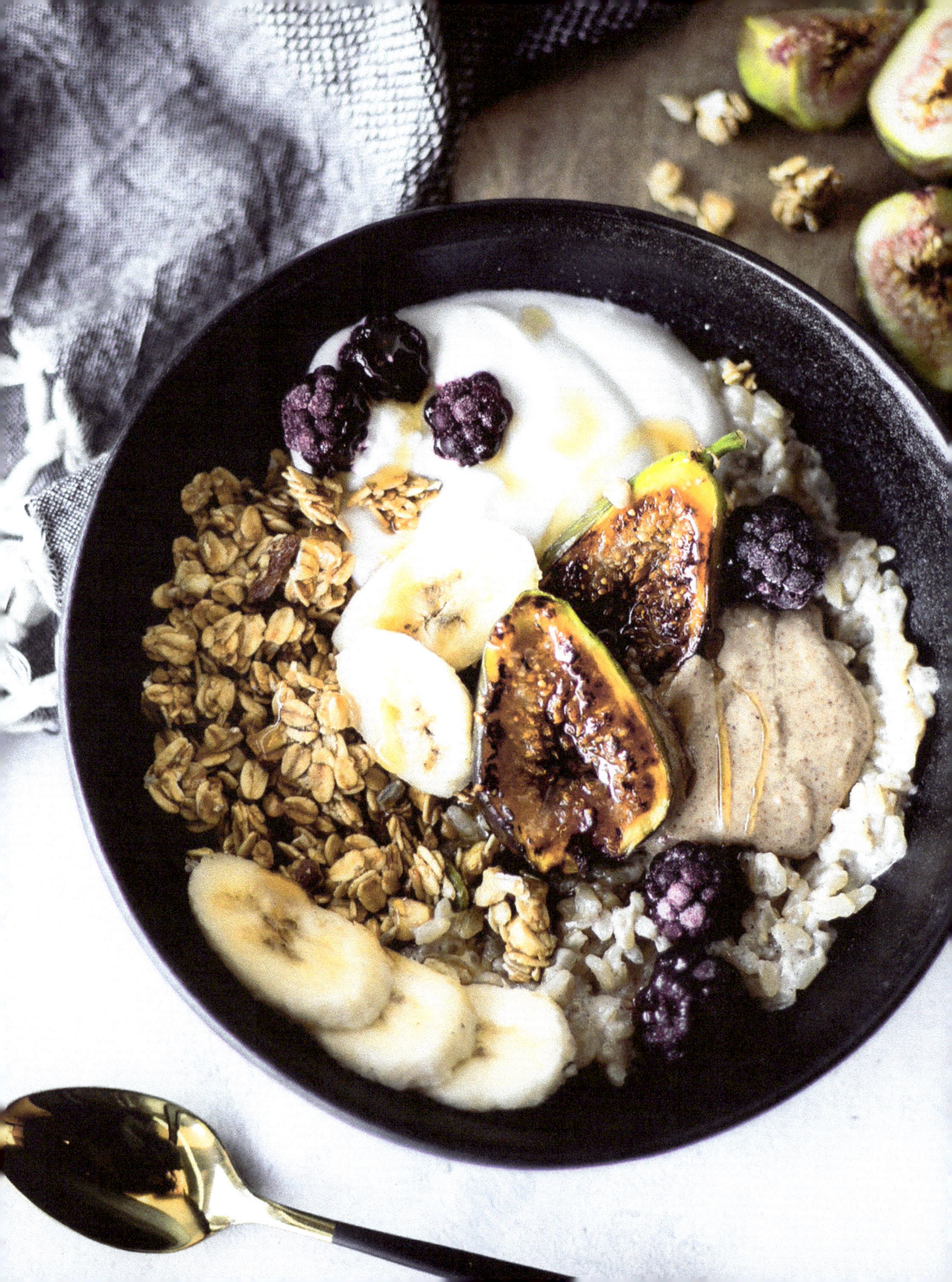

Cardamom Brown Rice Pudding with Burnt Figs & Maple

Miriam Haug @mealsbymiri

Imagine a cold morning in a Scandinavian cabin with your hands wrapped around this nourishing, spice-filled bowl of rice pudding. Well that was Miriam Haug's reality before moving to Melbourne in 2018. Despite our winter's being a little less intense than those of her home country, she still indulges in this bowl filled with the warming flavours of cardamom for breakfast, especially around Christmas.

'Rice pudding is a very common thing we eat in Norway, especially around Christmas and at large family gatherings,' Miriam says. 'I wanted to make a version that was a bit more extra - to take it to the next level.'

Topped with crunchy granola, sticky caramelised figs and sweet maple syrup, this is the perfect 'lazy Sunday morning' breakfast.

Vegan, gluten-free, dairy-free

Ingredients

50 grams (2 oz) medium grain brown rice

200 grams (7 oz) coconut milk

150 millilitres water

1 teaspoon raw sugar

½ teaspoon cardamom

1 teaspoon vanilla

Pinch of salt

1 fig

Optional toppings: muesli, coconut yoghurt, blackberries, maple syrup and banana slices.

Method

Add all your ingredients (except the fig) into a pot set over medium heat and bring to a simmer. Boil while stirring occasionally for about 40 minutes until your rice pudding is thick and creamy and any excess liquid has evaporated. Feel free to add some extra coconut milk or water during the cooking process if needed.

Cut the fig in half and place it face down in a non-stick fry pan over a medium heat. Cook it until the insides are slightly soft and charred.

Serve up your rice pudding topped with the charred fig, muesli, coconut yoghurt, blackberries, maple syrup and banana slices.

Serves 1

Savoury Porridge Breakfast Bowl

Sally O'Neil @thefitfoodieblog

After a trip to Japan, health enthusiast and recipe developer Sally O'Neil wanted to recreate congee, a rice dish often eaten for breakfast in Asian countries. The problem? She doesn't really like rice.

'I wanted to find an alternative to rice that was still warm and cosy, but didn't weigh me down,' she explains. 'I love oats, so I experimented with those and the result was delicious! I love to serve this on a cold winter morning to really warm me up.'

Sally recommends topping your savoury oats with whatever takes your fancy; roast tomatoes, mushrooms, feta cheese and bacon are delicious additions.

Vegetarian, dairy-free, refined sugar-free

Ingredients

1 cup quick oats

2 cups vegetable stock or water

2 eggs, poached or soft boiled

1 avocado, sliced

Salt and pepper

Tahini, to taste

Method

Add the oats to a pan over a medium heat and pour in the vegetable stock.

Cook for two minutes, stirring until the porridge is thick and creamy. Divide the porridge between two bowls.

Top your porridge with the sliced avocado and place one of the eggs in each of the bowls.

Drizzle over tahini and season to taste.

Serves 2

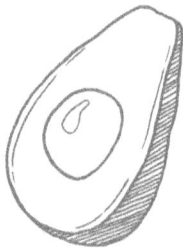
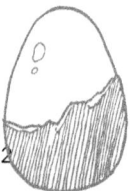
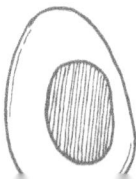

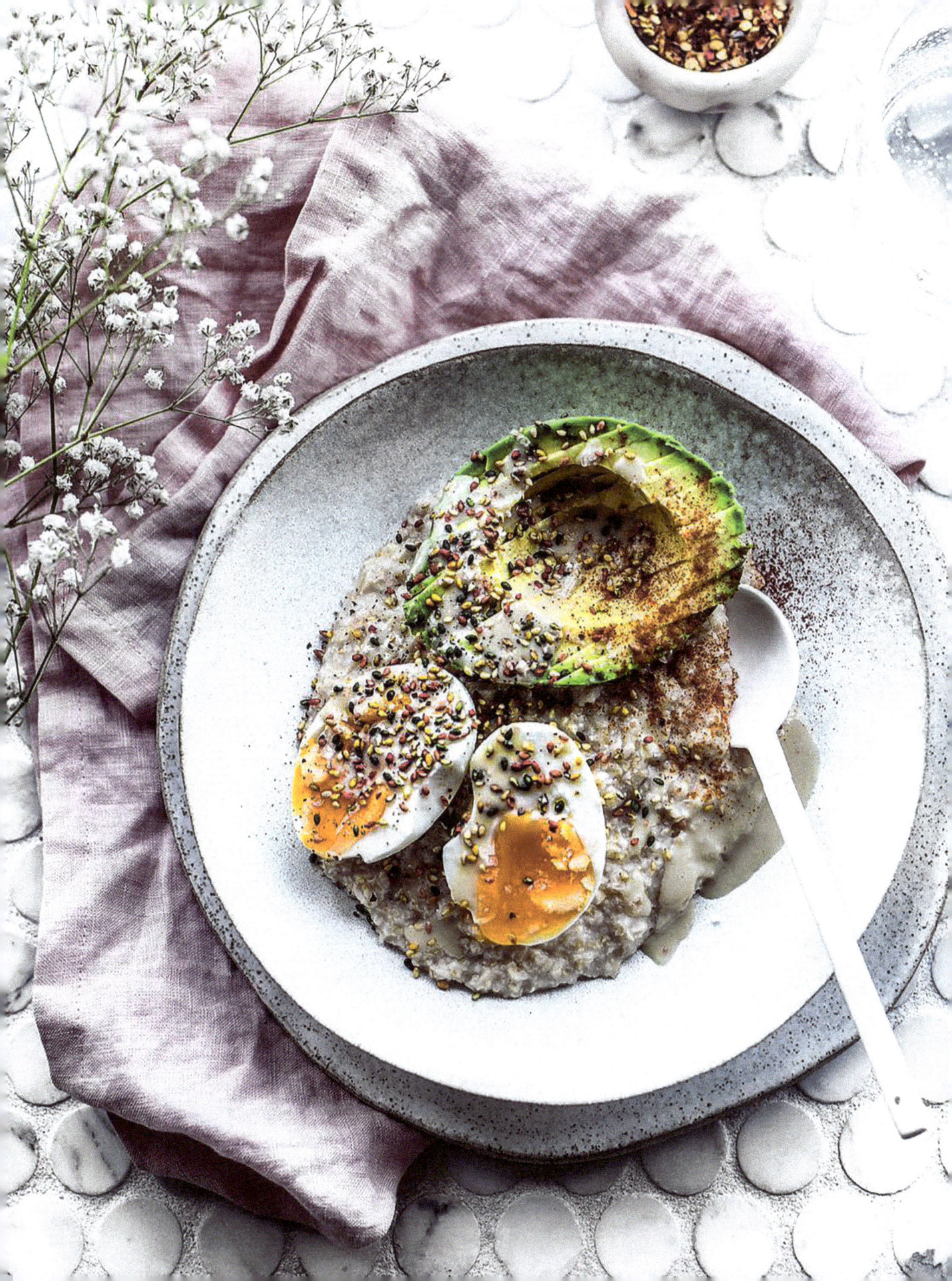

Sunday Morning Crepes

Chloe Munro @the_smallseed_

Plant-based recipe developer Chloe Munro will be the first to admit that her life is far from the picture perfect feed people see on her Instagram. So when you see this photo of her Sunday Morning Crepes, she wants you to know it's not often that she gets to slow down, unwind and have such a beautiful breakfast.

'I love to be able to unwind with my family on a Sunday morning, but in reality sometimes I'm running out the door with a piece of toast in my mouth!' she laughs.

Chloe's words are a reminder that the perfection you see on Instagram isn't always real world. But it can make those weekend mornings when you do get to relax over breakfast with loved ones all the more special.

In those moments, cook up a batch of these vanilla-filled crepes, put your phone away and enjoy your own little moment of perfection.

Vegan, gluten-free, dairy-free, refined sugar-free

Ingredients

160 grams (5½ oz) gluten-free flour

2 cups almond milk

1½ teaspoon pure vanilla extract

1½ tablespoon rice malt syrup

Coconut yogurt, fresh berries and maple syrup, to serve

Fresh berries (optional)

Method

Sieve flour into a bowl. In a separate bowl, combine the almond milk, vanilla extract and rice malt syrup.

Make a well in the centre of the flour and add the wet ingredients. Stir well with a hand whisk until a smooth batter forms and any lumps have disappeared.

Heat your pan (Chloe uses a 9 inch frypan) over a medium heat and add a little oil. Once oil is hot, add a ladle of the crepe mixture and tilt the pan with a circular motion until batter is evenly spread across the base of the pan.

Cook the crepe for approximately 2 minutes, then flip with a spatula and cook on the other side for a further 2 minutes.

Once cooked, place the crepe on a plate and cover to keep warm. Repeat with remaining batter.

Fill each crepe with coconut yogurt and fold over. Top with berries, drizzle with maple syrup and enjoy!

Makes 8-10 crepes

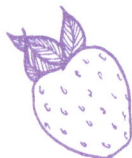

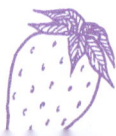

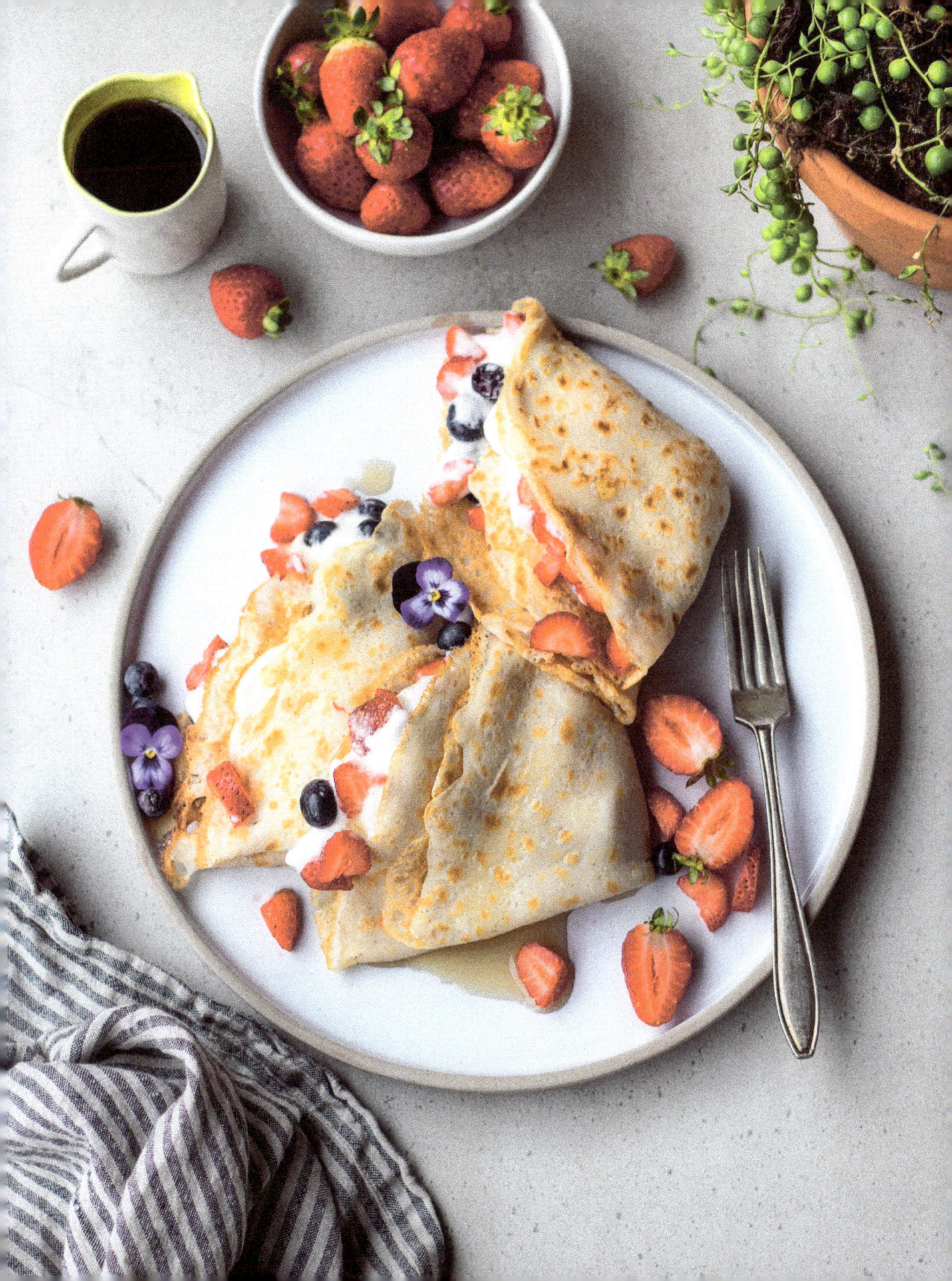

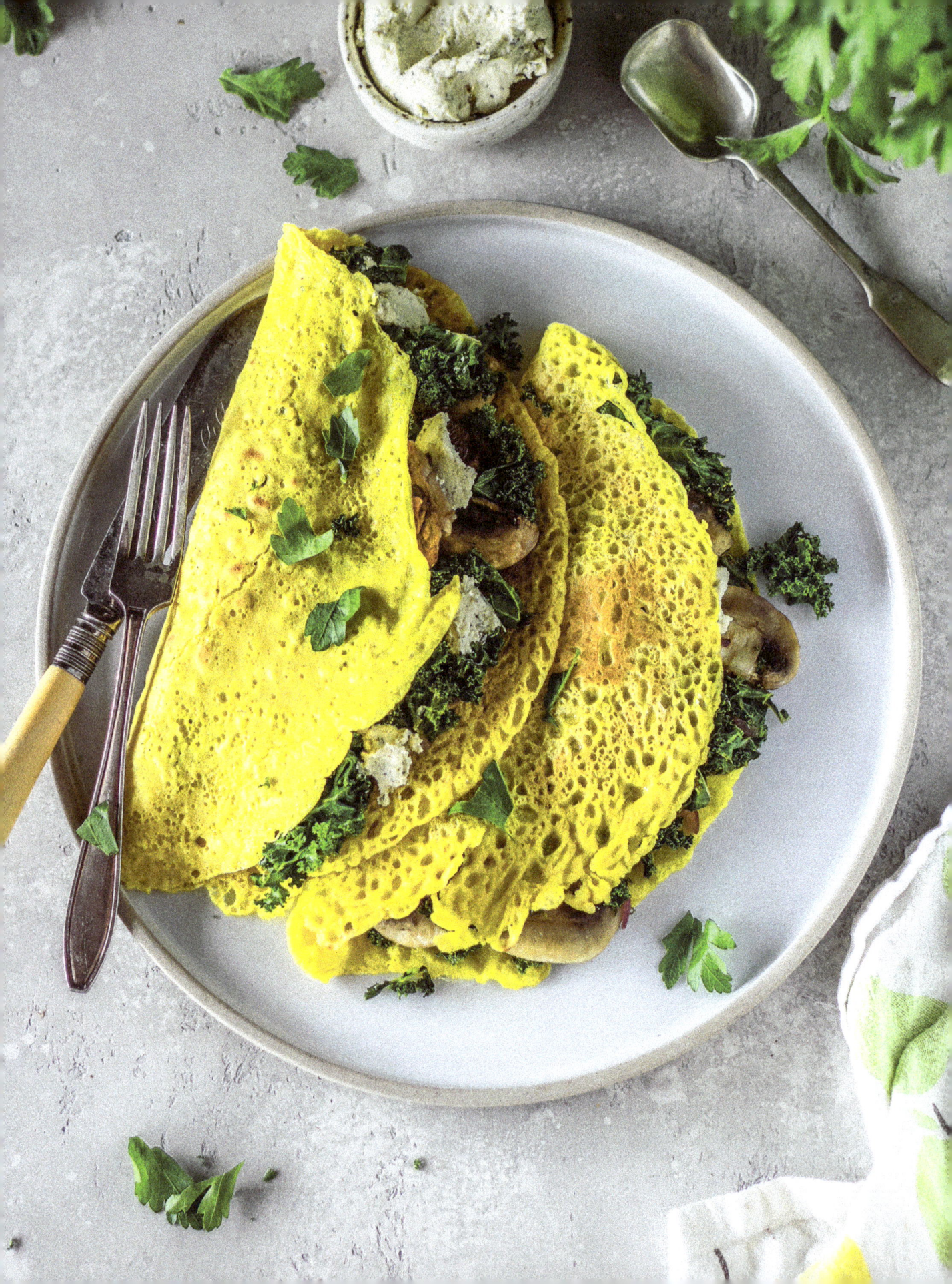

Savoury Chickpea Crepes Filled with Sauted Kale, Garlic Mushrooms & Cashew Cheese

Chloe Munro @the_smallseed_

When it comes to creating her recipes, Chloe Munro has a very relaxed approach.

'I play around with different ideas when I'm cooking,' she says. 'What do I fancy eating? What's in season? What looks good at the market? And then I get creative with the ingredients. Cooking doesn't have to be strict or regimented. For me it's a truly artistic outlet.'

These crepes were the result of an afternoon spent getting creative in the kitchen, and now make a regular appearance on Chloe's table.

Vegan, gluten-free, dairy-free, refined sugar-free

Ingredients

For the crepes

½ cup chickpea (besan) flour

155 millilitres cold water

1 tablespoon nutritional yeast

⅛ teaspoon turmeric powder

⅛ teaspoon garlic powder

⅛ teaspoon onion powder

Pinch of salt

For the filling

½ brown onion, thinly sliced

8 button mushrooms, sliced

1 garlic clove, finely sliced

2 handfuls of kale, roughly chopped

Cashew cheese, to serve

Hemp seeds

Method

Preheat your oven to 180°C (350°F). Start by making the crepe batter. Place all dry ingredients into a bowl and stir to combine.

Slowly pour the water into the dry ingredients while whisking. Whisk well to ensure that no lumps form. You want the batter to be completely smooth.

Heat a frypan over medium heat, spray lightly with oil and wait until it's hot. Turn the heat under the frypan down to low. Add a small soup ladle of the crepe batter to the pan and gently turn and tilt the pan until the batter evenly coats the base of the pan in a thin layer.

Cook the crepe for around 1-2 minutes, then flip and cook for a further minute or so on the other side. Once cooked, place the crepe on a plate and keep warm in the oven. Repeat with the remaining crepe batter.

For the filling, heat a lightly oiled frypan over a medium heat. Once hot, add the onion and saute for 1-2 minutes until translucent. Next, add the mushrooms, garlic and kale. Cook for around 3-4 minutes, or until mushrooms and kale are cooked through.

Remove crepes from the oven, fill with the kale and mushroom mixture, top with cashew cheese and serve.

Serves 2

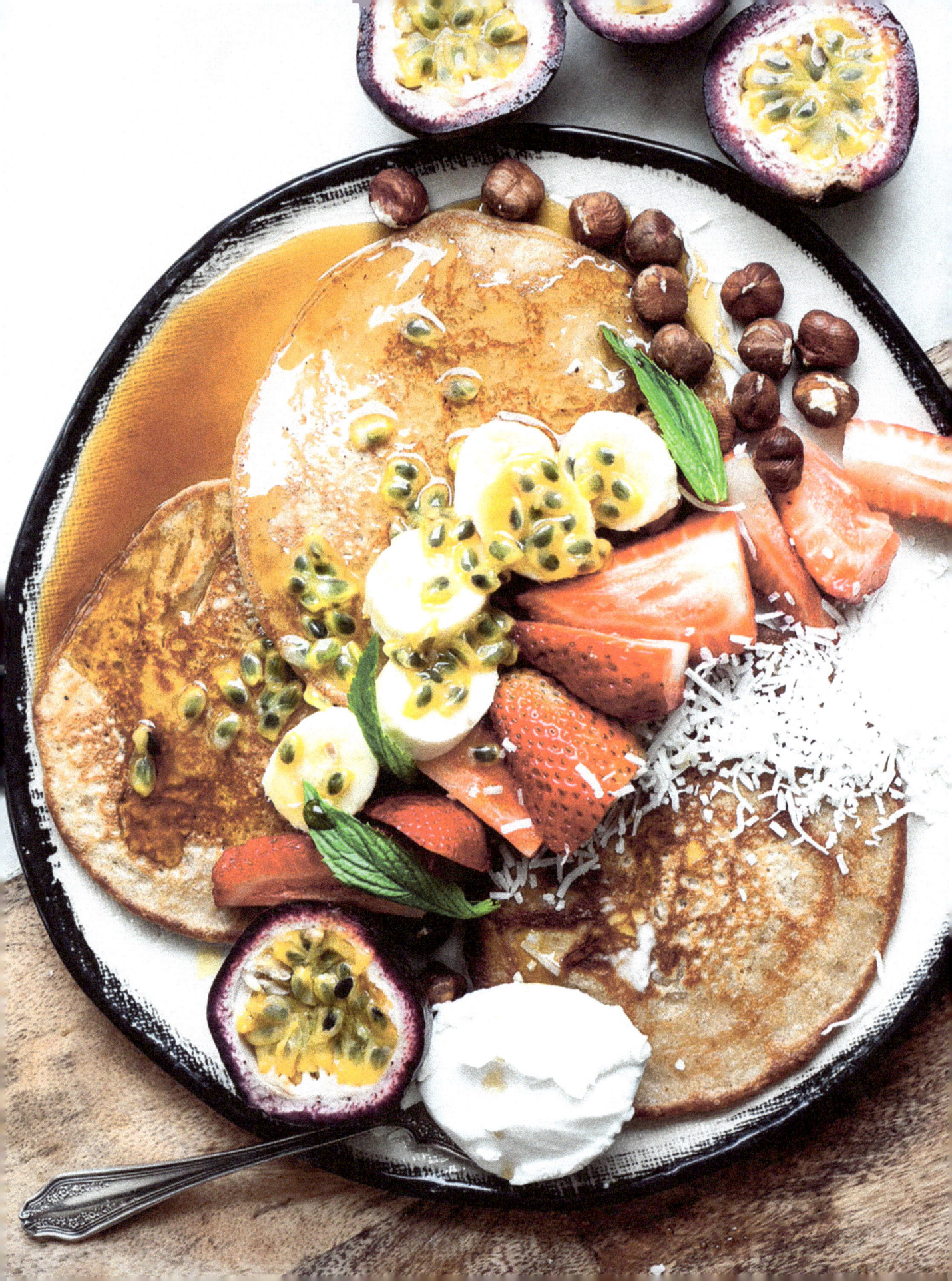

Coconut Banana Pancakes

Courtenay Perks @wholeremedy

In Courtenay Perks' home in Watsons Bay, Sundays are often spent baking with her four beautiful daughters. She lets her girls rifle through her cookbook collection - which numbers over 100 books! - to find something they'd like to make.

However, on certain occasions, this process is skipped and the girls immediately decide they want one thing, and one thing only. Mum's pancakes.

Filled with the can't-go-wrong combination of coconut and banana, these fluffy pancakes can be whipped up in minutes and are perfect to pile onto the middle of your table to let everyone help themselves to their favourite toppings.

Vegan, gluten-free, dairy-free, refined sugar-free

Ingredients

1 cup spelt flour (can substitute for other gluten-free flour)

¾ cup whole oats

¼ cup shredded coconut

3 tablespoons almond butter

1 cup organic coconut milk

3 bananas sliced

2 teaspoons vanilla extract paste

Toppings of choice: fresh fruit, pure maple syrup, coconut yogurt, vegan chocolate chips

Method

Blend all ingredients in a blender until smooth.

Heat a non-stick frypan over medium heat. Add a little olive or coconut oil. Add a ladle of pancake batter to the pan and cook pancakes in batches until golden brown on both sides.

Serve warm with pure maple syrup, passion fruit, berries and coconut yoghurt.

Serves 4

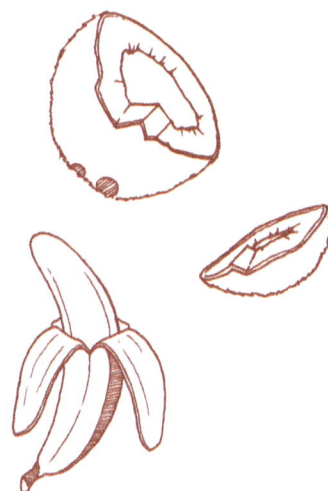

Baked Papaya with Lime & Coconut Yogurt

Lee Holmes @leesupercharged

Forget sad fruit salads with soggy apple and questionably brown banana. This brekkie is a true celebration of tropical, fruity flavours that tastes like summer on a plate.

The inspiration for this dish came to nutritionist, wholefoods chef and author Lee Holmes when she tasted something similar on a blissful holiday in Kerala, India.

Following many of the principles found in Ayurvedic cooking, Lee says this is a 'cooling' dish, so is perfect for warmer seasons.

While papaya isn't something you might use frequently, it's bursting with incredible flavour and digestive enzymes that boost gut health, so it's worth scouting out in your greengrocers.

Vegan, gluten-free, dairy-free, refined sugar-free

Ingredients

1 large papaya, cut in half, seeds removed

1 teaspoon ground cinnamon

zest and juice of 1 lime

250 grams (1 cup) coconut yoghurt

Method

Preheat your oven to 180°C (350°F) and line a baking tray with baking paper.

Place the papaya on the baking tray and sprinkle with cinnamon, lime zest and drizzle with the lime juice.

Place the papaya in the oven and bake for around 15 minutes, or until the papaya is lightly coloured. Remove from the oven and allow to cool slightly.

Serve topped with the coconut yoghurt and an extra drizzle of lime, if you like.

Serves 2

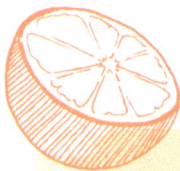

You can add some lime slices to the baking tray alongside the papaya to caramelise them. Then squeeze the juice over the papaya just before serving for an extra tropical punch.

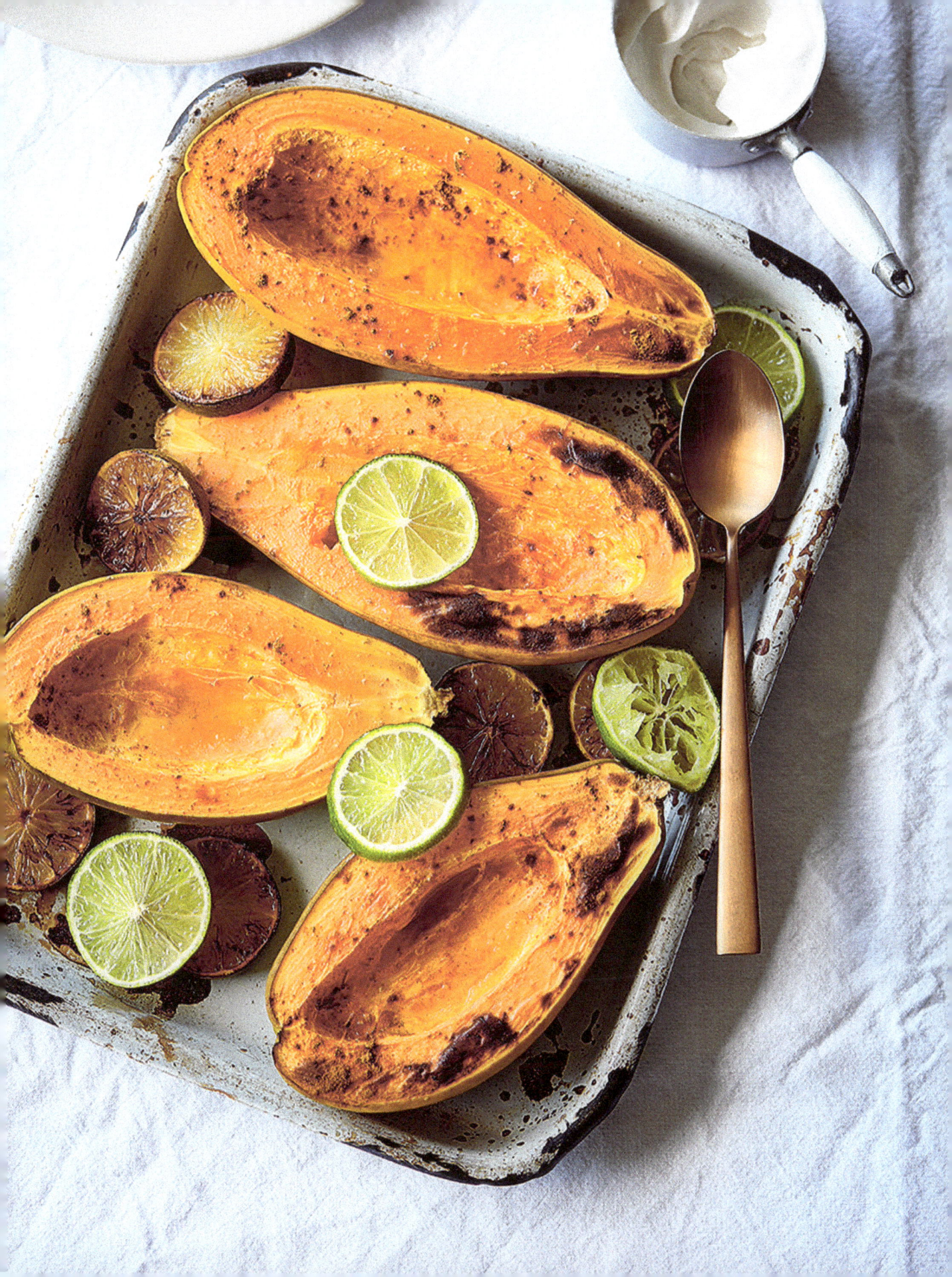

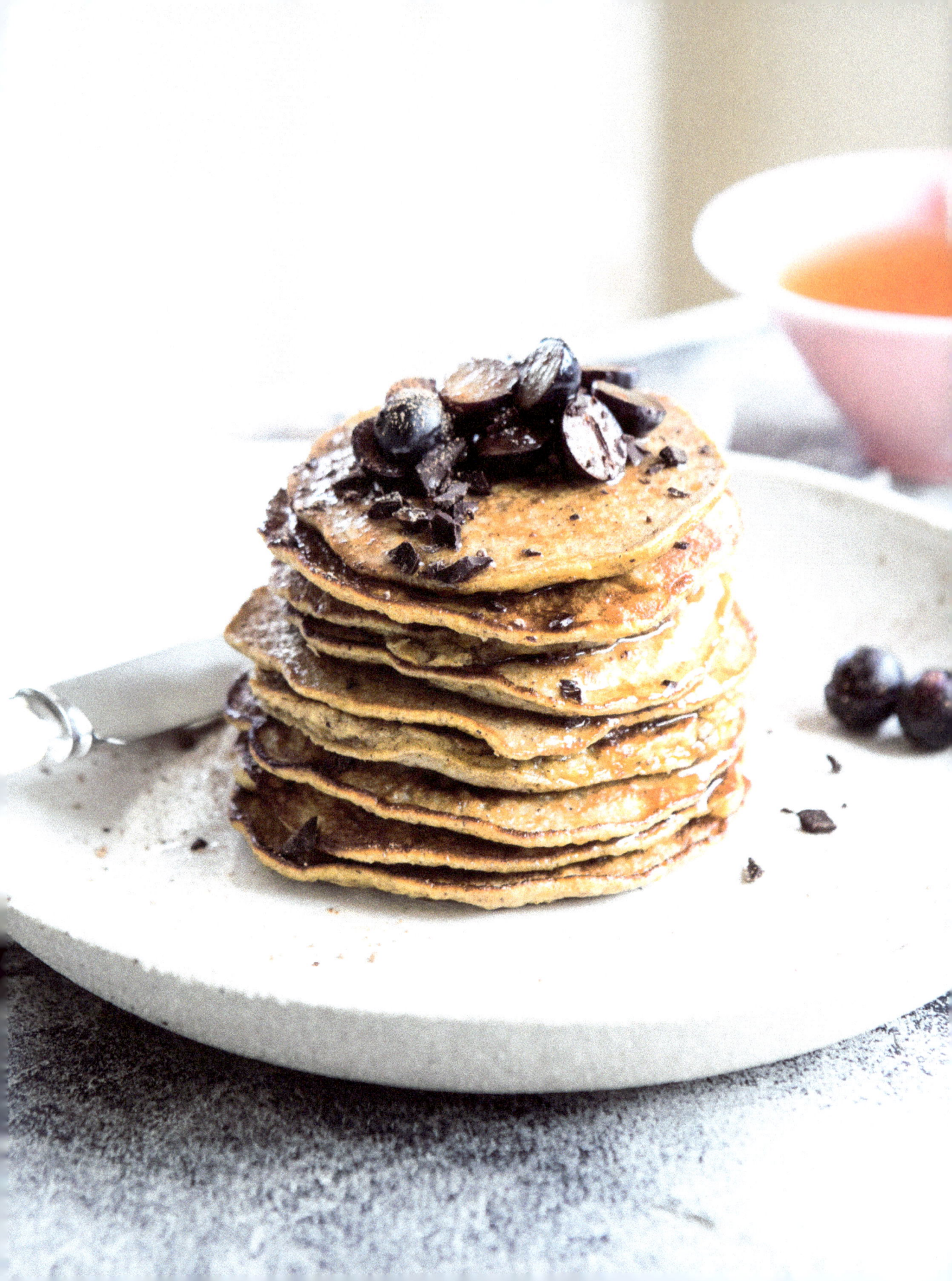

4-Ingredient Flourless Pancakes

Nadia Felsch @nadiafelsch

While she knows it may not be popular opinion, nutritionist Nadia Felsch has never been a huge fan of pancakes.

'I've always found that flour makes them too dense,' she admits. 'Which is why I've used eggs in place of flour in this recipe. It makes them so light and fluffy.'

These super quick and easy pancakes are, as Nadia puts it, 'un-stuffupable', and can even be whipped up before work. Her favourite way to enjoy these however, is on a special weekend morning, topping them with fresh fruit to cut through the sweetness.

Vegetarian, gluten-free, dairy-free, refined sugar-free

Ingredients

1 large banana

3 eggs

¼ cup dessicated coconut

1 teaspoon ground cinnamon

Extra-virgin olive oil, to cook

Berries and maple syrup, to serve

Method

Peel the banana and mash in a bowl with a fork. Crack your eggs into a large bowl, whisk and then combine with the mashed banana. Add all the remaining ingredients (except the oil) and stir well to combine.

Heat the oil in a fry pan over medium heat and spoon small portions of the mixture into the pan. Once a spatula can go cleanly under the pancake and it looks golden underneath, flip it over. Once both sides are golden brown, remove from the heat and place on a plate in an oven set at a low temperature to keep warm.

Repeat this process until all the mixture has been cooked, then serve your pancakes warm topped with maple syrup and berries.

Makes 9 pancakes

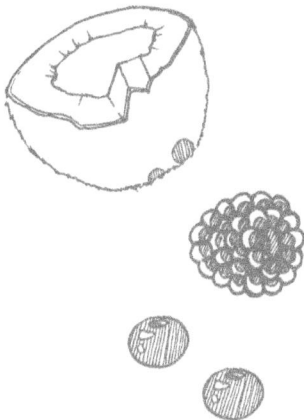

Shakshuka

Jen Murrant and Hannah Singleton @healthyluxe

With more than two serves of veggies and a good dose of protein from eggs, this rich shakshuka is a great breakfast. Or lunch... Or dinner.

'This is a regular meal in our house,' says nutritionist and naturopath Jen Murrant. 'And while we often have it for a quick midweek dinner, it's also a fantastic healthy breakfast. It's a simple recipe to use as a base, and then you just add whatever vegetables you have in your fridge.'

Mother and daughter duo, Jen and Hannah, recommend serving this shakshuka with toasted sourdough, fresh herbs, chilli, a sprinkle of cumin and parmesan cheese.

Vegan alternative, vegetarian, dairy-free, refined sugar-free

Ingredients

1 tablespoon olive oil

1 red onion, finely chopped

2 small capsicums, chopped

2 small zucchinis, chopped

1 small red chilli, finely chopped

400 grams (14 oz) fresh or tinned organic tomatoes

⅓ cup filtered water

1 pinch of turmeric

1 teaspoon cumin

1 teaspoon paprika

Pinch of Himalayan salt and pepper

2-3 organic eggs

Basil leaves, micro herbs, fresh chilli and parmesan, to garnish

Sourdough toast, to serve (optional)

Method

Place a deep sided fry pan or saucepan over low-medium heat. Add the oil and onion and sauté for a few minutes until the onion is translucent.

Add in the remaining chopped vegetables, tinned tomatoes, water and spices. Lower the heat under the pan and simmer for approximately 30 minutes, stirring occasionally.

Add the eggs to the pan, cover and leave to cook for 5-10 minutes, depending on how well-cooked you like your eggs.

Top with basil and/or micro herbs, and season with your choice of spices, Himalayan salt and pepper. Serve this alongside sourdough toast.

Serves 2

To make this dish vegan, simply swap out the eggs for your favourite legumes (chickpeas or cannellini beans work well) or tofu.

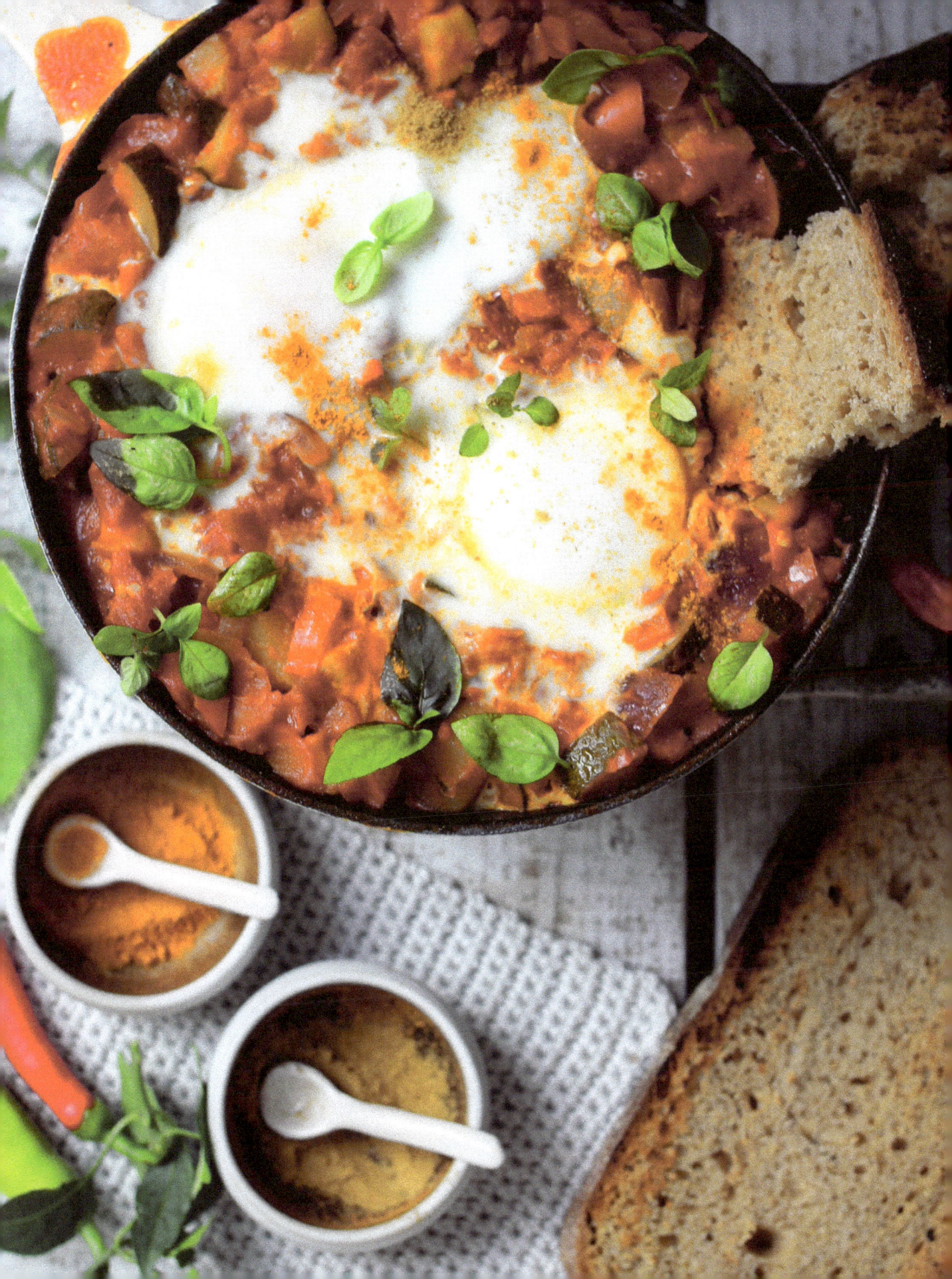

Stuffed Mushrooms with Pesto

Stephanie Geddes @nutritionist_stephgeddes

When developing her 21-Day Detox program, nutritionist Steph Geddes, who also heads up nutrition for 28 By Sam Wood, wanted to create a dish that encouraged her clients to eat more legumes.

'I think a lot of people are scared of cooking with legumes, because they don't know what to do with them,' Steph says. 'In this dish mushrooms are the perfect vessel to carry the beans that's easy, tasty and gives you all their nutritional benefits.'

If you're using store-bought pesto rather than making your own, Steph suggests looking for brands that contain as few preservatives and additives as possible.

Vegan, gluten-free, dairy-free, refined sugar-free

Ingredients

4 large stems of kale, stalks removed

2 x cans cannellini beans, drained

4 x spring onion, finely chopped

1 tablespoon olive oil

1 tablespoon of lemon juice

¼ cup water

¾ cup walnuts, roughly chopped

Handful of parsley, chopped

4 portobello mushroom, stalks removed

2 bunches of asparagus

12 mini roma/cherry tomatoes (or any kind)

Store-bought pesto, to serve, or use the recipe below for Steph's pumpkin seed pesto.

Method

Preheat the oven to 180°C (350°F).

Place a colander over a pot of boiling water. Place the kale in the colander, ensuring it's not touching the boiling water, and steam your kale until just wilted. Drain, squeeze out excess water and finely chop.

Use a food processor/high speed blender to blend the cannellini beans, spring onion, olive oil, lemon juice. Add the water a little at a time, stopping before the mixture is totally smooth - you want a bit of texture. Add the kale, parsley and walnuts and pulse a few times to combine.

Place your mushrooms top-side down on a tray covered with baking paper. Fill each mushroom with the bean mixture and bake in the oven for 15 to 20 minutes, or until starting to crisp or go brown on top. You can finish them off under the grill if they are not browning enough.

While your mushrooms are cooking, grill the asparagus and tomatoes on a grill pan for approximately 5 to 10 minutes, or until asparagus is cooked through and chargrill marks have appeared.

For the pesto

1 packed cup of basil leaves

¼ cup olive oil

1 clove garlic

¼ cup pumpkin seeds

½ long green chilli (optional)

1 tablespoon lemon juice

Once cooked, remove the mushrooms from the oven and serve on a plate alongside the grilled vegetables and some pesto.

For the pesto

Combine all ingredients in a food processor or high speed blender and blend until you reach your preferred consistency.

Dollop over your roasted mushrooms and grilled vegetables and serve.

Serves 4

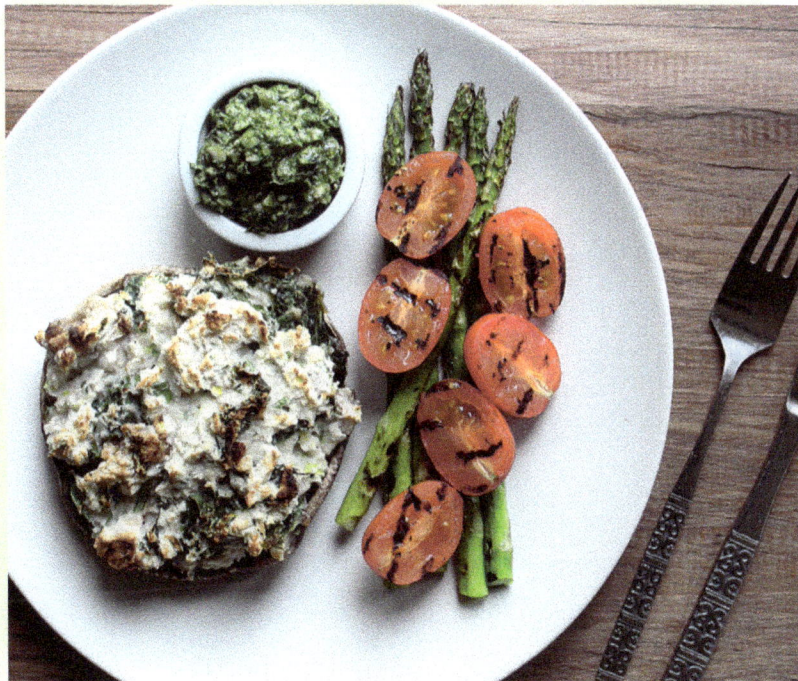

Breakfast Tofu Scramble

Sami Bloom @samibloom

When clinical nutritionist Sami Bloom began her journey into plant-based eating, eggs were what she thought she would miss most. So when looking for a vegan alternative to her favourite breakfast scramble, she turned to tofu and began experimenting.

'I was a shitty cook growing up,' Sami laughs. 'I just didn't make time for it and was looking at it all wrong. Vegan cooking now allows me to be creative, but not necessarily complicated. If you use the right spices and salt, tofu is a really good alternative to eggs, as it's high in protein and, when scrambled, can have a similar consistency.'

Vegan alternative, vegetarian, dairy-free, refined sugar-free

Ingredients

4 tablespoons coconut milk

100 grams (3½ oz) firm tofu, finely chopped/diced

1 handful of button mushrooms, sliced

2 stalks shallots or chives, sliced

1 clove garlic, minced

2 cups of leafy greens, kale and spinach work best

1 ½ tablespoons nutritional yeast

½ teaspoon sea salt

Additional nutritional yeast, salt and pepper, wholemeal toast and avocado, to serve (optional)

Method

Throw one tablespoon of the coconut milk and the tofu into a fry pan over a medium heat, breaking the tofu apart with a spatula to form a scramble-like consistency.

After about 3 minutes, once the tofu is starting to brown slightly, add your chopped mushrooms, shallots and garlic to the pan. Place lid on the pan to steam-fry for around three to five minutes, stirring occasionally.

Add in the greens, remaining three tablespoons of coconut milk, nutritional yeast and sea salt and warm in the pan for three to four minutes, stirring to ensure it doesn't stick to the pan.

Transfer the scrambled tofu to a plate with any additional nutritional yeast or cracked pepper you desire. You can serve this with a side of wholemeal toast and 1/4 avocado for a balanced breakfast.

Serves 1

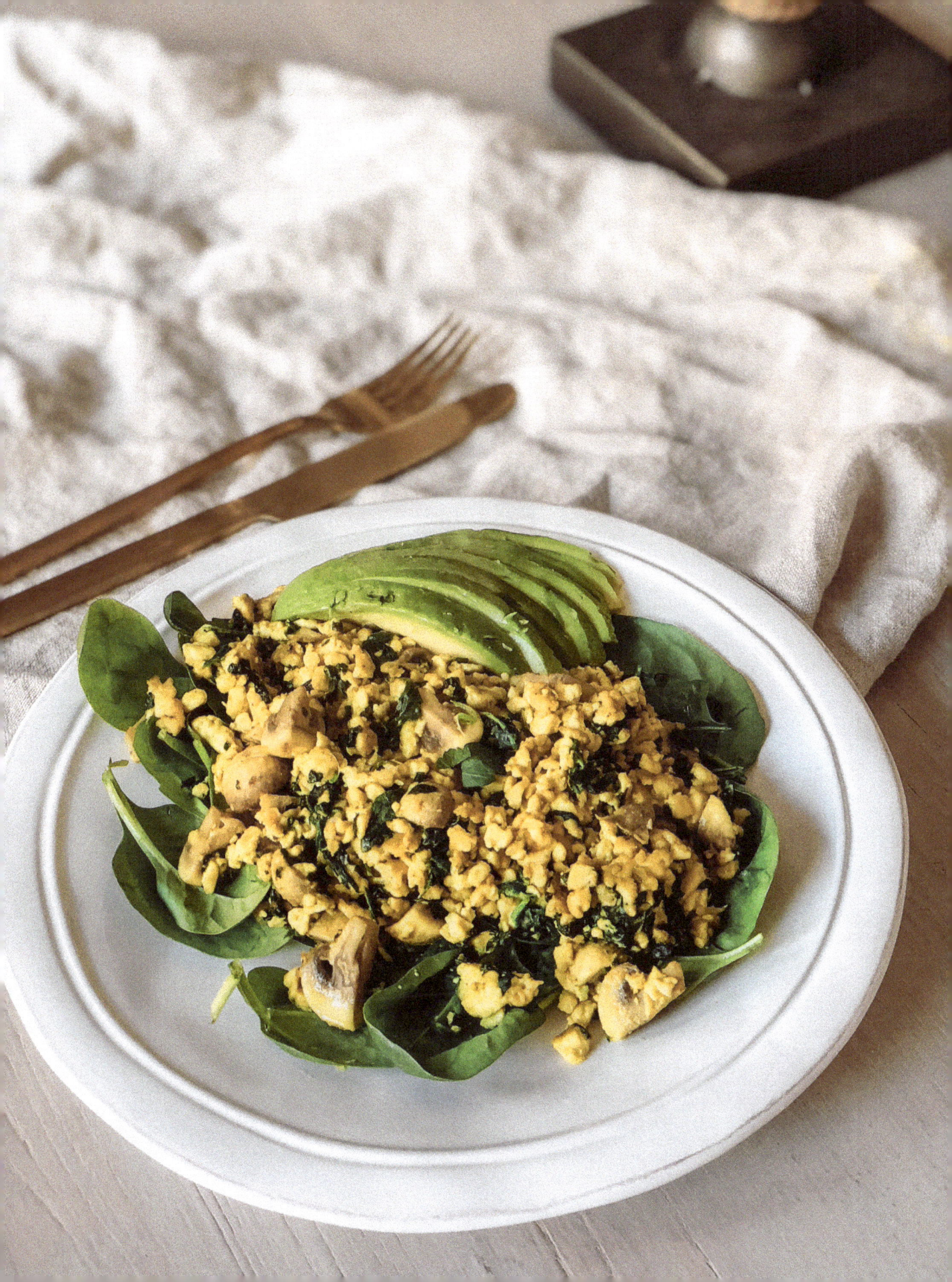

Sarah Holloway on Finding your Way & Seizing your Yay

Sarah Holloway @spoonful_of_sarah

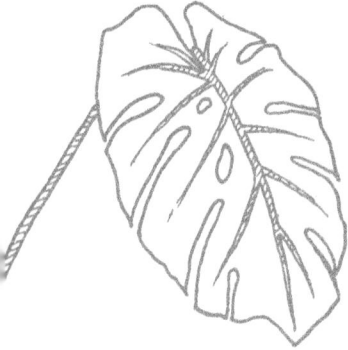

They say a spoonful of sugar helps the medicine go down... but when it comes to finding joy in the everyday, we think a spoonful of Sarah Holloway (AKA @spoonful_of_sarah) is enough to inspire you.

At just 30 years of age, Sarah is perhaps best known for taking a leap of faith that saw her leave her high-paying job as a lawyer to co-found green tea empire Matcha Maiden and vegan cafe Matcha Mylkbar. She has since gone on to become one of Australia's most loved business women, attending panels and events to share her insights alongside other industry professionals, and has even begun an incredibly popular podcast, Seize the Yay.

Just like most of us, Sarah's story starts off with humble beginnings. Growing up in Melbourne's South Eastern suburbs, both Sarah and her brother were adopted from South Korea at a young age. It was a culture that she says was always celebrated and encouraged within her family home. Both Sarah's parents were raised in regional areas, seeing much of her childhood spent running around on farmland, forging a strong sense of family and community that she feels she might have otherwise missed had she been raised a "city girl".

It is perhaps this grounded upbringing that makes Sarah so humble, loveable and disarmingly charming, despite her impressive and somewhat intimidating professional bio. She's quick to acknowledge her normalcy and isn't shy to have a laugh at herself.

Sitting in her favourite Melbourne cafe, she's decked out in black leggings, Nike runners (she's training for the Melbourne Marathon) and her fiance Nic Davidson's oversized fluffy jumper. With bright eyes and long dark hair that falls around her shoulders, she radiates an openness and warmth that puts all those in her presence at ease.

'I think I'm the most down to earth person in the world,' laughs Sarah. 'And I'm a total oversharer, so there's not a lot that people don't know about me! I wear my Qantas pajamas everywhere and I wear a mouthguard to bed, so it's really not a sexy time!'

It's small, wonderfully human details such as these that Sarah manages to coax from many of her podcast guests, which makes you realise that all of the well-known entrepreneurs and acclaimed personnel that frequent her show aren't that different from you and I.

'That's my favourite part about the Seize the Yay podcast,' Sarah explains. 'You get to see that everyone's just a person. If you read interviews, it can be hard to see how normal someone is, but when you hear their voice and hear them laugh - it makes them human.'

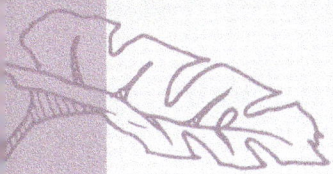
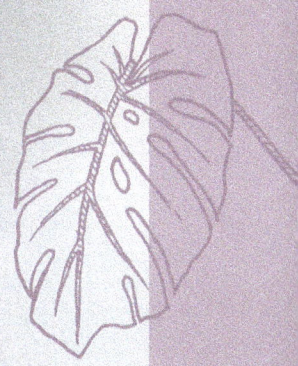
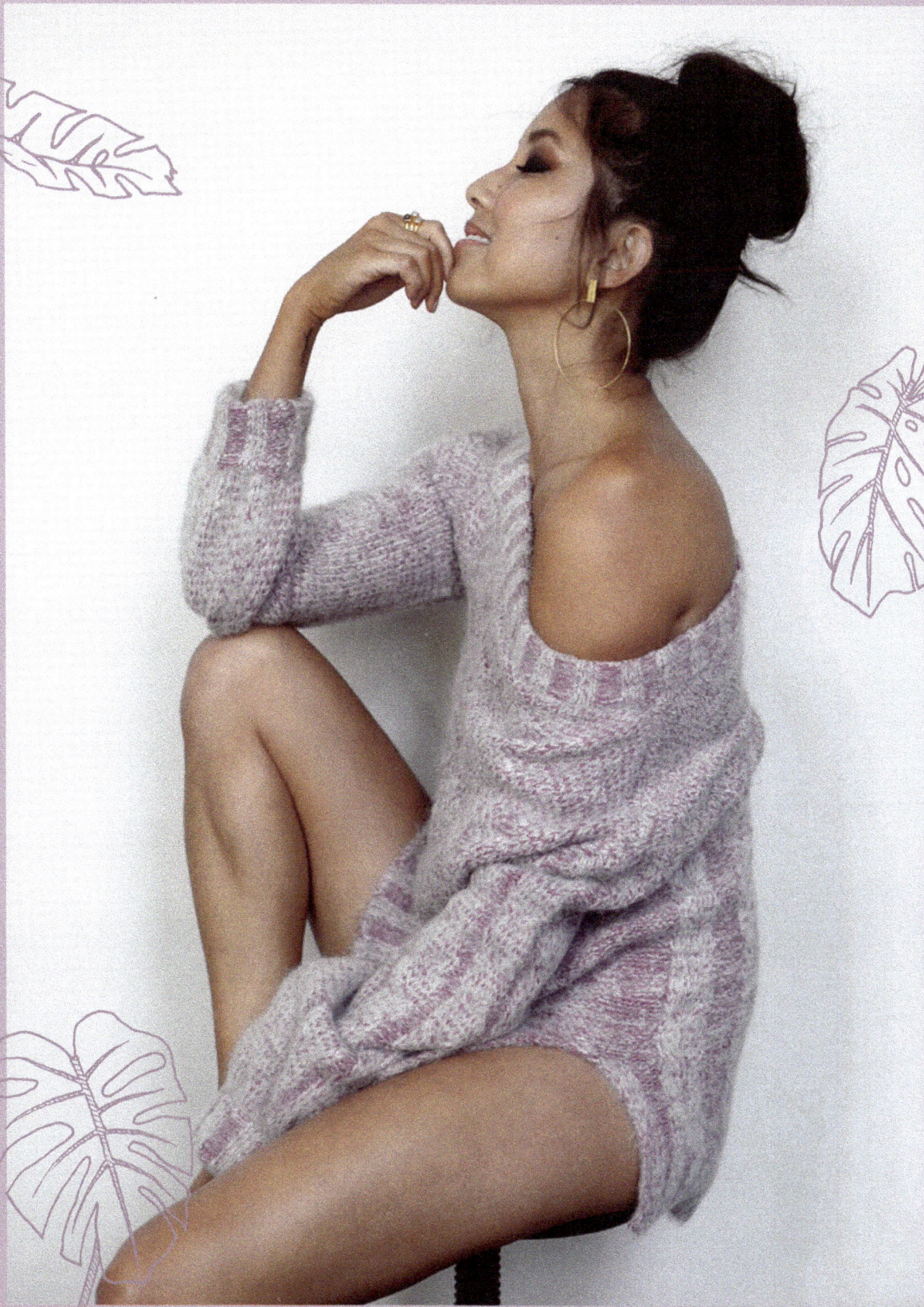
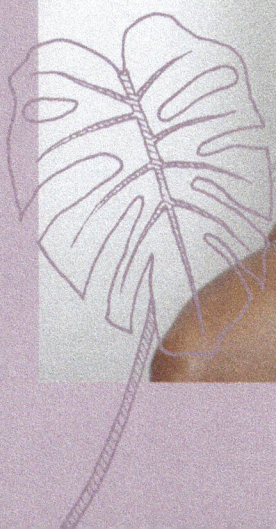

The aim of Sarah's podcast is to move beyond a person's professional bio, taking the emphasis off what they do and instead focus on who they are. Her conversations reveal the real, raw and unglossed version of a person's life, and delve into what really makes them tick. She encourages her audience to look past the suits and success to see that each one of these impressive, high-flying professionals needs an element of light-heartedness and creative play in their day.

It's an ethos that balances two notions: that of taking every opportunity and getting the most out of life, with the need to take time to engage in the things you love doing, so you can live your happiest life.

Help! I Don't Know What I'm Doing With My Life

These days, there's an incredible amount of pressure on people to follow a linear career progression: finish high school with good grades, graduate university and then go into full-time work for the next 40 years of your life. And while this stereotype is slowly being broken down with the increasing number of start-ups and side hustles, we can't help but see there's still pressure, whether internally or from external sources, that makes us feel the need to conform to this pattern of behaviour. As though we need to have our 10 year life plan figured out.

After a slightly shaky start to high school (Sarah admits she had a rebel stage), she was able to achieve the grades she needed to undertake a Law/Arts degree at Monash University, following which she landed the 'dream job' as a mergers and acquisitions lawyer at a leading international law firm in Melbourne. But even at this point in her life, Sarah says she still wasn't completely sure that this was what she wanted from her career.

'I just thought I'd try my best to get into a really good law firm and see if I liked it once I was there,' she says, taking a sip of her chai tea. 'I realised that it might not be my forever job, but I just wanted to do my best and see how it went.'

'I think as humans we really like certainty and want to know where we're going with regards to our careers. But I believe that we just have to get comfortable with not knowing exactly what direction we're travelling in. It can often feel like there's an enormous pressure to choose what career path you should take, but if you don't know what you want to do, that's ok – most of us don't! The best thing you can do is keep learning and discovering as much as you can from your experiences, until you find out what you love.'

'And it's funny what happens when you're open to new opportunities, they sometimes just hit you, as long as you're open to them.'

From Lawyer to Entrepreneur

And hit her these opportunities did.

While in Hong Kong on a work trip in 2014, Sarah found herself hooked on, of all things, matcha green tea. After acquiring a horrendous stomach bug in Rwanda earlier that year, Sarah had sworn of caffeine, but she found that matcha gave her a similar energy boost to coffee along with additional health benefits.

After returning to Australia, both Sarah and Nic became increasingly frustrated with the lack of quality matcha tea available on the market, and so Matcha Maiden was born. Well, it wasn't quite that simple, as Sarah explains.

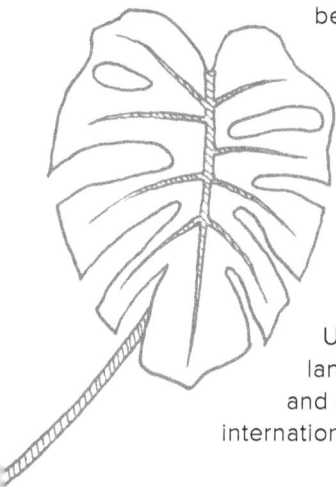

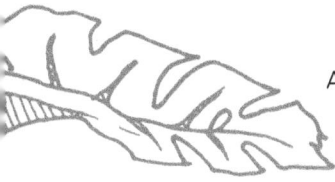

At the time the company launched, both her and Nic were still working intense full time jobs. They would then scurry home after a long day and bury themselves in website development, creating marketing collateral, building a social media following and dealing with Australian customs as they imported their product from Japan.

It's very easy to think that the transition to entrepreneurship happens easily - that it's the "overnight success" that people so often talk about. But what many people don't realise is the self-learning, dedication and often very unglamorous hours of labour that go into starting your own business.

'Every entrepreneur, influencer or noted industry professional I've spoken to has faced setbacks or adversity in their lives,' confirms Sarah. 'They haven't just made it straight to the top without hardships, and that's what's made them resilient. I think when you hear these people's struggles it can help to validate the difficult times in your own journey. It allows you to see that the difficulties and setbacks you face along the way are all part of the process.'

Doubt Kills More Dreams than Failure Ever Will: Combatting Your Inner Critic

If you feel like you're alone when it comes to experiencing self-doubt, know that this is a very natural human impulse that plagues even the most successful of entrepreneurs.

'When I took the leap of faith to quit my job and start Matcha, it was by no means an easy jump,' Sarah admits. 'I'm indecisive at the best of times, so I agonised over the decision and was plagued by doubt and negative self-talk.

I nearly talked myself out of it altogether so many times along the way!'

'Overcoming self-doubt in any area of your life can be difficult because it's the most natural reaction that humans experience when we're faced with stepping outside our comfort zone and confronted with doing something new. It's a protection mechanism.'

'We have the thoughts: what if it's shit, what if I look stupid, what if it feels uncomfortable? The biggest thing for me has been learning to view discomfort as a sign that I'm doing something good, instead of a sign that I should avoid something. I still doubt myself all the time, but I acknowledge those fears and then let them go, because I've chosen to take action.'

When talking about self-doubt, Sarah, a self-confessed quote queen, relays one of her favourite mantras: 'doubt kills more dreams than failure ever will'. She explains that while it's totally natural to experience self-doubt, it's so important not to let it dictate your decisions. If you choose not to move forward because of negative self-talk, then you risk never reaching your full potential. Whatever it is you want to do, whether it's leaving your job, starting a side hustle, making new friends or starting a new project, we love Sarah's practical advice: 'book it into your calendar and just go!'

You Are(n't) What You Do

You walk into a party filled with people you've never met before. Awkward.
What do you do? Naturally, you paste a smile on your face and start talking to the least threatening looking people there.

'Oh hi, I'm....' and you introduce yourself with a little wave.

'Oh hey! And what do you do?'

This is a question that we're confronted with all too often, and while it seems like a very natural part of modern interaction, we're starting to ask the question - is it beneficial? Does it help you understand who the other person really is at their core? Sarah thinks not.

'That question is literally the reason why I started the Seize the Yay podcast,' she explains. 'I just noticed how much people define themselves and others based on their career and what they do for work; No one asks what your hobbies are, what you do for fun and what lights you up, and I think we're really starting to lose our sense of self as a result.'

If you've ever listened to the Seize the Yay podcast (and if you haven't, PSA you really should!), you'll most likely have had Sarah's incredibly catchy intro song stuck in your head at some point. If you haven't, let us enlighten you:

'Busy and happy are not the same thing, we too rarely question what makes the heart sing. We work then we rest, but rarely we play and often don't realise there's more than one way. So this is a platform to hear and explore, the stories of those who found lives they adore. The good, bad and ugly, the best and worst day will bear all the facets of seizing your yay.'

This song explores the notion that in today's society, there's so much emphasis placed on "doing" and productivity. So much so that it's become a measure of our self worth and intrinsically tied up in our identities.

'We put people in boxes based on what they do for work, and we define our own worth by how productive we are,' says Sarah. 'That's why so many people are burning out, because they don't feel like they have value when they're not doing something that achieves a successful outcome.'

This sentiment highlights a trap that so many of us find ourselves caught in - the need to be successful in order to feel "enough". In striving for this success, we all too often forget to stop and ask ourselves if what we're doing is actually providing us with a sense of fulfillment.

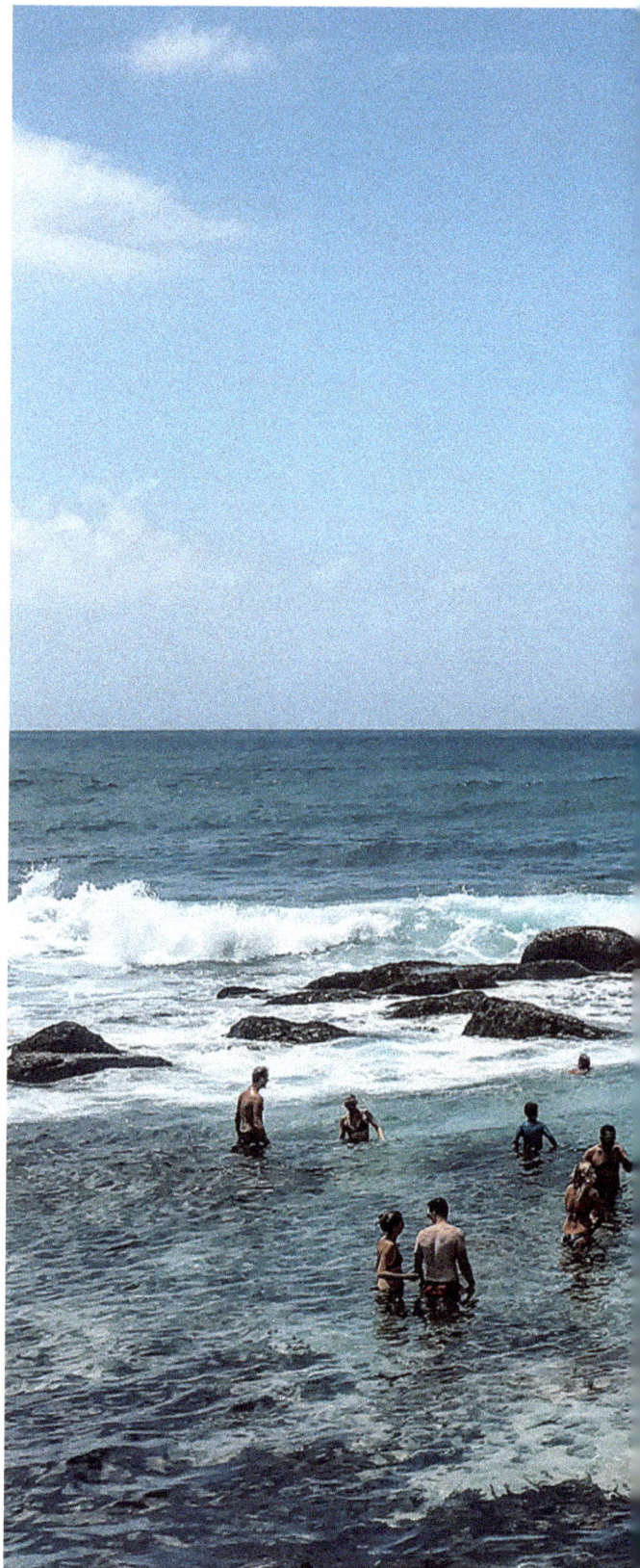

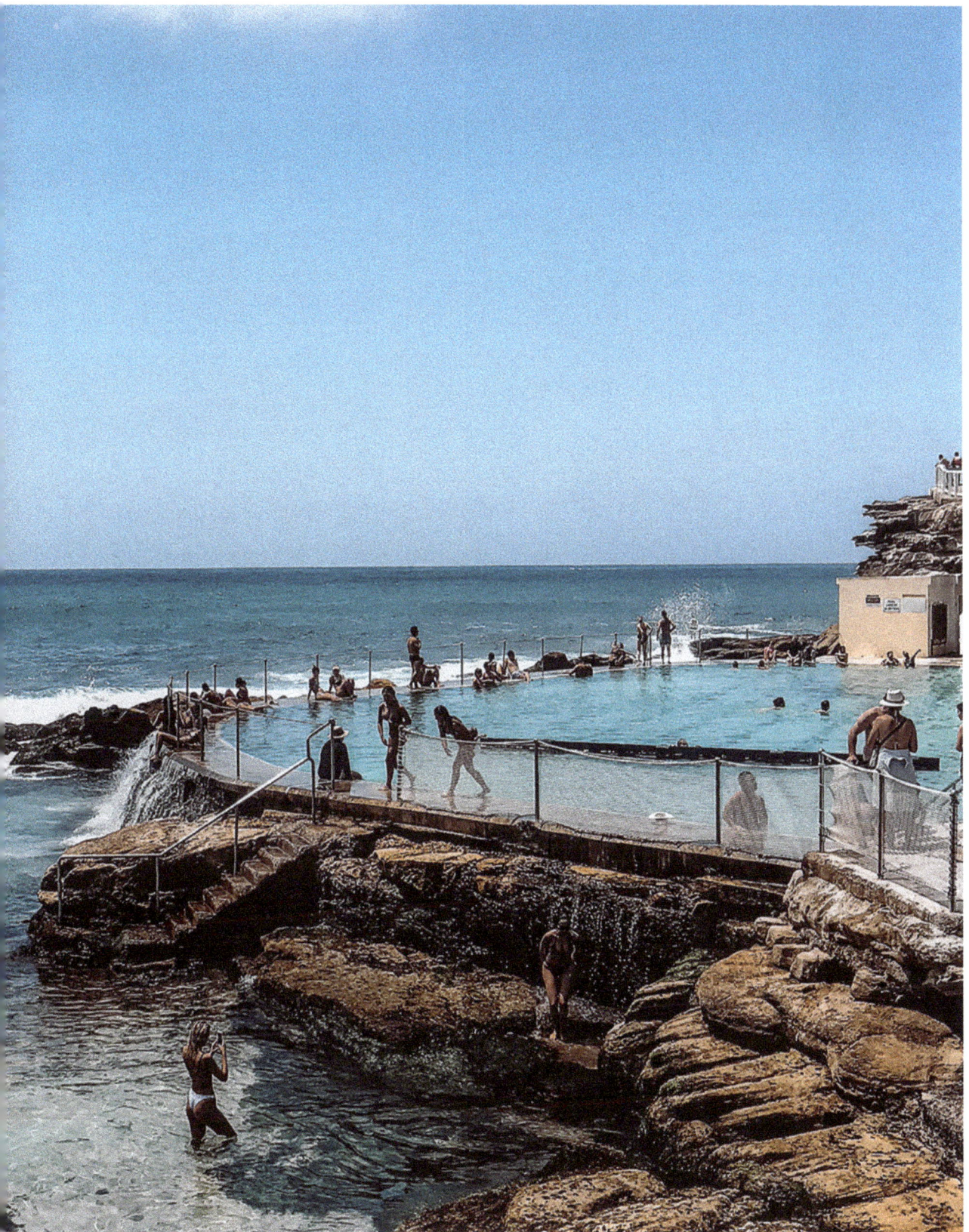

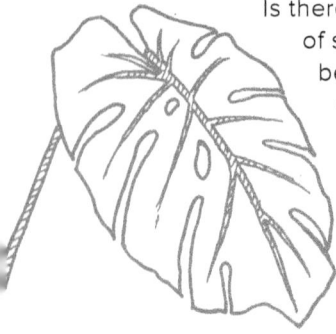

Is there room for joy within this algorithm of success? Or does happiness simply become unimportant and inevitably cast aside, along with play, silliness and our sense of wonder? Have we allowed the all-consuming daily grind and performance-driven society that we live in to dictate - not just our schedules - but how we perceive the world and ourselves?

These are all big questions to be sparked by just one little podcast jingle, but they're questions Sarah urges us to ask ourselves.

'Life can't just be about being busy, hustling and kicking goals,' Sarah says throwing her hands up. 'That kind of life is to the exclusion of joy, fulfillment and excitement, and if what you're doing doesn't light you up then what's the point?'

A-fucken-men.

Find Your Way to Yay

So then, just how do we pull ourselves out of this hard-core hustling lifestyle? Below you'll find some of Sarah's practical tips to help you avoid getting caught up in the daily grind and truly make the most of your day by finding your own kind of yay.

1. Find a Hobby

One thing that all of Sarah's interviewees seem to have in common is having a hobby that allows them to counterbalance their extreme productivity and fulfills them in a way their work can't. Even if you're not planning on being the next Steve Jobs or starting your own business, Sarah says that finding a creative outlet that simply brings you joy is the key component to seizing your yay.

'It should be something that makes you forget what time it is and just makes you feel happy,' she says. 'It doesn't have to have an outcome - you don't even have to be good at it! But it shouldn't be related to your job and shouldn't have anything

to do with self-development or learning. It needs to be something that releases you from the productivity mindset.'

This could be knitting, gardening, playing the guitar or collecting stamps! Whatever it is, you have to find something that is only for enjoyment's sake and then allow yourself to do it. Do this and you'll find yourself more relaxed, motivated and happier because you have some joy in your life.

2. Find a Crew that Supports You

Another of Sarah's most beloved quotes, and one that she believes wholeheartedly is from the late American entrepreneur, author and motivational speaker Jim Rohn: *You are the sum of the five people you spend the most time with.*

'I absolutely believe the environment around you is the key to success,' says Sarah, who makes sure she keeps herself in good company. 'Sometimes we need to do a little clean out and re-evaluate our circle, just to make sure you're surrounding yourself with people who take you higher and support you every step of the way.'

Surround yourself with amazing people, because no one has done it on their own. You can't live a positive life with a negative mind or a negative environment, so create a space that's going to push you in the right direction and help you live a thriving life.

3. Just Do It

Done is better than perfect, so just DO it ya'll. Don't agonise over the process of getting things 100 percent right because then you'll never start. Just begin the process and trust that you'll figure it out along the way. Rip the bandaid off and don't give yourself too much of a chance to talk yourself out of it. Yes, you'll make mistakes along the way, but you'll learn from these and come back more resilient as a result.

4. It Is Just Work, After All

While we might all have dreams of falling into (or creating) the job of our dreams, in reality not all of us are going to absolutely love our 9-5. But that's totally ok!

'I think people believe they have to be completely happy in their job all the time - but it's called work for a reason,' laughs Sarah. 'In fact, it's a huge privilege to be able to find something that you might love to do!'

Sometimes you might have to accept that you might not love your job, but seizing your yay isn't just about finding joy in your working life, but in your life generally. As long as you have another source of happiness, creativity and excitement flowing into your life from somewhere then that's all that matters.

5. Avoid Burnout

Whether you're a uni student in the throws of exams or an office worker struggling with daily deadlines, scheduling in time to do the things you love is critical. Give relaxation and your hobbies the same level of priority as your work.

'Permanent marker that shit into your diary,' says Sarah enthusiastically. 'That's the only way I've been able to shift my mentality from thinking of things like rest and joyful activities as being optional to things that are necessary.'

This could be making time to get a massage on the weekend or going to a sewing class one night a week. Whatever it is, make sure that you hold yourself to account by writing it in your schedule, because once the stress and pressure of daily life sets in it's all too easy to ignore.

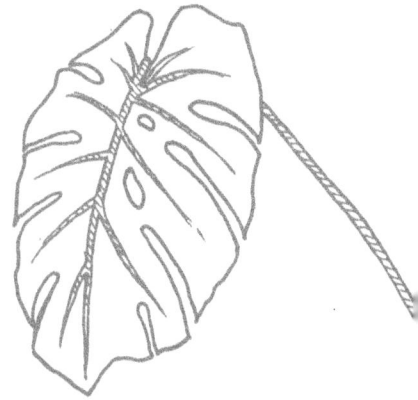

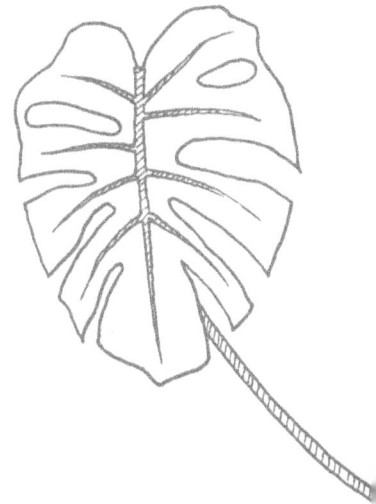

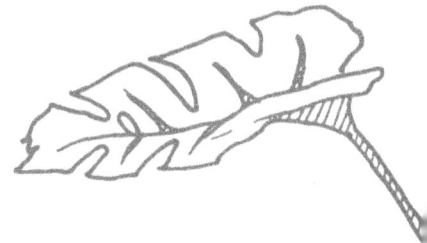

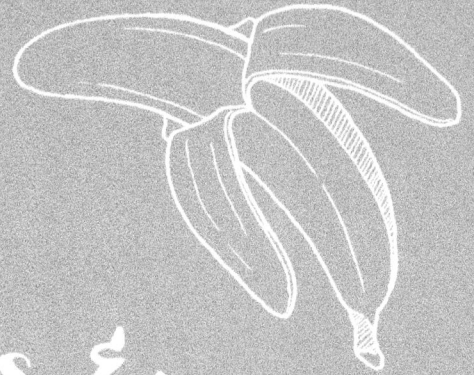

Smoothies &
Smoothie Bowls

It's hard to pinpoint when smoothies
and they're bowl equivalent began to
dominate our Instagram feeds, but my
gosh we're glad they did.

Perfect for breakfast, lunch or dinner
(no judgement), these delicious recipes
hit the spot when you're craving
something sweet and refreshing. Based
on bananas, fresh berries and even with
a few sneaky veggies thrown in for good
measure, we're certain you'll love these
recipes just as much as we do.

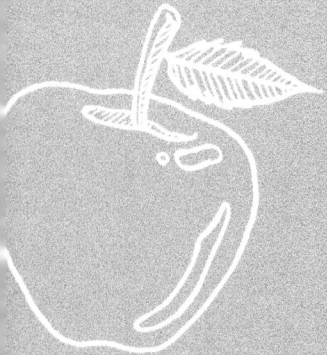

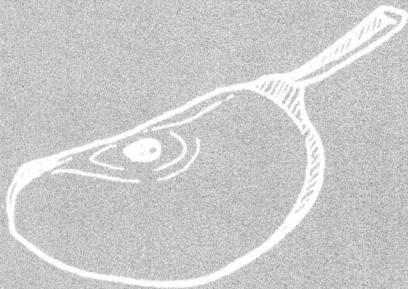

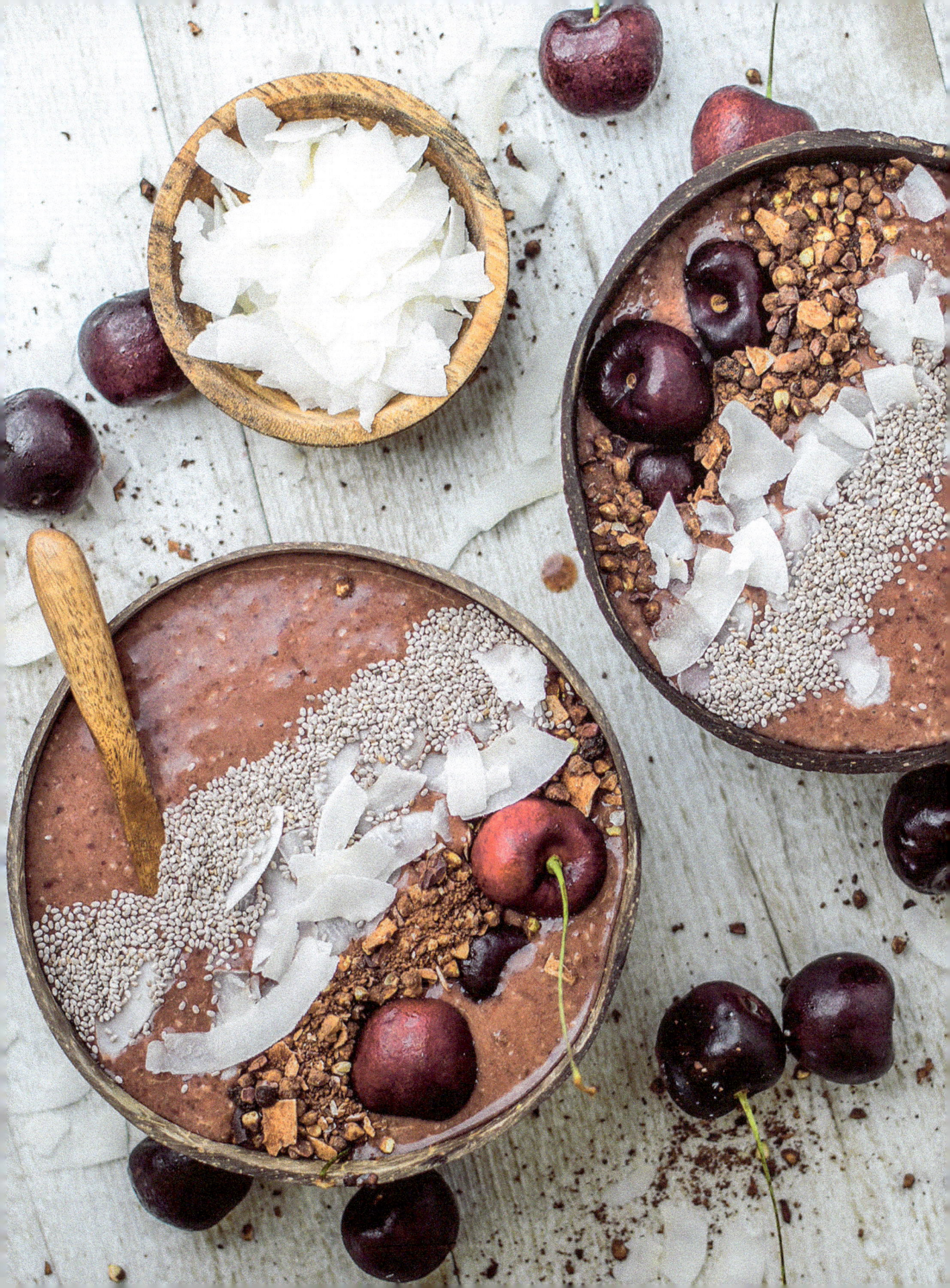

Acai Bowl with the Lot

Phoebe Conway @Pheebsfoods

After studying nutrition, Phoebe Conway felt herself moving away from the calorie-focused, weight loss-obsessed idea of food and discovered a new way of looking at health.

'I now see food as fuel, something that nourishes my body and mind. It helps me think, sleep and move in the ways I want and need,' she says. 'Finding a healthy balance is when you're feeding your body things that make you feel good, but you're still enjoying life at the same time.'

This Acai bowl is one of the first recipes Phoebe created when she began her health journey and satisfies her sweet tooth with the natural goodness of acai and fruit.

Eat this on a warm summer morning after a good sweaty workout and you'll feel refreshed in no time.

Vegan, gluten-free, dairy-free, refined sugar-free

Ingredients

2 frozen acai packs

1 frozen banana

½ cup frozen blueberries

1-2 tablespoons coconut milk or water

1 serving (scoop) vanilla protein powder

Granola, nut butter, berries, banana, dried coconut and goji berries, to serve

Method

Place all of the smoothie ingredients into a high powered blender or food processor except the coconut milk. Add one tablespoon of coconut milk and blend until smooth, scraping down the sides when necessary. If you want to loosen the mixture a bit, add more coconut water.

Pour the mixture into 2 bowls, smooth with the back of a spoon and top with your favourite toppings.

Serves 2

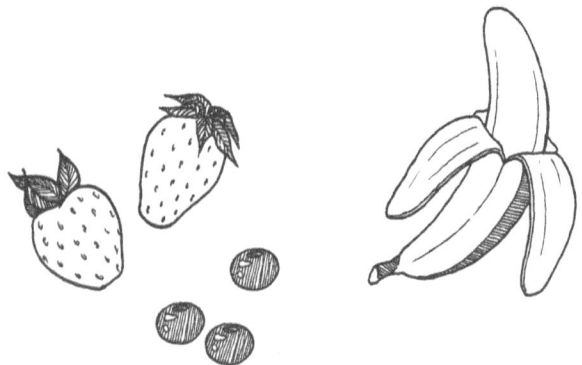

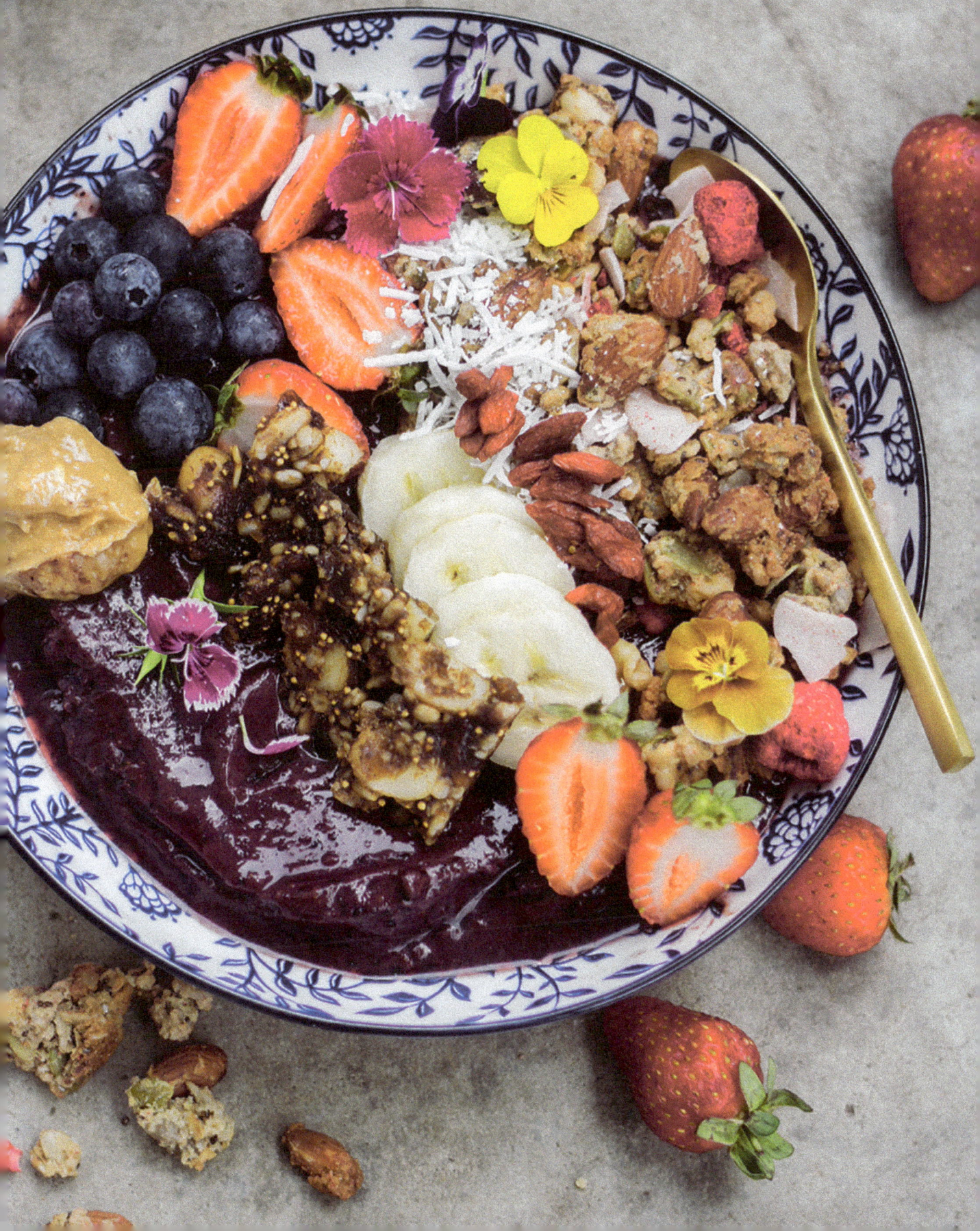

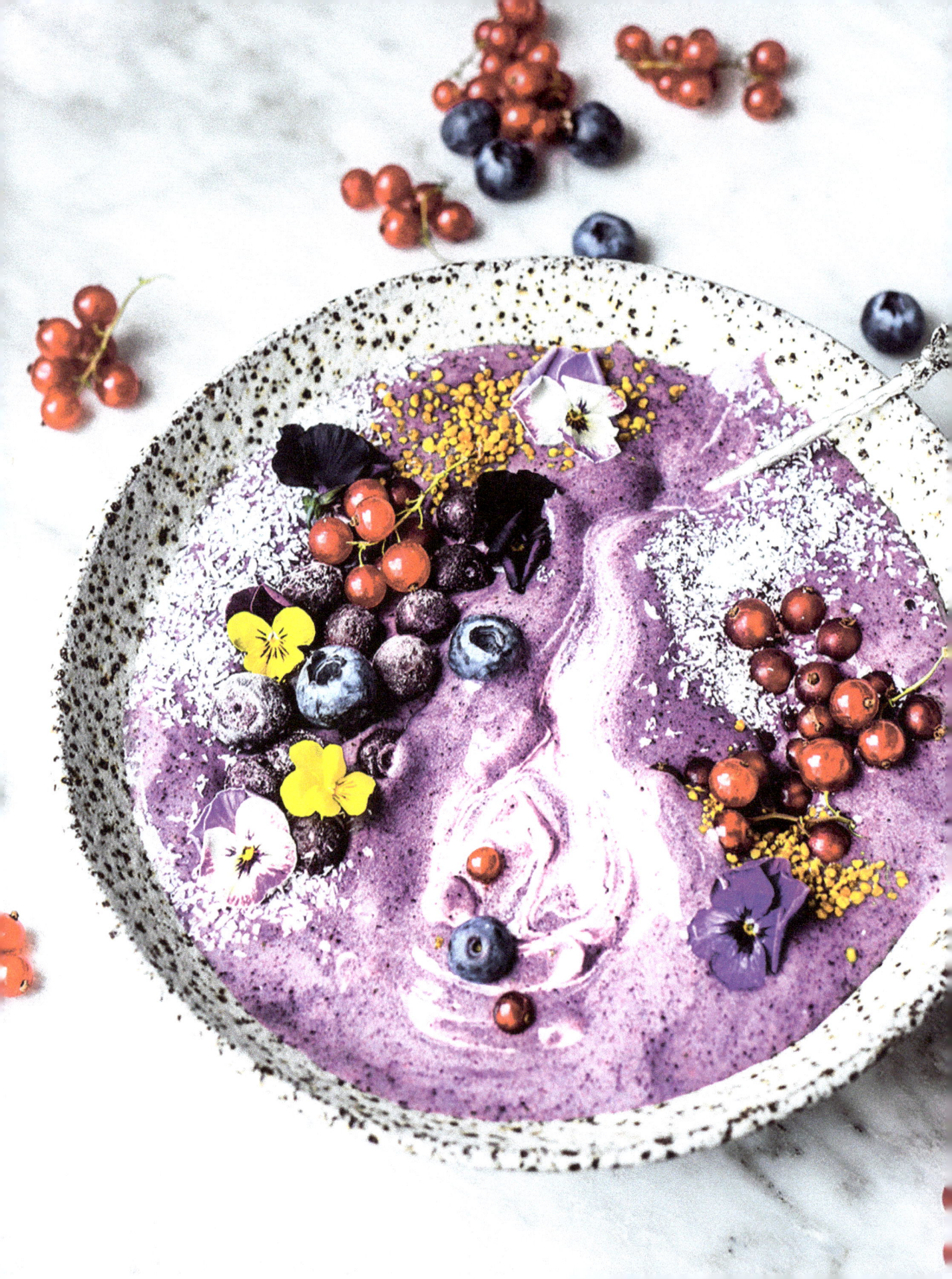

Blueberry Bliss Bowl

Sally O'Neil @thefitfoodieblog

Nutrition undergrad and recipe developer Sally O'Neil calls this dish her 'ode to Australian summer', as blueberries are in abundance in Aus during the warmer months. Used to the fruit from the UK where she grew up, Sally says she created this recipe to make the most of our deliciously sweet Aussie blubes.

'This bowl honestly tastes like it's been injected with this amazing blueberry flavour,' Sally says. 'Berries and bananas are amazing here, so I try to utilise them in every which way possible, and this dish is one of my favourites!'

Blueberries are packed with antioxidants and vitamin C, making them excellent for skin health and boosting your immunity. As well as this, they contain natural sugars but are low in calories, making them a healthy way to curb sugar cravings.

Vegan option, gluten-free, dairy-free, refined sugar-free

Ingredients

1 frozen banana

½ cup blueberries (fresh or frozen)

1 scoop (30g) vanilla pea protein (use vegan if desired)

1 tablespoon psyllium (optional)

1 tablespoon maca powder

Pinch Himalayan pink salt

½ cup coconut water or filtered water

Additional blueberries, bee pollen, desiccated coconut, red currants, coconut yoghurt, edible flowers (pretty but not necessary!), to serve

Method

In a blender, add all the ingredients (except the toppings – duh!) and blend until thick and smooth. You may need to use a spoon to get the mixture into the blades and to scrape down the sides. At this stage, don't be tempted to add more liquid – or else you'll end up with fruit soup!

Transfer the mixture to a bowl and add all your favourite toppings, swirl in some coconut yoghurt for creaminess and then go for gold.

Serves 1

To keep this smoothie bowl vegan, simply omit the bee pollen and use vegan protein powder.

Green Smoothie Bowl

Tarni Deutsher @healthywholefood

If the idea of consuming a bowl of sweet green goo doesn't appeal to you then you clearly haven't had a great green smoothie bowl. Until now.

'Anyone that knows me knows I'm a green superfood fiend,' says passionate food blogger and photographer Tarni Deutsher. 'I'm all about getting as many greens as possible into my diet, which is why I wanted to create a recipe that loads up on the stuff.'

After testing around 80 greens powders for this smoothie bowl, Tarni swears by the brand she's recommended here, though she says you can use your favourite. If you're new to green smoothies, she also suggests using more neutral-flavoured greens, such as spinach and cucumber, rather than going too hard too fast with something like kale.

Vegan, gluten-free, dairy-free, refined sugar-free

Ingredients

Base Ingredients

150 grams (5 oz) frozen banana

80 grams (3 oz) frozen mango

80 grams (3 oz) frozen zucchini

100 grams (3½ oz) spinach

1 heaped teaspoon Greens Powder (Tarni recommends Green Nutritionals Green Superfoods)

1 teaspoon cinnamon powder

3-4cm (1"-2") chunk of fresh aloe vera gel (optional. If you can source this it's a great addition for your gut!)

½-1 cup water, coconut water or your favourite plant-based milk

Smoothie superchargers

1 teaspoon maca powder

1 teaspoon high quality manuka honey for its antiviral and antibacterial properties

1 teaspoon high quality chaga and/or reishi mushroom powder

Method

Put all base ingredients into a high-speed blender with half a cup of your liquid of choice and blend on low, gradually increasing the speed while scraping down the sides of the blender. Add any additional smoothie superchargers here if desired.

Add more liquid until you reach your desired consistency. Use less liquid for a smoothie bowl, and more if you want a pourable smoothie.

Once everything is fully blended and incorporated, pour into a bowl and top with your favourite fruits, muesli, nuts or seeds.

Serves 1

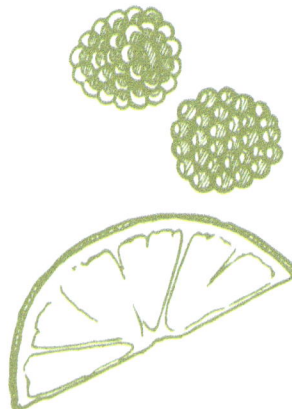

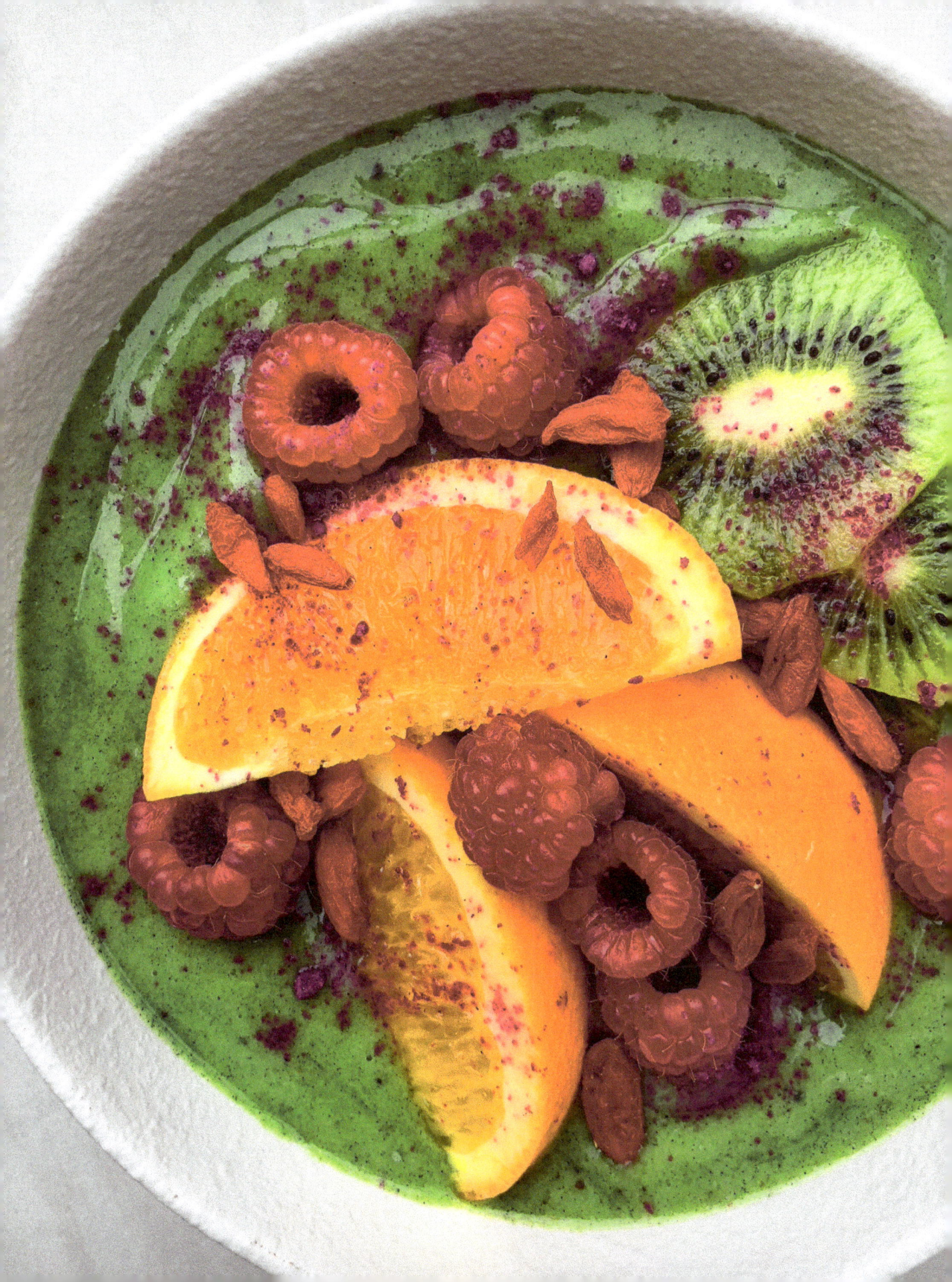

Mango & Banana Smoothie Parfait

Cassidy Bates @healthiielife

Beaches, blue skies and sunshine are a constant backdrop for Gold Coast-based vegan recipe developer Cassidy Bates. And while we can't all be lucky enough to wake up to a tropical paradise, when you start your day with her mango and banana parfait, you'll feel like you're almost there. If you close your eyes.

This refreshing, fruity concoction is the perfect summer breakfast. Get creative with your toppings and add the flavours you love. Coconut flakes, cacao nibs, buckinis and additional fresh fruit are all delicious options.

Vegan, gluten-free, dairy-free, refined sugar-free

Ingredients

For the base

½ cup puffed rice

2 tablespoons coconut yogurt

For the smoothie

1 frozen banana

1 cup frozen mango

½ cup plant-based milk

For the toppings

2 tablespoons coconut yogurt

4-5 strawberries

Method

Add the puffed rice to the base of your jar and top with the coconut yogurt.

In a blender, add the frozen banana, mango and milk, and blend until smooth and creamy.

Pour the smoothie mixture into your jar over the puffed rice and coconut yogurt.

Top your parfait with the remaining coconut yogurt and strawberries.

Serves 1

Chocolate Banana Smoothie Bowl

Sabrina Lu @nourishfulsabrina

Smoothie bowls are an easy way to pack a lot of nutrients into your morning. They're the perfect sweet treat, with the texture and flavour of ice cream, but with all the added benefits of fruit, protein and a good dose of healthy fats from the toppings.

'I created this because I love the idea that you can turn something as simple as frozen bananas into a healthy ice cream alternative that's just so much more beneficial for your body,' says Melbourne-based food blogger Sabrina Lu.

This is a great recipe to satisfy your sweet tooth on a warm summer morning, and Sabrina recommends getting creative with your toppings until you find your favourites.

Depending on how thick and creamy you like your bowl, you may need to play around with the amount of milk you add to achieve your desired consistency.

Vegan, gluten-free, dairy-free, refined sugar-free

Ingredients

3-4 medium frozen bananas

1 tablespoon cacao powder

¼-⅓ cup of almond, or plant based milk of choice

⅓ scoops vegan chocolate protein powder

Toppings of choice: cacao nibs, shredded coconut, caramelised buckinis, sliced banana

Method

Add all your ingredients except the toppings to a powerful blender and blend until thick and creamy.

Spoon the mixture into a bowl, smooth out the top with the back of your spoon and top with desired toppings.

Serves 2

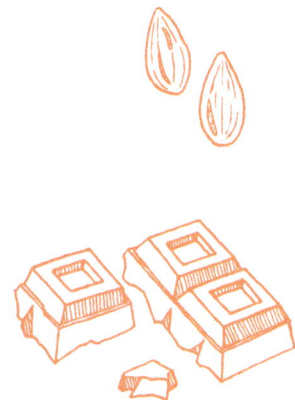

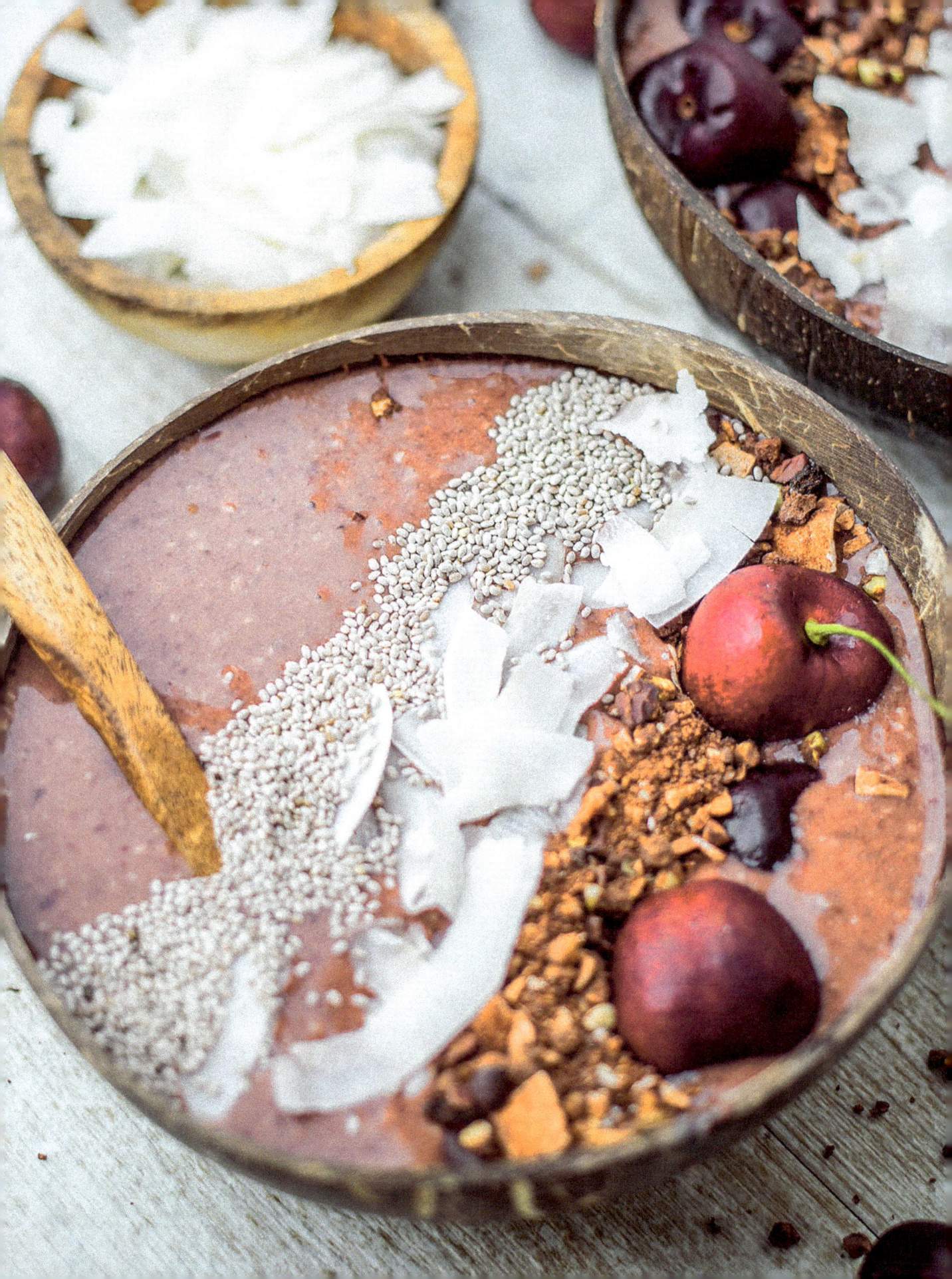

Cherry Ripe Acai Smoothie Bowl

Talida Voinea @Hazel_and_cacao

'I always get so excited about cherry season every year, and yet I never seemed to take full advantage of it,' says health food blogger Talida Voinea. 'But I saw a cherry-inspired smoothie bowl pop up on my instagram feed from my friend Summer who goes by @nutri_mum, and I decided to create my own version.'

After changing her diet in order to recover from severe hormonal imbalances, Talida aims to include as many nutrients - particularly healthy fats - into her diet as possible. The almond butter, cherries, acai and cacao provide an incredible array of antioxidants, vitamins and minerals.

Vegan, gluten-free, dairy-free, refined sugar-free

Ingredients

1 banana

1 cup frozen cherries

1 frozen açai pouch

1 tablespoon cacao powder

1 tablespoon almond butter

2 tablespoon shredded coconut

2 tablespoon maple syrup

Splash of almond milk

Topping: Chocolate granola, coconut flakes, fresh cherries, chia seeds

Method

Place all the smoothie ingredients in a high-speed blender and blend until smooth. Add just a little milk and keep adding until you achieve your desired consistency.

Pour into a bowl and top with desired toppings.

Serves 1

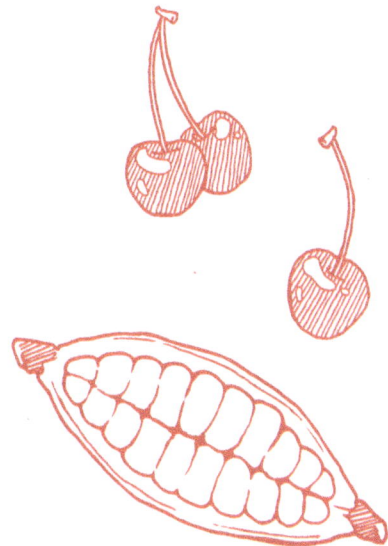

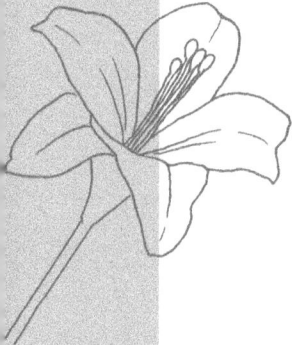

Leanne Ward on Body Acceptance & Cherishing Your Space Suit

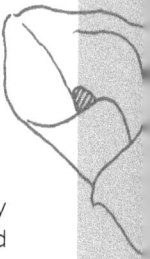

Leanne Ward @the_fitness_dietitian

Nurturing important relationships in our lives is something that most of us prioritise. Whether it's the relationship you share with your mum, sister, brother, best friend, cousin or work-wife. We tend to these relationships, water them, feed them and watch them grow. Carefully nurturing them to help them flourish. But how much attention do we place on the relationship we have with ourselves? And perhaps even moreso, how much care do we place in having a positive relationship with our bodies?

Our bodies are our space suits. They carry us through this world, allowing us to dance, run, skip and move our way through life in whichever way we so choose. But strangely enough, rather than respecting these vessels, we seem to turn against them, picking and prodding, desperately trying to change them.

It can be challenging and uncomfortable to be in a body that you judge or dislike, something that nutritionist and dietitian Leanne Ward knows all too well. From the age of just 14, Leanne stood at six feet tall, seeing her tower over her friends and making her a spectacle among her peers.

'My relationship with health and nutrition was wonderful growing up, I had such a great healthy environment,' says Leanne. 'But when I hit high school, it dawned on me how different my body was compared to those around me. I became so self conscious of my body and appearance, because I just wanted to fit in with everyone else.'

'People started calling me a "big girl", and while they meant tall, that's not necessarily the way I interpreted it,' Leanne says sadly.

Ashamed of her body, Leanne began trying to obscure it from the world, swathing herself in oversized, baggy clothes. Rather than holding herself proudly, she would stoop over, seeing her develop terrible posture and back pain as a teenager.

When she was 16 years old, Leanne describes a pivotal moment in her life that really began the horrible cycle of body shame and self-punishment that would last throughout her teenage years and into early adulthood.

'One day one of my friends made a throwaway comment; "You'll always be tall, but at least you can make yourself be skinny," 'and from that moment I became obsessed with the notion of being thin,' says Leanne. 'I became so preoccupied with nutrition and exercise that I dedicated myself to learning everything I could about food and calories. I was doing cardio six or seven days a week, I wanted a six-pack and a thigh gap. My whole worth was tied up in being thin.'

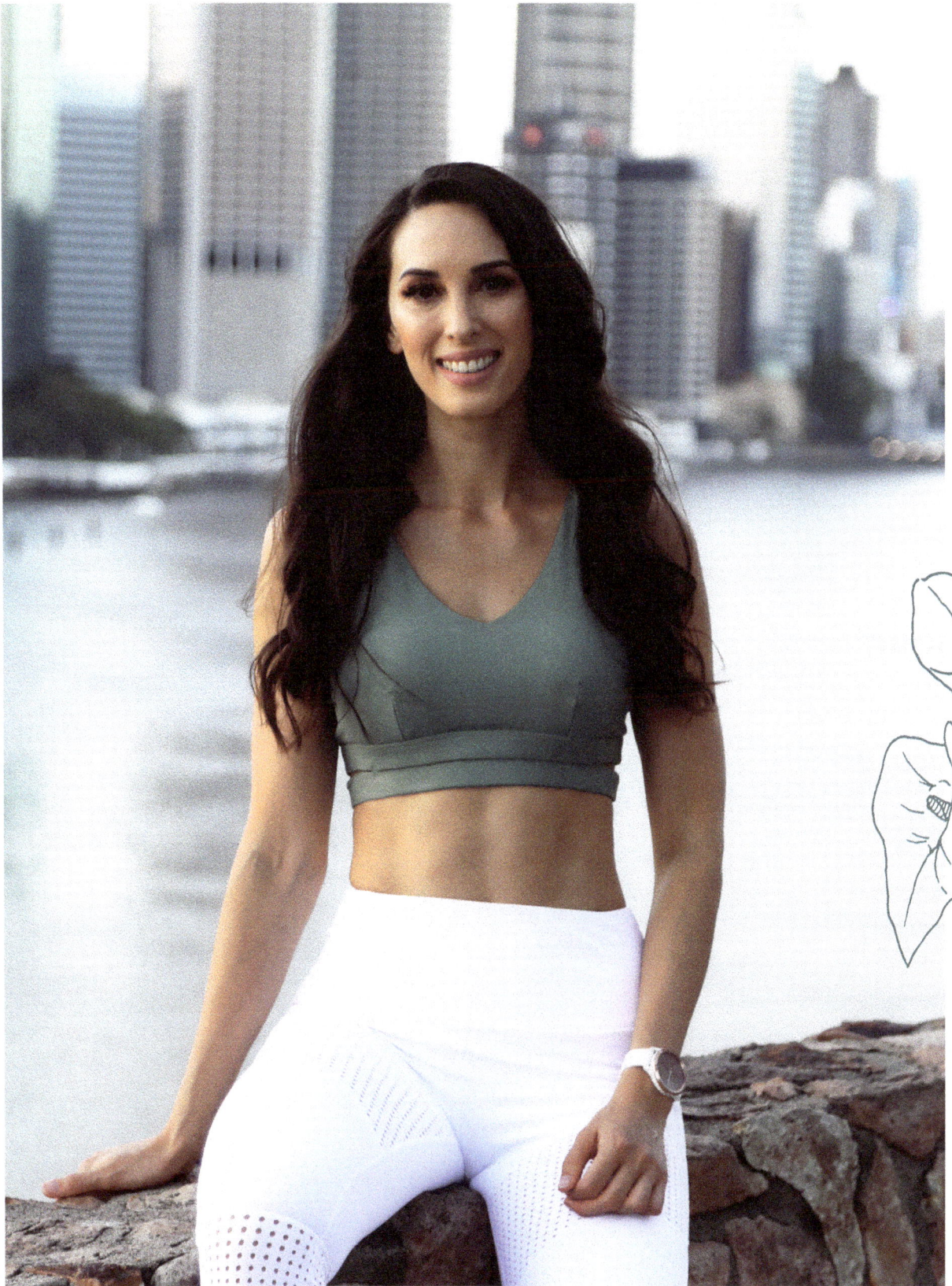
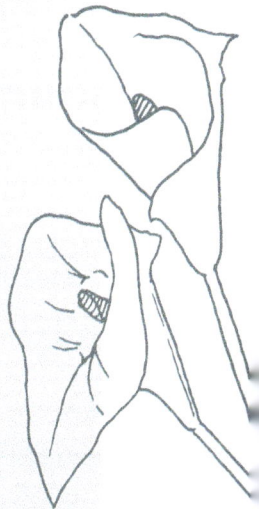

Leanne's story is by no means an uncommon one amongst women of any and all ages. We feel compelled to change our bodies to fit in or fulfill the "perfect" body shape that's dictated to us by the society we live in. As a qualified dietitian and nutritionist, Leanne now treats many women in her Brisbane clinic who struggle with their relationship with their bodies, fighting against them rather than accepting the form they were born with.

'Most of the women I work with want to lose weight, whether they're overweight, unhealthily underweight or maintaining a healthy size. But the message I keep hearing is that they want to be thinner,' says Leanne. 'They believe that once they achieve their ideal weight they'll be happy and confident.'

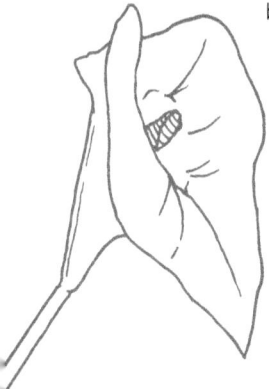

This is the trap that so many of us fall into: believing that once we look a certain way, happiness will follow. We abuse our bodies in the hopes of finding something better, rather than finding joy and appreciation for the amazing body we have that's staring right back at us in the mirror.

'What these women don't understand, is that they can be happy, confident and worthy regardless of their weight,' Leanne says, flicking her long dark her behind her shoulder. 'The pressure to lose weight stems from the modern society we live in. I see young girls posting #inspo and #fitspo on images of women who are clearly underweight and unhealthy, and it scares me now. But I understand because I was that girl once too.'

A Coming of Acceptance

One fateful day, Leanne found herself sitting with her mother in their car with tears rolling down her face, talking about how much she hated her body. At that moment, an incredibly short woman walked across the road in front of them and Leanne lamented how she wished her feet were as small as that womans.

Her mother turned to her, 'If you had feet that

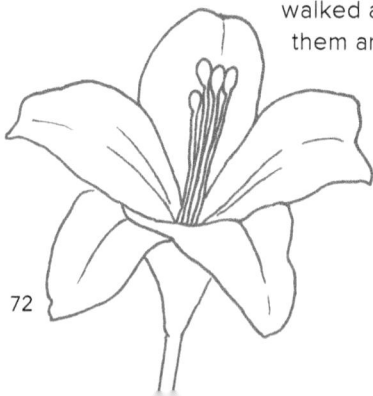

small,' she said, 'you would literally fall over!' 'We both burst into fits of laughter, because I knew she was right,' giggles Leanne. 'I guess I'd never really thought about it, but my feet were completely in proportion to the rest of my body. I was exactly the way I was for a reason, and in that moment I realised that was OK. From then on, I promised myself I would learn to appreciate everything about my body.'

'I don't want to sugar coat it and say that I wake up every day completely in love with my body, but I do wake up every day and appreciate everything my body does for me. Self-love starts with appreciation and gratitude for your body, and that was the lesson I learnt that day.'

Leanne's Tips for Respecting your Body

So, just how do you begin to relinquish years of body shame and dissatisfaction when it's something that might be so innately ingrained into your way of thinking? Leanne has given us her pointers to begin making peace with your beautiful, one-of-a-kind space suit.

1. Block out Social Body Braggers

While Leanne believes the pressure to have the "ideal" body has always been forced upon women, she says social media has exacerbated the problem.

'Young women are looking at Instagram and seeing these perfect photos of women's bodies, but they're forgetting that they're edited,' she says. 'Social media is a highlight reel, it's not the reality of what's really going on. But we stare at photoshopped and airbrushed images every single day to the point where we believe looking that way is normal.'

For the record, it's not.

For this reason, like many other of our contributors, she recommends a social media detox as a good starting point if you're struggling with accepting your body as it is.

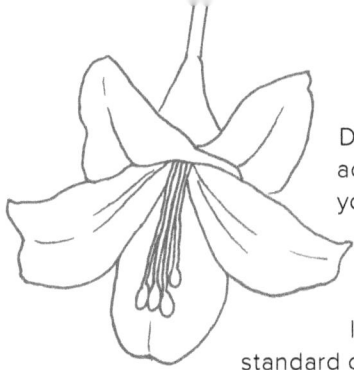

Delete or mute any accounts that make you feel insecure about the way you look or that promote an unattainable (and likely unrealistic!) standard of beauty. And, for heaven's sake, unfollow any skinny tea, calorie counting or ridiculous fad dieting accounts. Trust us, that shit is poison.

2. Clean Up Your Environment

We're not talking about recycling here (though you should do that too!). We're referring to the world in which you surround yourself - the content you consume, what you read, listen to and watch. But perhaps most importantly, think about the people you surround yourself with and consider how they affect the way you think about and perceive your body.

'Spend time with people who respect you for who you are, not what you look like,' suggests Leanne. 'Having a healthy environment is just as important as putting healthy food into your mouth when it comes to feeling good about yourself physically.'

3. Seek Professional Guidance

You can come up with a million excuses to avoid this one: 'I don't have time, it's too expensive, my cat ate my car keys' (trust us, we've heard them all), but when it comes to beginning your journey to body acceptance, Leanne strongly recommends seeking professional help.

'It's your health, so it's worth the investment,' she says firmly. 'I would have come to terms with my body much earlier if I had reached out to a professional for help, and I think most women would find the same. It's strange that we see a dentist to fix our teeth, or a mechanic to fix our car, but when it comes to our minds we don't take the same care.'

So make sure you take the time to see a mind mechanic to help you sort through any negative thoughts you might be having. Yes, it can be a little scary and intimidating, but it's worth it for the

space it will free up in your mind. That's space you can fill with positive thoughts instead!

4. Put Pen to Paper

So often we dwell on things in the past or worry about the future that we lose sight of what's happening now, in the present. We can become so caught up in negative thoughts about ourselves and our bodies that it can be hard to break out of this way of thinking.

'Journaling has been a game changer to help me release any negative thoughts about myself from my head,' says Leanne. 'Once they're on paper, they're so much easier to rationalise and see as untrue or ridiculous.'

We're often much better at giving advice and talking kindly to our friends, so Leanne recommends looking at your thoughts on paper, then writing advice to yourself just as you would give to your BF.

5. Be Patient

Just like any relationship, the one with your body will take time, so don't expect to be completely accepting of yourself straight away. Some days you will look in the mirror and think, 'DAYUM GIRL!', and there will be times when all you can focus on is the cellulite on your thighs or your bloated stomach. And that's ok. The relationship you have with your body will always be a work in progress, but the good news is that you have your whole life to work on it.

If you're having a bad body image day, take the time to appreciate everything it does for you. Thank your strong legs for being able to carry you, thank your tummy for protecting your organs and, yes, even thank your god damn cellulite, because it means your body's fibrous tissue is working on point!

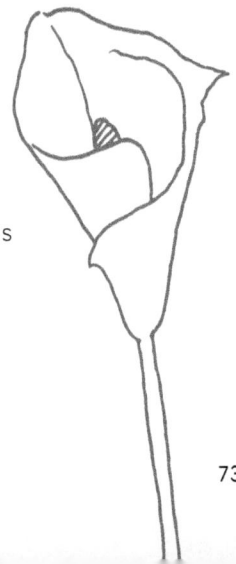

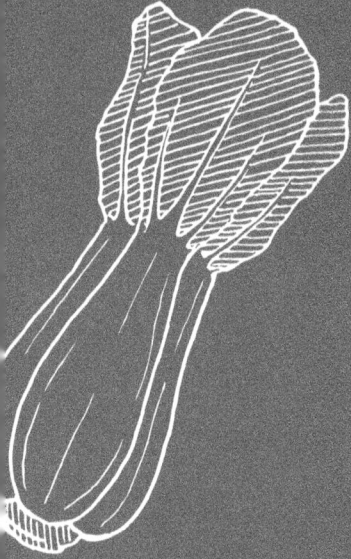

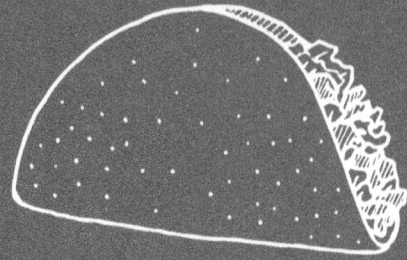

Mains

These recipes can be eaten for lunch or dinner and have been chosen because they're quick, easy and will make you feel good from the inside out. Each of these dishes will give you an incredible injection of nutrients that will feed your body, but more than that, they will enrich your soul.

We suggest that you slow down and enjoy the process of cooking and eating them. Share Sami Bloom's eggplant parmigiana with your family, bring a plate of Olivia Kaplan's tacos to a friend's fiesta, or else let a bowl of the Healthy Luxe's vegan mac and cheese warm your soul while curled up on your couch watching Netflix.

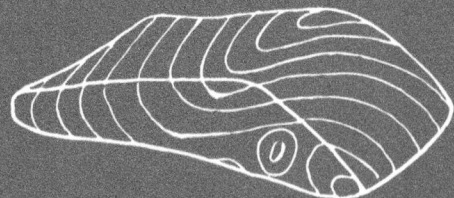

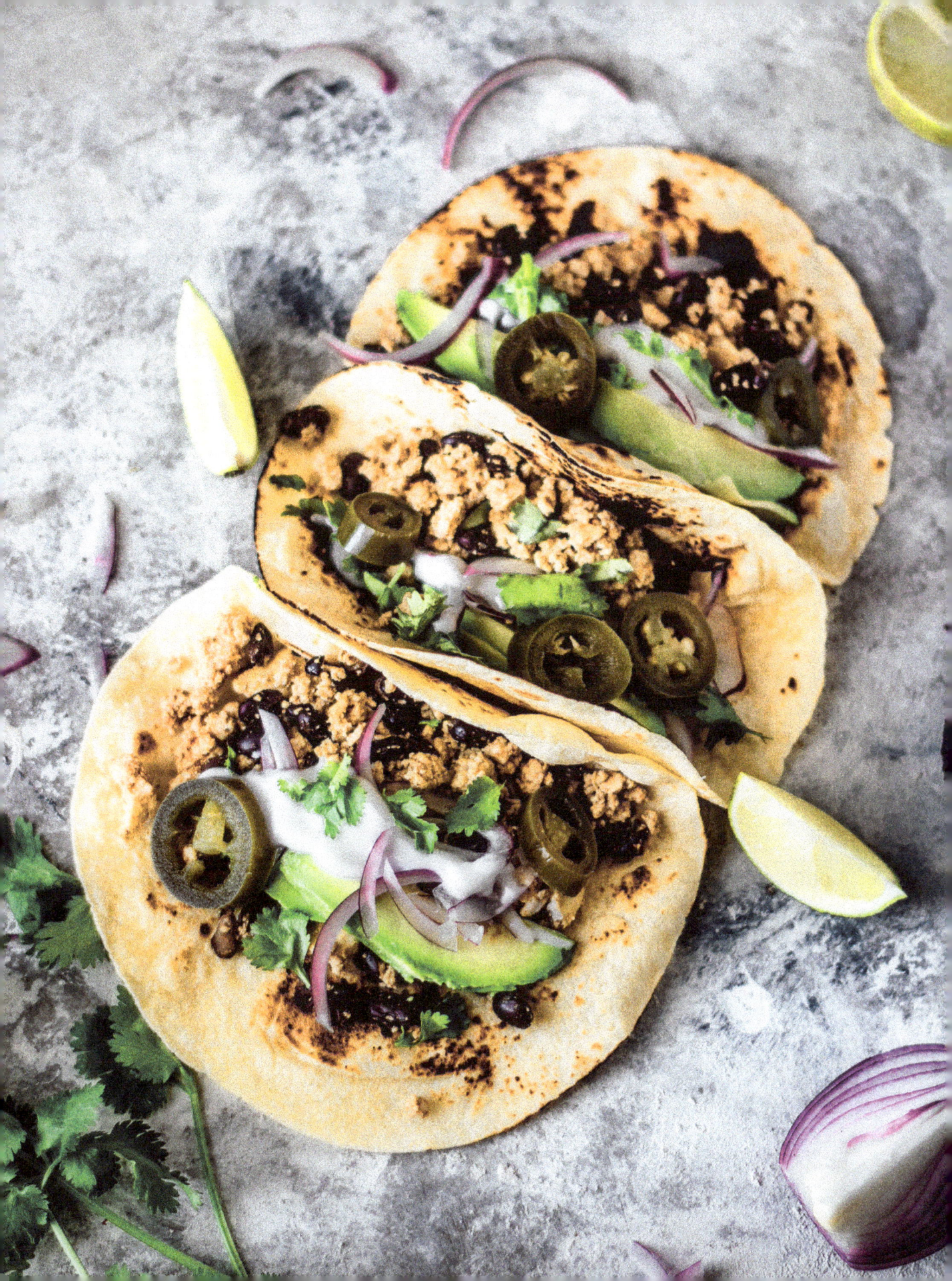

Tofu Black Bean Tacos

Sasha Back @earthlingsassha

16-year-old Sasha Back will be the first to admit that these tacos aren't 'traditionally Mexican', but by using smoked paprika, cumin and cayenne they certainly have a good dose of the Mexican flavours we all know and love.

Being cheap, quick and easy, this dish is perfect for students or those who are new to cooking. Of course, they're also great for those with a bit more experience in the kitchen, because they're just damn delicious!

Vegan, gluten-free, dairy-free, refined sugar-free

Ingredients

360 grams (12½ oz) medium-firm tofu block

400 grams (14 oz) black beans, drained and rinsed

½ tablespoons olive oil

1 teaspoon ground cayenne

½ teaspoon ground garlic

½ teaspoon onion powder

1 ½ tablespoon soy sauce

1 teaspoon ground cumin

1 teaspoon smoked paprika

½ teaspoon salt

For the vegan sour cream

½ cup natural coconut yoghurt

2 teaspoons vinegar

1 teaspoon salt

To serve

Corn tortillas, warmed

1 avocado, sliced

Sliced jalapenos

Lime

Red onion, sliced

Method

Begin by pressing the tofu. Place your tofu block onto some paper towel and place a wooden chopping board or heavy plate on top to weigh down the tofu and press out the liquid. Let this sit for 10-15 minutes while you prepare the other ingredients.

To make the vegan sour cream, mix all the ingredients together in a small bowl until well combined. Put aside.

Set a fry pan over medium-high heat and heat olive oil. Finely crumble the pressed tofu block with your hands into the pan. Add the rinsed and drained black beans and let this cook for 2-3 minutes, continuously stirring to make sure the tofu doesn't stick to the pan.

Add all the remaining spices and soy sauce to the fry pan and mix until incorporated. Let this cook for a further 3-5 minutes.

To assemble your tacos, fill your tortillas with the tofu and bean mixture, sliced avocado, jalapenos and red onion. Top with vegan sour cream and lime juice.

Makes 6-7 tacos

Top tip: If you make the vegan sour cream the night before, the sour cream will be tangier and more sour.

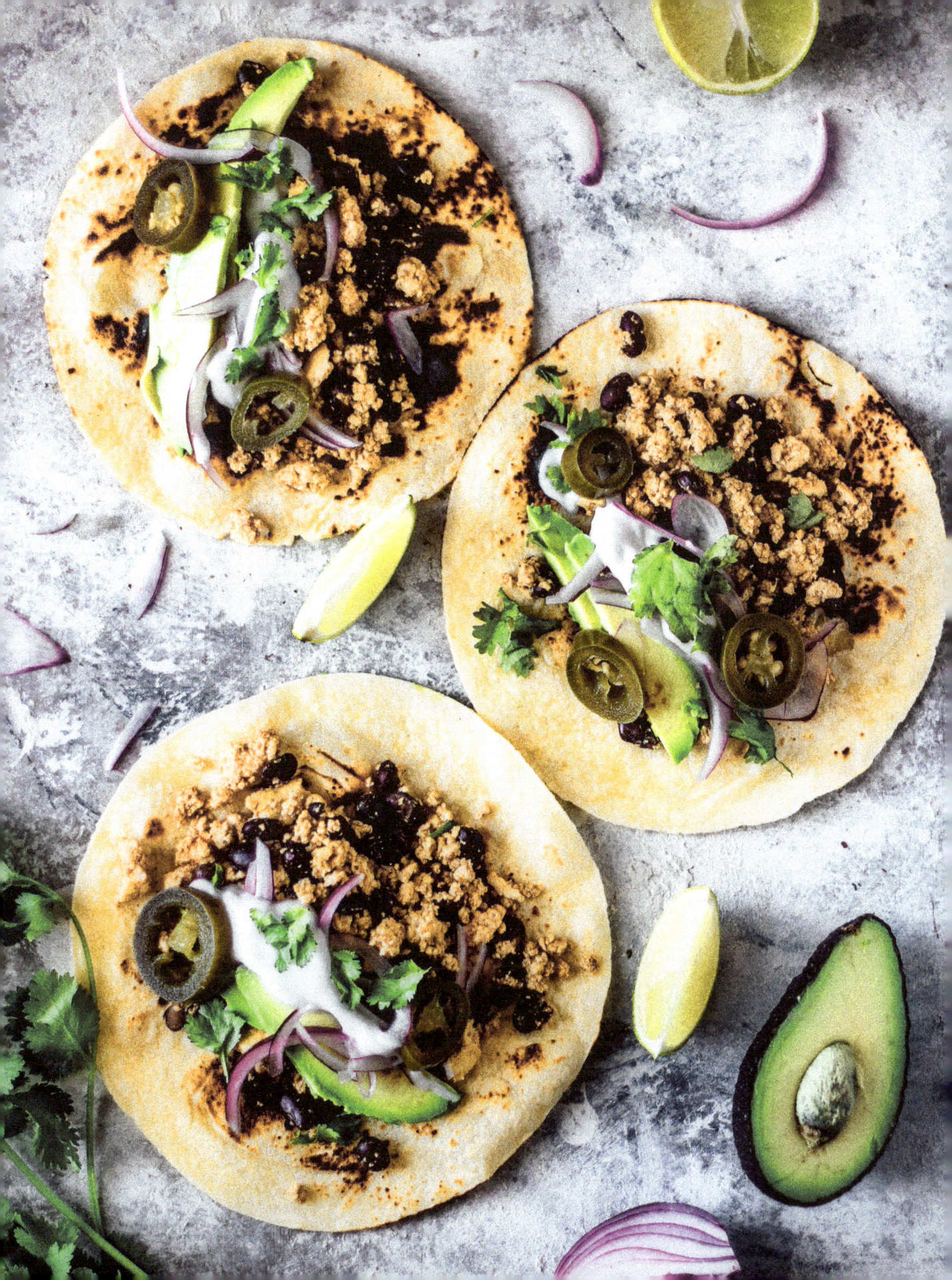

Smoky Eggplant Tacos

Olivia Kaplan @livinbondi

If you don't like eggplant, listen up. Cooked badly, it can be slimy, bitter or flavourless. But we're going to say something controversial that you might not like.

You've probably just never eaten it cooked well. There, we said it.

In its element, eggplant is smokey, creamy and basically a sponge for any flavour. This dish, explains Sydney-based nutritionist and presenter Olivia Kaplan, is what she uses to get people on board the eggplant train - next stop, delicious-ville.

'This is the recipe I make for people when I'm trying to convert them to eggplant lovers, and so far I've had a 100% success rate,' she laughs.

'It's a great dinner party recipe. Simply place everything in a beautiful big bowls in the centre of the table, top with fresh coriander, sesame seeds, extra lime and a sprinkle of fresh paprika - these little touches really take a dinner spread to the next level.'

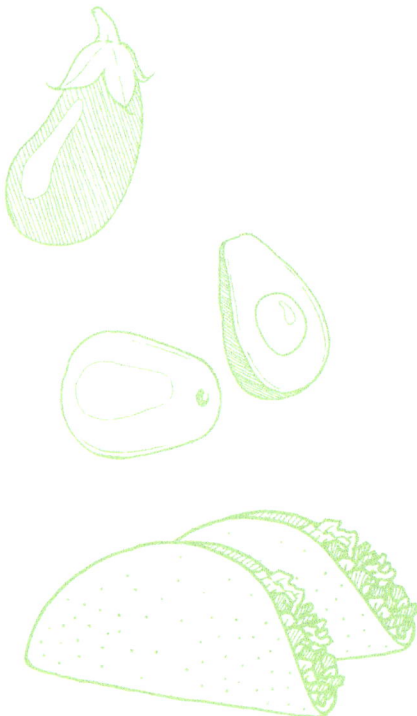

Vegan, gluten-free, dairy-free, refined sugar-free

Ingredients

1 large eggplant (or 2 small eggplants), cut into chunks

2–3 tablespoons olive oil

2 tablespoons organic tamari

2 teaspoons smoked paprika

1 clove garlic, crushed

¼ head red cabbage, finely shredded

2 tablespoons apple cider vinegar

2 avocados

4–8 fresh corn tortillas or coconut wraps

1 jar cashew cheese or dairy-free cheese alternative

4 limes, sliced into wedges

¼ bunch coriander (cilantro), leaves picked

1 red chilli, fresh, sliced

Sea salt and black pepper

Method

Preheat the oven to 200°C (400°F). In a large bowl, combine the eggplant, olive oil, tamari, paprika and garlic. Toss together to coat, and lay out in a single layer on a baking tray.

Place the tray in the oven to bake for 30 to 40 minutes, or until eggplant is soft but crispy on the outside.

Meanwhile, prepare the remaining ingredients. Place the shredded cabbage in a large bowl with the apple cider vinegar, a generous pinch of sea salt and a good drizzle of olive oil. Toss to coat and set aside in a large bowl for serving.

Mash the avocado with a fork to make the guac. Add a pinch of salt and some diced chilli and lime juice, if you like. Set aside for serving.

Place all other ingredients in bowls for a self-serve taco party.

Prior to serving, place the tortillas in the oven for a couple of minutes to heat through, or microwave according to packet instructions.

To assemble tacos, spread with guac, top with cabbage, eggplant, chilli, coriander, a dollop of cashew cheese and a squeeze of fresh lime.

Serves 4

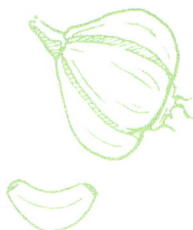

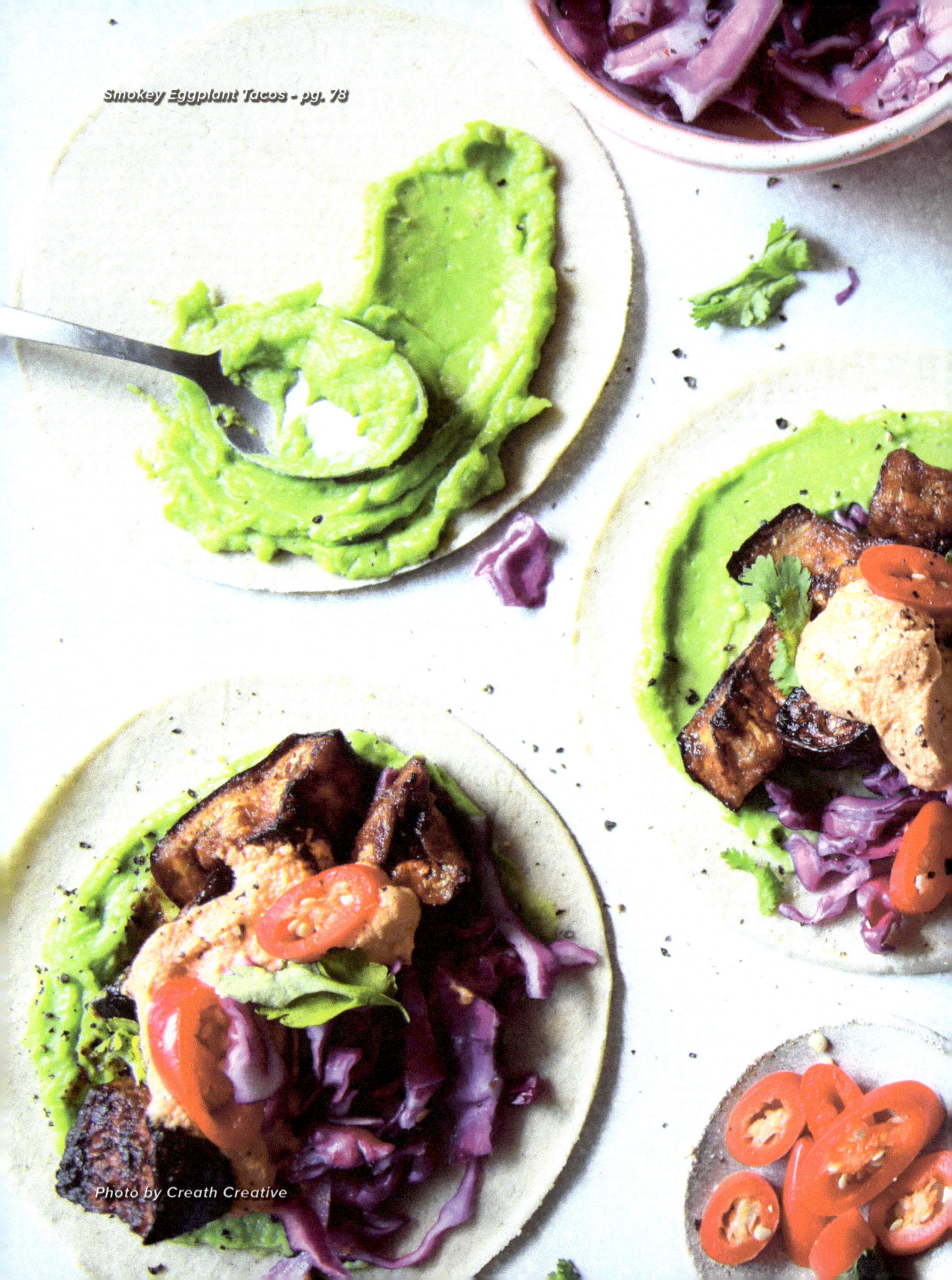

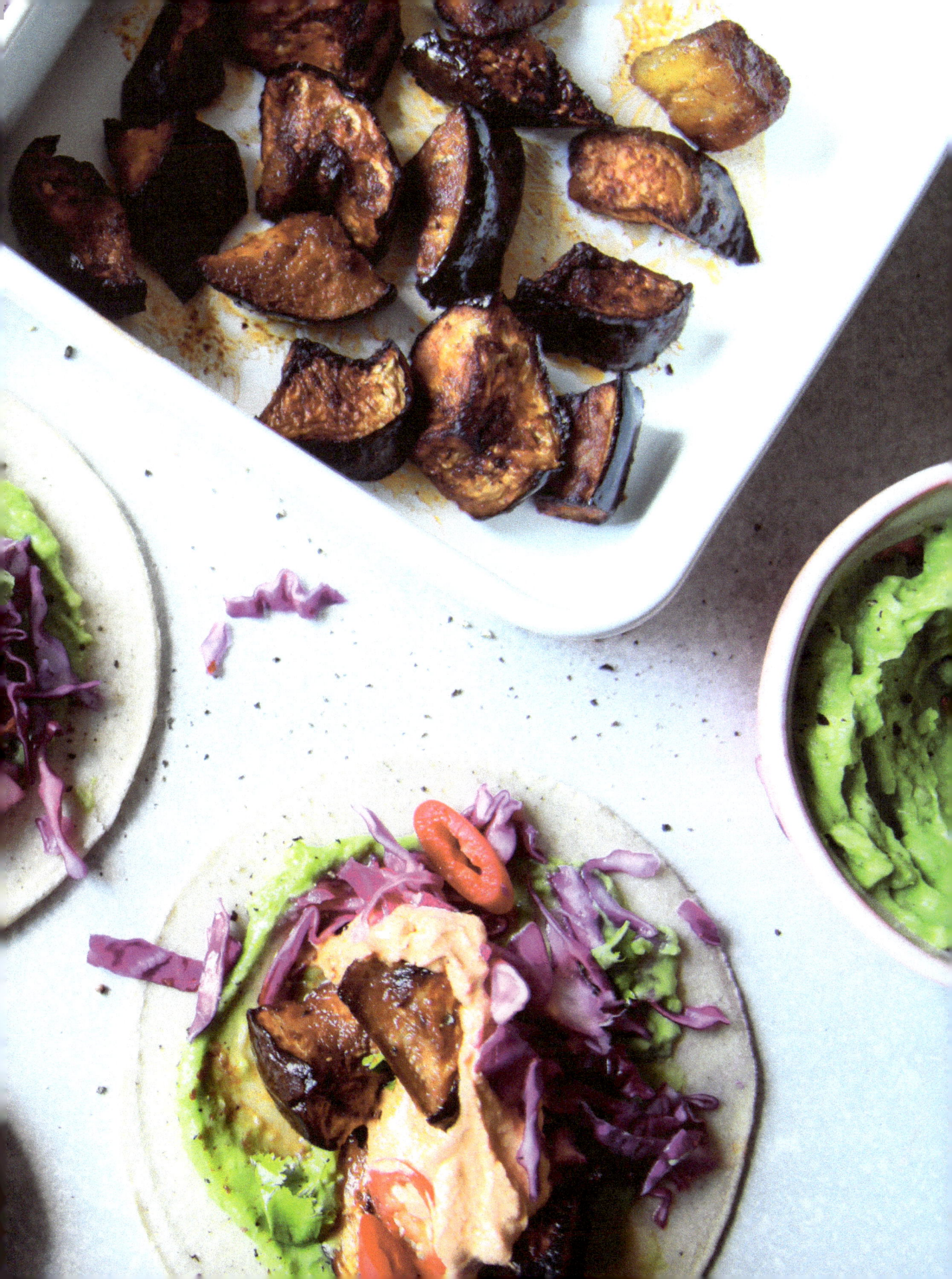

Smokey Jackfruit Burrito Bowl & Nacho Cheeze Sauce

Aliza Strock @shaktifresh

While the ingredient list might seem intimidating at first glance, personal chef Aliza Strock promises this dish is deceptively simple. 'It may seem like a laborious dish, but it's just a matter of timing,' she says. 'The more you make it, the more you'll get comfortable with the different elements - I reckon I can make the cheeze sauce with my eyes closed!'

This meal is now a staple weeknight dinner for Aliza, seeing her use whatever vegetables she has on hand. 'I use this dish to clean out my fridge,' she laughs. 'Sometimes I even add sliced mango and shredded purple cabbage for an extra colourful punch.'

If you don't have jackfruit readily available (most Asian grocery stores carry it) you can substitute it with any other plant-based protein such as tofu, tempeh, or TVP (textured vegetable protein).

This recipe will probably give you leftover cheeze sauce, which you can store in an airtight jar or container in the fridge for up to five days. Use it on pasta, as a dip with corn chips or eat it with a spoon. No judgement.

Vegan, gluten-free, dairy-free, refined sugar-free

Ingredients

For nacho cheeze sauce

1 small butternut pumpkin, peeled and cubed

1 cup raw cashews

1 cup nutritional yeast

1 cup of soy milk or unsweetened almond milk (plus extra if needed)

1 teaspoon each of garlic powder, onion powder, smoked paprika, turmeric, salt, pepper

For pico de gallo salsa

250 grams (8½ oz) cherry tomatoes

Method

To prepare the cheeze sauce, soak cashews in a bowl of boiling water for 30 minutes and boil or steam your pumpkin until soft.

Add cooked pumpkin and blanched cashews to a high-powered blender along with the remainder of the sauce ingredients and blend until smooth and creamy. You may need to add more liquid as you blend to achieve a thick creamy consistency.

To prepare the pico de gallo, quarter the cherry tomatoes, dice onion and chop coriander. Toss in a small bowl with lime, salt and pepper and set aside.

To prepare the guacamole, scoop avocado into a bowl. Add the lime, diced onion, coriander, lime and seasonings. Mash it all together with a fork and set aside.

Cook your rice or quinoa according to packet directions.

½ small red onion

½ cup chopped coriander
(cilantro)

Juice of 1 lime

Salt and pepper to taste

For guacamole

1 large avocado

½ cup chopped coriander

½ small red onion, diced

Juice of 1 lime

Salt and pepper to taste

For burrito bowl

1 cup white or brown rice, or
quinoa

1 x 565 gram (4 oz) can of
jackfruit in brine

1 teaspoon each of: smoked
paprika, ground cumin, Salt
and pepper

1 red capscium, chopped

1 green or yellow capscium,
sliced

1 x 400 gram (14 oz) can
of black or kidney beans,
drained and rinsed

1 small head cos lettuce,
washed and chopped

¼ -½ teaspoon cayenne
pepper

Drain and rinse the jackfruit. Cut off the hard part of the
jackfruit pieces and, using your fingers, start to break
the jackfruit apart into a bowl. Combine with smoked
paprika, cumin, salt, pepper and one tablespoon of
olive oil.

Add the slices capsicum to a pan along with one
tablespoon of olive oil and heat over a medium-high
heat and and sauté for 10–12 minutes, or until softened.
Set aside.

In the same pan, sauté the jackfruit for 8–12 minutes.
Set aside.

To serve, add desired amount of grains to half a
bowl, and your lettuce on the other half. Top with
cooked jackfruit, sautéed capsicums, beans, salsa and
guacamole. Drizzle with a healthy amount of the nacho
cheeze sauce and enjoy!

Serves 2

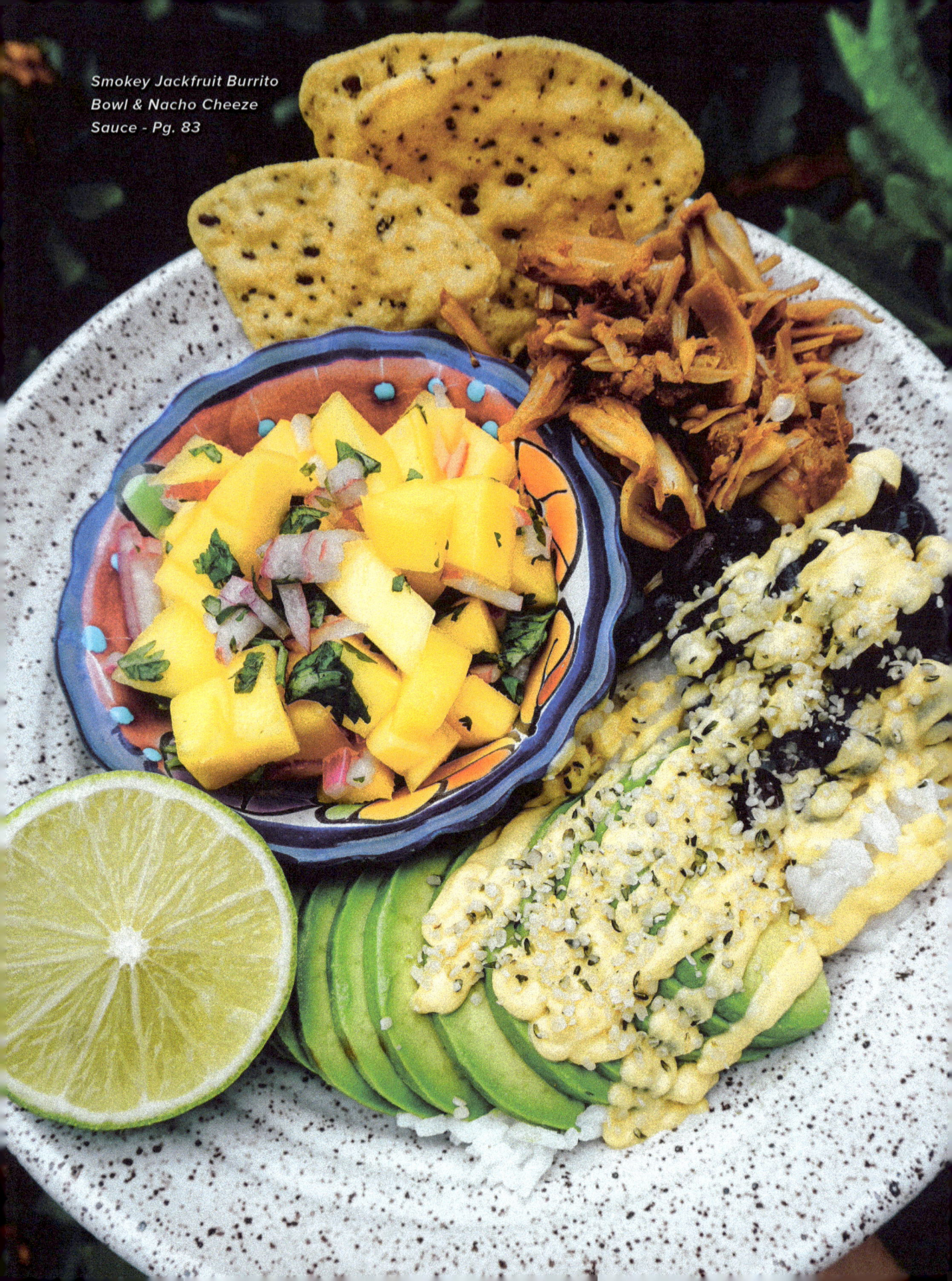

Smokey Jackfruit Burrito Bowl & Nacho Cheeze Sauce - Pg. 83

Mexican Burrito Bowl

Lauren Mariano @lm_nutrition

Having pantry staples such as spices, tinned legumes and tomatoes on hand makes whipping up a quick, nourishing and filling lunch or dinner easy. This healthy Mexican-inspired bowl created by practising dietitian Lauren Mariano is one of her go-to favourites and sees her using whatever vegetables she has on hand to create a satisfying meal.

'I start with pantry staples and then add spices to add depth of flavour,' she explains. 'This recipe makes six portions, so you can have heaps of leftovers for lunch or when you get home late from work.'

'I also love sharing it with friends. I put everything in the middle of the table and let everyone build their own bowls, adding more of the ingredients they love.'

Vegan, gluten-free, dairy-free, refined sugar-free

Ingredients

1 tablespoon olive oil

1 onion, diced

2 teaspoons garlic, minced

150g (5 oz) mushrooms, sliced

1 green capsicum, sliced

2 zucchinis, grated

3 carrots, grated

500 grams (1lb) broccoli (fresh or frozen)

1 tablespoon cumin

2 tablespoons smoky paprika

1 tablespoon ground coriander

2 x 400 gram (14 oz) tins diced tomatoes

2 x 400 gram (14 oz) tins kidney beans

1 x 400 gram (14 oz) tins corn

120 grams (4 oz) spinach (fresh or frozen)

Brown rice, fresh coriander (cilantro), chilli and Greek yoghurt, to serve

Method

Heat olive oil in a pot over medium heat. Add onion and garlic and saute until they start to brown.

Add the mushrooms, carrot, zucchini, capsicum, broccoli and spices and stir until evenly coated and the vegetables start to brown slightly.

Add the tinned tomatoes and simmer for 15 minutes until the sauce starts to thicken and reduce.

Stir in the kidney beans, corn and spinach and simmer for a further 10 minutes.

Add salt and pepper to taste and serve with brown rice, chilli, coriander and Greek or coconut yoghurt.

Serves 4-6

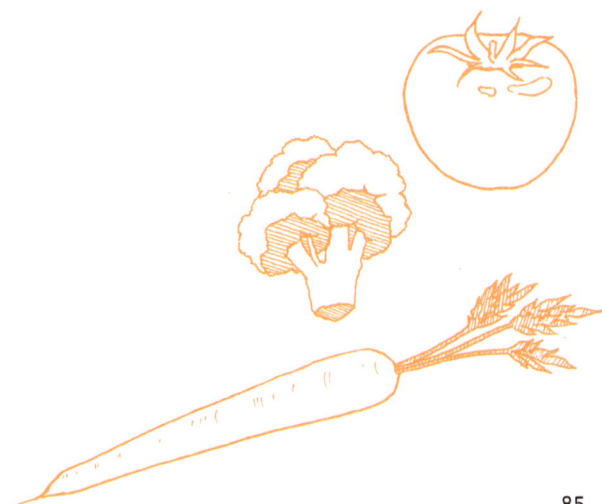

Low Fodmap Cypriot Grain Salad

Laura Ford @laurafordnutrition

This incredible, vibrant salad from Melbourne-based dietitian Laura Ford is based off her favourite Cypriot Grain Salad from George Calombaris' Hellenic Republic restaurant. Laura's made her version FODMAP friendly, so it can be enjoyed by those who struggle to digest the naturally occurring carbohydrates and sugars that are found in certain types of foods.

'This dish is so delicious, so I wanted everyone to be able to enjoy it,' Laura says. 'I think a lot of people think they have to stick to a recipe and that might make it off-limits to people who struggle with FODMAP intolerances. But I want to help people feel confident in making changes and substitutions they need to.'

Laura has included veggies, crunchy nuts and juicy pomegranate seeds to add texture and sweetness. You can serve this dish as part of a banquet, or else have it as a side with a portion of your favourite protein.

Vegan option, vegetarian, gluten-free, dairy-free alternative, refined sugar-free

Ingredients

For the salad

¾ cup quinoa, rinsed

¾ cup black rice

1 bunch silverbeet, stalks removed and finely sliced

1 bunch coriander (cilantro), chopped

½ bunch parsley, chopped

3 tablespoons toasted pumpkin seeds

3 tablespoons toasted slivered almonds

3 tablespoons toasted pine nuts

2 tablespoons baby capers

¼ cup currants

Juice of 1 lemon

4 tablespoons extra virgin olive oil

Method

Cook quinoa and black rice separately in boiling water with a pinch of salt until both are just cooked. Refer to packet instructions for best cooking time. Drain well and allow to cool.

Heat 1 tablespoon of olive oil in a pan on medium heat and add silverbeet. Cook for 3 minutes until slightly wilted. Remove from heat.

Combine the yogurt, ground cumin and maple syrup in a small bowl and set aside.

In a large bowl, place the coriander, parsley, quinoa, rice, toasted nuts and seeds, capers, currants, cooked silverbeet, baby spinach, lemon juice and the remaining 3 tablespoons of olive oil. Mix well and season to taste.

Place the salad into a serving dish and top with cumin yogurt and pomegranate seeds. Place in the middle of the table and let everyone help themselves!

Serves 6-8 as a shared dish

Salt and pepper to taste

120 grams (4 oz) washed baby spinach, to serve (more if you like)

1 pomegranate, deseeded or 1 packet of pomegranate arils, to serve (see note)

For the yogurt dressing

1 cup lactose-free** yogurt (see note)

1 teaspoon ground cumin

1 tablespoon maple syrup

Pomegranate may be high in fructose, however less than a ¼ cup per serve is usually a well tolerated amount.

If you're making this dish for coeliacs make sure that the yogurt you're using doesn't contain gluten. Liddell's is a lactose-free variety but it does contain gluten. If you're not avoiding lactose, we suggest using a thick Greek yogurt in place of the lactose-free variety - it's super yummy!

To make this dish vegan, simply omit the yogurt dressing.

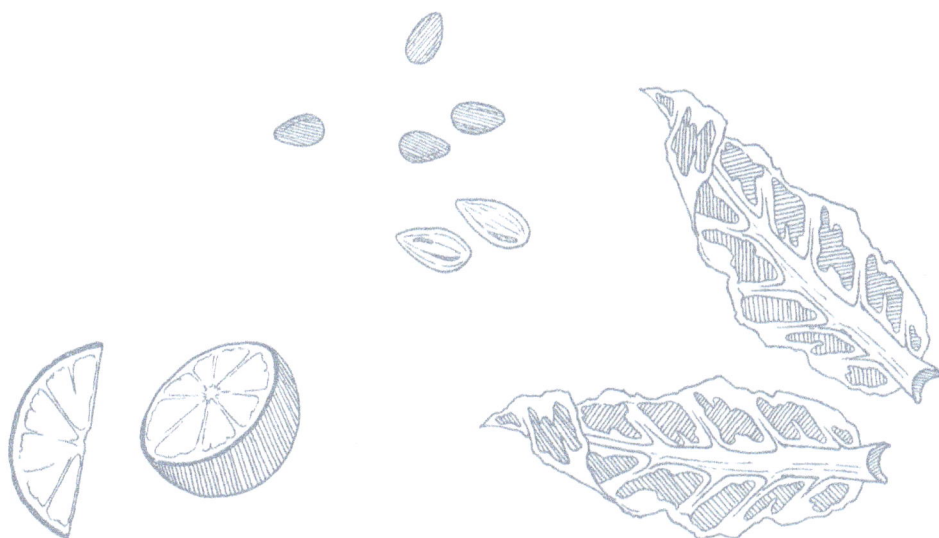

Sushi Nourish Bowl

Cassidy Bates @healthiielife

Who loves sushi? We do!

But we all know it's not the most convenient thing to prepare. With all the filling and rolling - it seems like a lot of effort just for lunch. Especially when the rolls often end up a little flacid and sad because you're in a rush.

16-year-old recipe creator Cassidy Bates was sick of flacid sushi, so she brought a bowl into the equation, allowing her to keep all the flavours she loved while getting rid of the hassle.

'This dish is the perfect way to enjoy sushi without having to spend ages making it,' she says. 'The best part is getting creative with your ingredients, you can add whatever flavours you love the most, so you end up with something delicious and wholesome that's the perfect lunch time meal.'

Vegan, gluten-free, dairy-free, refined sugar-free

Ingredients

⅓ cup brown rice

½ an avocado, sliced

4 tomatoes, chopped

¼ carrot, grated

¼ of pumpkin, chopping into 2-inch pieces

¼ cup beetroot, shredded

¼ block of tofu or tempeh

Handful of lettuce, chopped

½ a lemon

Sesame and edamame beans for topping

Method

Preheat oven to 200°C (400F). Boil the brown rice according to package instructions.

Place pumpkin on a tray covered with baking paper, lightly spray with olive oil and bake in the oven for 35-40 minutes, or until soft and cooked through.

In a fry pan set over medium heat, add the tofu or tempeh and lightly fry in a little olive oil until golden brown.

Place the cooked rice in a bowl. Then add the pumpkin, vegetables and tofu. Top with lemon juice sesame and edamame beans.

Serves 1

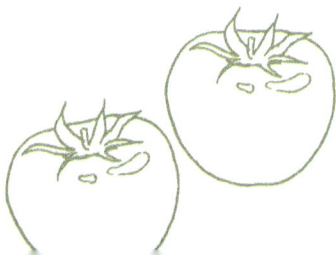

Chinese Garlic-Braised Eggplant

Liz Miu @itslizmiu

'An avocado takes 15 years to grow from a sprout to a tree, and yet most of us don't even understand the incredible processes and effort involved in getting it to our tables,' explains social entrepreneur and vegan YouTuber Liz Miu.

Listening to Liz talk about her love of food is nothing short of inspiring. Her passion for sharing food and educating others about its origins is addictive. Almost as addictive as her Chinese garlic-braised eggplant.

'So many people don't like eggplant because they don't know how to prepare it correctly,' says Liz. 'This is a really easy, flavoursome way to cook eggplant if you're trying to get to know it, because it'll most definitely turn you into an eggplant lover.'

Vegan, gluten-free, dairy-free

Ingredients

500 grams (1lb) eggplant

¼ cup cornflour

½ teaspoon salt

¼ teaspoon ground white pepper

¼ teaspoon ground black pepper

1 cube fermented bean curd

5 cloves garlic

2 sprigs spring onion, chopped

1 teaspoon black bean sauce

1 tablespoon vegetarian oyster sauce

1 tablespoon sugar

Fresh chilli, finely sliced (optional)

Method

Chop eggplant into large chunky pieces and soak it in a bowl of lightly salted water for at least 30 minutes. You can use a heavy plate to submerge the pieces if need be.

Remove the eggplant from the water and pat dry with a tea towel.

In a separate bowl, mix the cornflour, salt, white and black pepper.

Toss your pieces of eggplant in the cornflour mixture so every piece is coated very generously with flour.

Next, fry the eggplant by first heating a few centimeters of frying oil in a deep pot or wok. You'll know the oil is hot enough when you put a wooden chopstick in and lots of bubbles rise rapidly out of the chopstick.

Fry the eggplant pieces in small batches of 5-7 pieces for about 3 minutes, turning so that the pieces cook evenly. Once the eggplant is nicely browned, remove your eggplant from the pot and drain on paper towel and set aside.

Continued over page.

Oil for deep-frying (e.g. rice bran)

Spring onions and sesame seeds, to serve

To make the sauce, mix black bean sauce, oyster sauce and sugar together in a small bowl and set aside. Heat 1 tablespoon of oil in a pan on medium heat. Add spring onion to the pan and cook until shiny, then add the garlic and cook for 12 minutes.

Add the black bean sauce mixture to the pan along with your fermented bean curd until it has dissolved. Add the eggplant and fresh chilli to the pan and stir until the eggplant pieces are evenly coated with the sauce.

Garnish with freshly sliced spring onions and toasted sesame seeds and enjoy with freshly steamed rice.

Serves 2-4

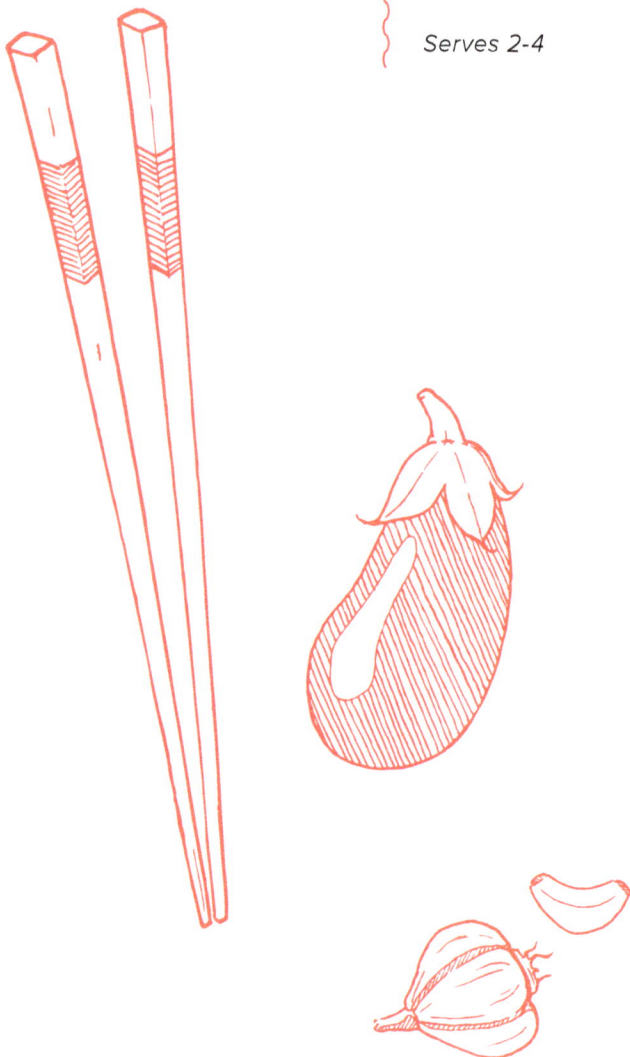

Sticky Tofu Lettuce Cups with Satay Sauce

Gabrielle O'Dea @nourishtheday

While not a born tofu fan, practising dietitian Gabrielle O'Dea has learnt to love this wonderful source of vegan protein. For her, it's all about the way you cook it, which is what led her to create this deliciously fresh dish that heros crispy, caramelised tofu.

'The trick is to cut the tofu into bite-sized pieces and fry it until it's crispy,' she says. 'Then you add a sticky sauce and the sesame seeds to give it a really caramelised, rich depth of flavour.'

'This recipe is one way I've been able to convert people to loving tofu, so if you have a friend who's hesitant to try it, definitely serve this up for them!'

Vegan, gluten-free, dairy-free

Ingredients

For the Tofu

400 grams (14 oz) firm tofu

2 tablespoons olive or canola oil

2 teaspoons sesame oil

3-4 tablespoons oyster sauce (use vegetarian oyster sauce if needed)

3 tablespoons sesame seeds

For the satay sauce

¼ cup smooth peanut butter (look for brands with only peanuts or peanuts and salt as the ingredients)

Juice of 2 small limes

½ teaspoon maple syrup

2 teaspoon tamari

¼-½ teaspoon sriracha sauce or other hot chilli sauce (optional)

Method

For the tofu

Chop the tofu into small bite sized pieces. Heat olive oil in a fry pan or wok over medium-high heat until hot. You'll know it's hot enough when you place a piece of tofu in and it sizzles straight away.

Add the tofu and sesame oil to the pan and pan fry for a few minutes, turning the tofu occasionally. You want most of the pieces to be lightly golden and slightly crisp.

Add the oyster sauce and sesame seeds (the oyster sauce may bubble and spit a little, so be careful). Stir to coat all the tofu in the sauce then continue to cook for a few minutes until the sides begin to caramelise. This is essential, so don't rush the process! Once cooked, remove from the pan.

For the satay sauce

Place all the ingredients for the sauce in a small bowl and mix until well combined. Add a little of the water to thin out if necessary.

Continued over page.

1-2 teaspoon water if needed

For the Lettuce cups

2 little gem lettuces, leaves washed and separated

1 lebanese cucumber, spiralised

1 carrot, shredded

1 red capsicum, finely sliced

1 cup red cabbage, finely shredded

Cooked brown rice, to serve

Peanuts, fresh coriander (cilantro) and mint, to garnish

To assemble, grab a lettuce cup and add in your shredded and spiralised veggies, and some brown rice. Top with the tofu and a drizzle of satay sauce.

Garnish with fresh mint, coriander, extra sriracha and sesame seeds as desired.

Serves 4 as a light starter

Substitutes and variations:
For a more substantial main meal, ditch the lettuce cups and cook up some rice vermicelli noodles instead. Toss the noodles with the cooked tofu, vegetables and top with satay sauce, peanuts and herbs for a refreshing noodle bowl.

If oyster sauce isn't your thing, any sticky sauce will do - try a mix of sweet soy and sweet chilli sauce, hoisin sauce, teriyaki sauce or combine some tamari, maple syrup and ginger for a different spin.

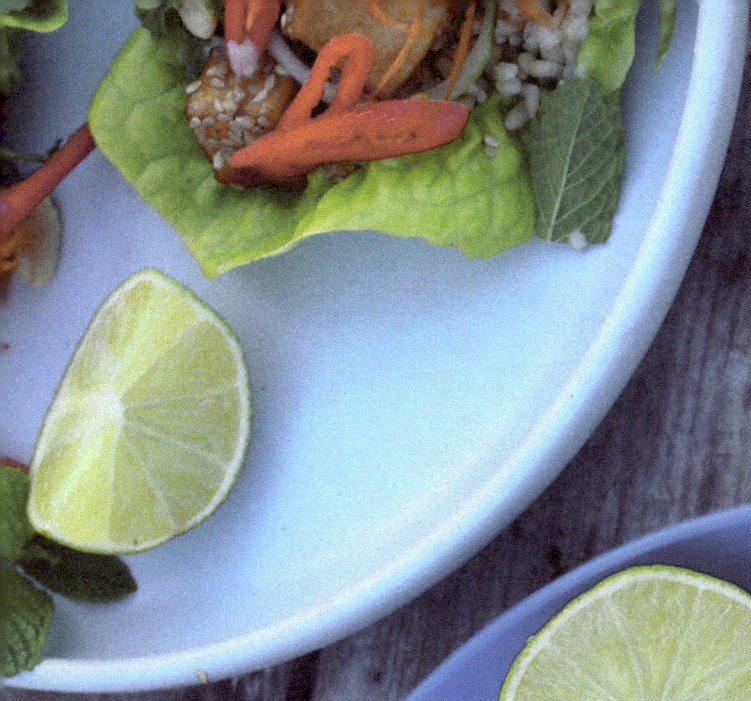

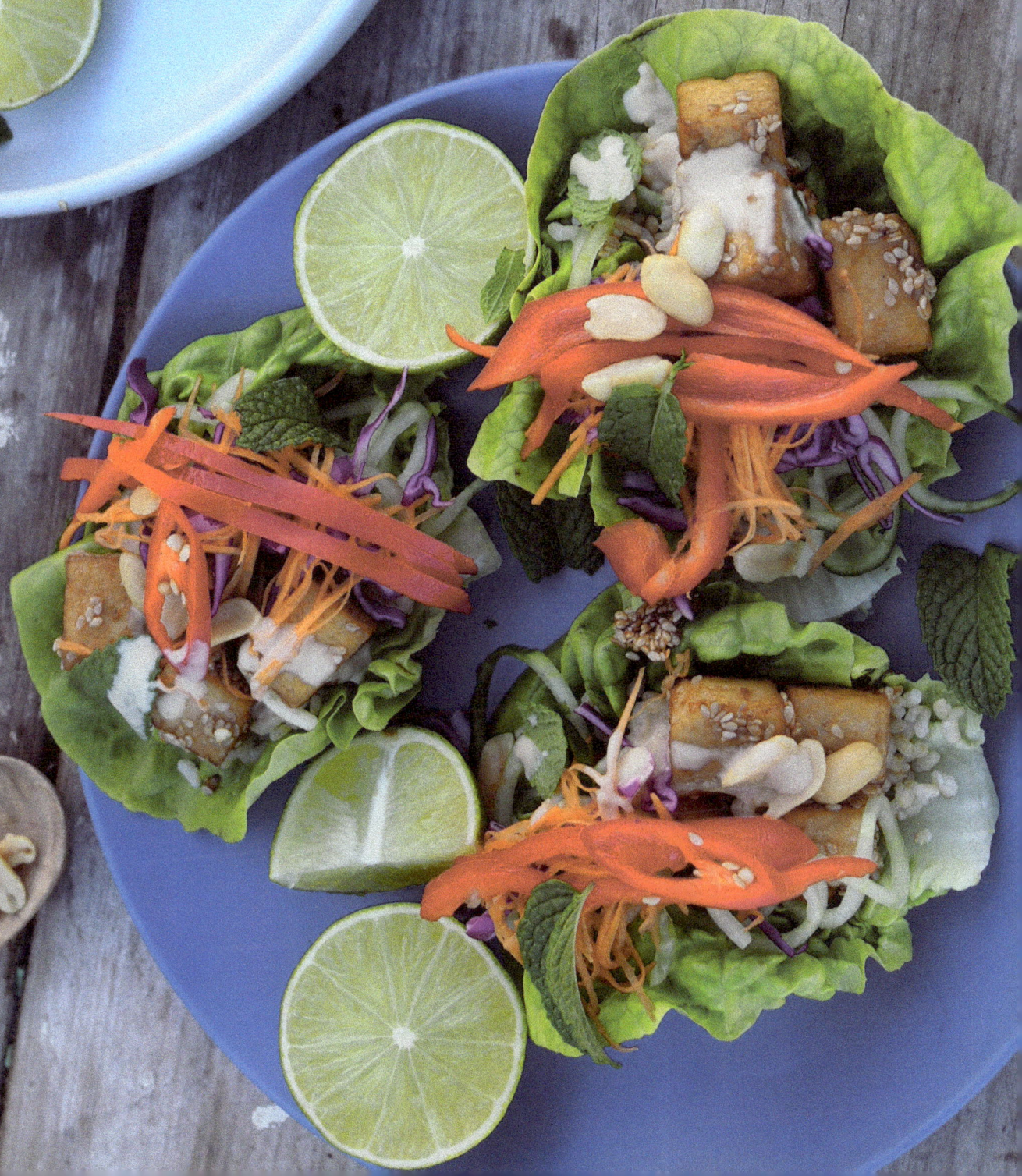

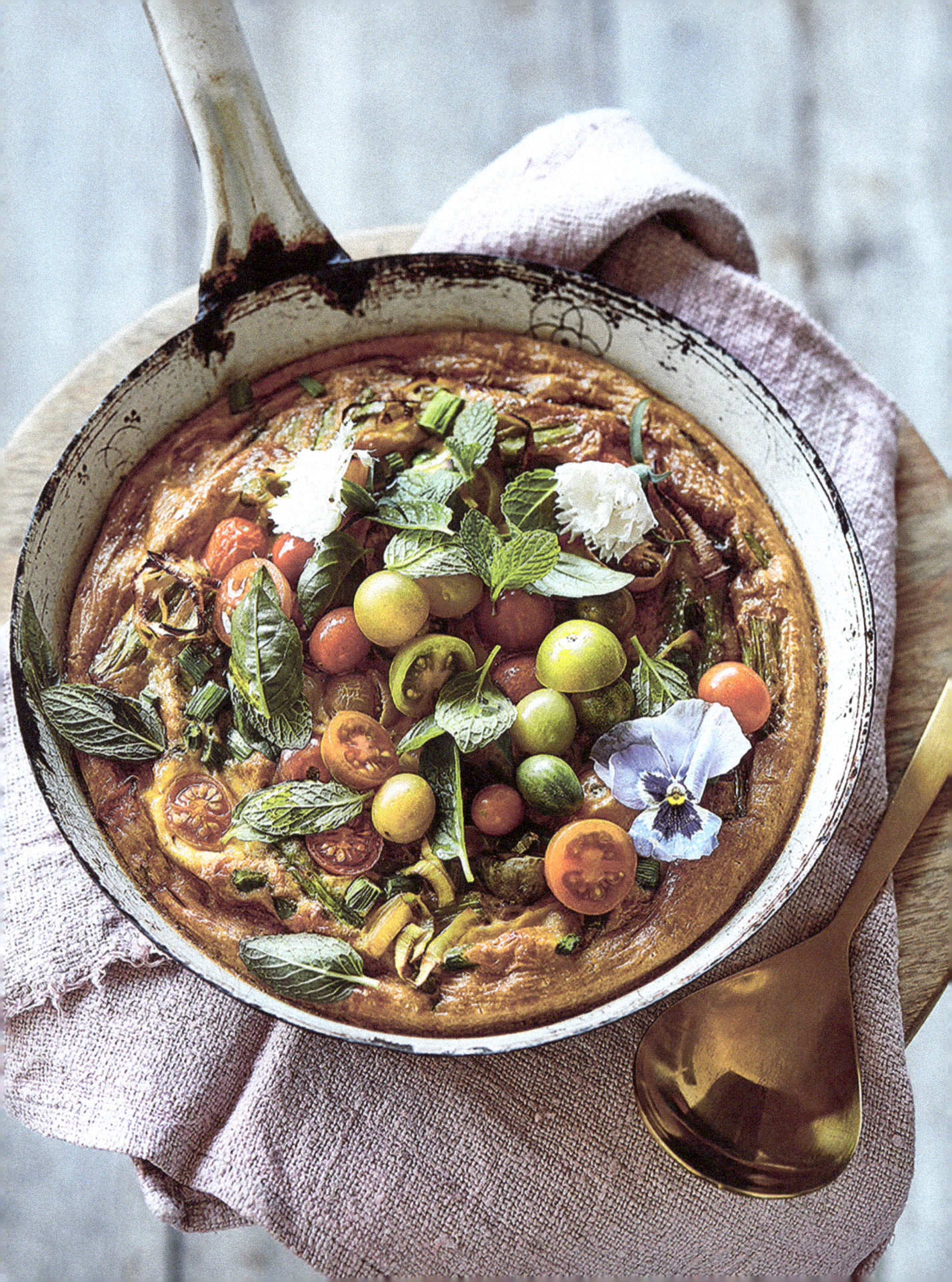

Crustless Vegetable Quiche

Lee Holmes @leesupercharged

After being diagnosed with an autoimmune disease, Lee Holmes radically changed her diet in order to improve her symptoms. This change has since led her into a career as a wholefoods chef, wellness educator and author who's passionate about sharing quick and simple recipes.

'I always had trouble navigating my way through complex gourmet recipes from magazines and cookbooks, and most of them contained ingredients I had never heard of before,' Lee admits. 'Some of the recipes left me thinking I'd bitten off more than I could chew and that there must be an easier way to prepare and cook nutritious food.'

It was this struggle that gave rise to recipes such as this simple, delicious crustless quiche, which is the perfect speedy weeknight meal or packed lunch.

Vegetarian, gluten-free, dairy-free

Ingredients

8 free-range eggs

125 millilitres (4 fl oz) almond milk

1 handful of basil leaves

1 thyme sprig, leaves picked

1 teaspoon ground cumin

½ teaspoon Celtic sea salt

2 tablespoons nutritional yeast flakes

10 asparagus spears, cut into 2.5cm (1") lengths and lightly sautéed

1½ cups sautéed chopped mixed vegetables such as leek, red onion, garlic, baby English spinach, zucchini, red capsicum, cherry tomatoes and rocket (arugula)

Mint leaves, to garnish (optional)

Method

Preheat the oven to 180°C (350°F) and grease a 22cm (9") pie dish or ovenproof frying pan.

Whisk the eggs well in a large bowl, then whisk in the almond milk, herbs, cumin, salt and nutritional yeast flakes.

Evenly scatter the asparagus and sautéed vegetables around the pie dish and pour the egg mixture over the top, ensuring the vegetables are evenly covered.

Transfer to the oven and bake for 25–30 minutes, or until the quiche is set in the middle and the top is puffy and lightly browned.

Enjoy warm or at room temperature, garnished with mint if desired.

Serves 4

Coconut Bacon Caesar Salad

Aliza Strock @shaktifresh

After turning plant-based in her early twenties, personal chef and founder catering company Skakti Fresh, Aliza Strock, was challenged with cooking her favourite dishes without animal products. The result, in this instance, is this light and crispy Caesar salad that's packed with flavour and plant-based goodness.

'I used to be a big fan of Caesar salad and was really craving those flavours', Aliza says. 'I used cashews for the dressing, as I feel they give a really creamy consistency.'

While coconut bacon might sound intimidating to make from scratch, Aliza promises it's deceptively easy and a wholefoods alternative to processed faux meat options.

'Over the last few years I've been trying to make everything from scratch - my sauces, pestos and marinades - because that's a really important ethos behind my food,' she explains. 'I'm a firm believer that energy and spirituality go hand-in-hand with food, and that we should all try to eat more of the food Mother Nature has provided for us.'

Vegan, gluten-free, dairy-free, refined sugar-free

Ingredients

For the coconut bacon

2 cups unsweetened coconut chips

1 cup tamari or coconut aminos

2 tablespoons maple syrup

1 tablespoon hickory liquid smoke

For the Caesar dressing

1 cup raw cashews

¼ cup soy or unsweetened almond milk (+ extra if needed while blending)

1 tablespoon Dijon mustard

1 tablespoon garlic powder

1 tablespoon onion powder

¼ cup nutritional yeast

Method

Preheat oven to 180°C (350°F).

To make the coconut bacon, marinate the coconut chips by combining them with the liquid ingredients in a sealable container. Shake well to coat the chips, and let marinate in the fridge for 20-30 minutes.

Meanwhile, to begin the Caesar dressing, soak the cashews in a bowl of boiling water for 30 minutes.

Bake marinated coconut chips in the oven for 10 minutes. Stir, then bake for another 5 or until just crispy. Be careful, there's a fine line between just crispy and burnt, so keep checking!

Once the cashews are soaked, blend them in a high-powered blender with the remainder of the dressing ingredients until smooth and creamy. You may need to slowly add more plant milk as you blend to reach that thick and creamy consistency.

Next, prepare the salad ingredients and place them in a large salad bowl.

Juice of 1 lemon

Salt and pepper to taste

For the salad

1 large head of organic cos lettuce, chopped

250 grams (8½ oz) cherry tomatoes, halved

2 avocados, diced

1 small red onion, diced

1 large cucumber, sliced

¼ cup pumpkin seeds

¼ cup hemp seeds

Optional: ½ cup roughly chopped parsley or mint

Place all the salad ingredients in a large bowl and add the coconut bacon and dressing. Toss everything together until well combined.

Serves 4

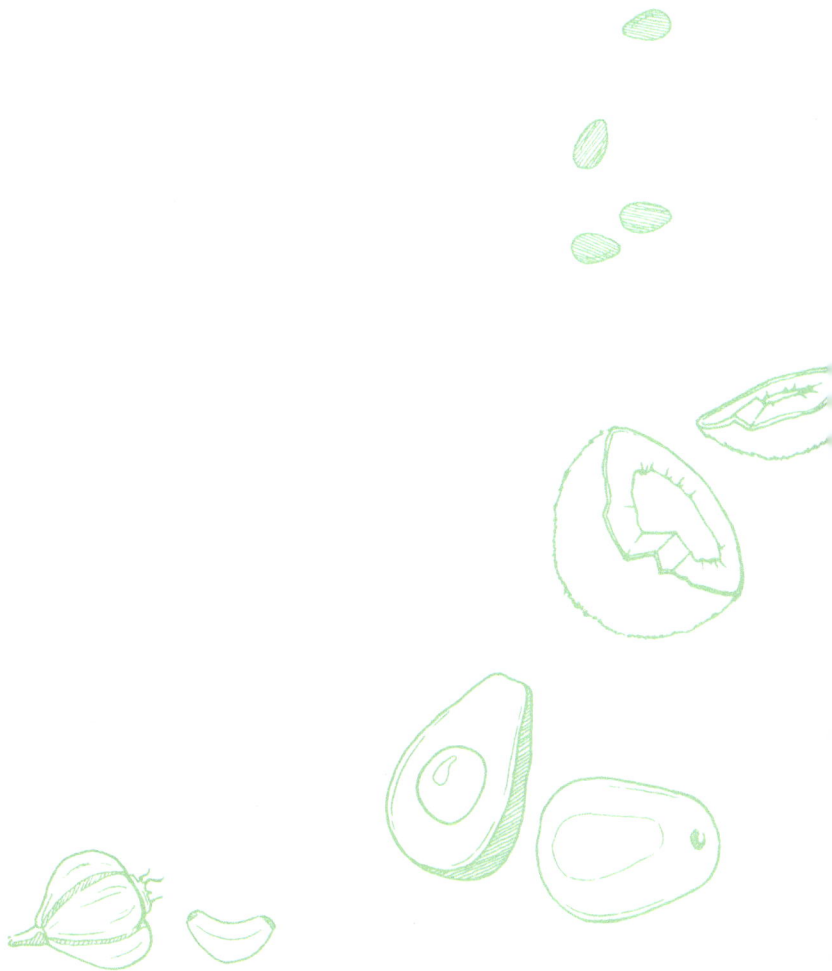

Easy Throw Together Bowl

Nadia Felsch @nadiafelsch

If a tin of tuna and some lettuce leaves come to mind when you hear the word 'salad', this filling, nutrient bomb of a bowl by food-lover Nadia Felsch will change the way you look at salads forever.

After being diagnosed with an auto-immune disease and PCOS, Nadia began experimenting with cooking more nutrient dense food as a way to help reduce her symptoms. This bowl (and its many variations) is something she took to making regularly and is still her go-to lunch of choice.

'This is how I eat most of the time,' she says. 'It's whatever's in the fridge and there's no hard and fast rules - so use whatever you've got on hand! To make this salad really satisfying, think about all the textural elements and how they work together; the smooth guacamole, the crunchy vegetables... that's what will make it really delicious.'

Vegan option, gluten-free, dairy-free, refined sugar-free

Ingredients

For the rice

½ cup cooked brown rice

1 tablespoon red onion, finely chopped

2 tablespoon fresh mint leaves, finely chopped

Extra-virgin olive oil, to dress

Salt and pepper, to taste

For the guacamole

½ medium avocado

1 tablespoon fresh coriander (cilantro) leaves, finely chopped

Fresh lemon and fresh lime juice, to taste

Salt and pepper, to taste

Method

Combine rice, onion and herbs together in a small bowl and mix well. Dress with olive oil and season to taste.

For the guacamole, add avocado to a small bowl and mash with a fork until smooth. Add the rest of the guacamole ingredients, mix to combine and season to taste.

Add all salad ingredients to a bowl along with the rice. Top with guacamole and boiled eggs.

Serves 1

For the salad

½ cup diced roast pumpkin

Handful snow pea sprouts

½ handful alfalfa sprouts

2 small red radishes, thinly sliced

1 small tomato, sliced into thin wedges

¼ cup red cabbage, thinly sliced

1-2 hard boiled eggs, halved

Use what's on hand and in your fridge. Leave things out, add things in. There is no perfect way to make this and in fact, it's more fun to make it your own!

For a vegan alternative, use your favourite legumes, tofu or tempeh as your protein source.

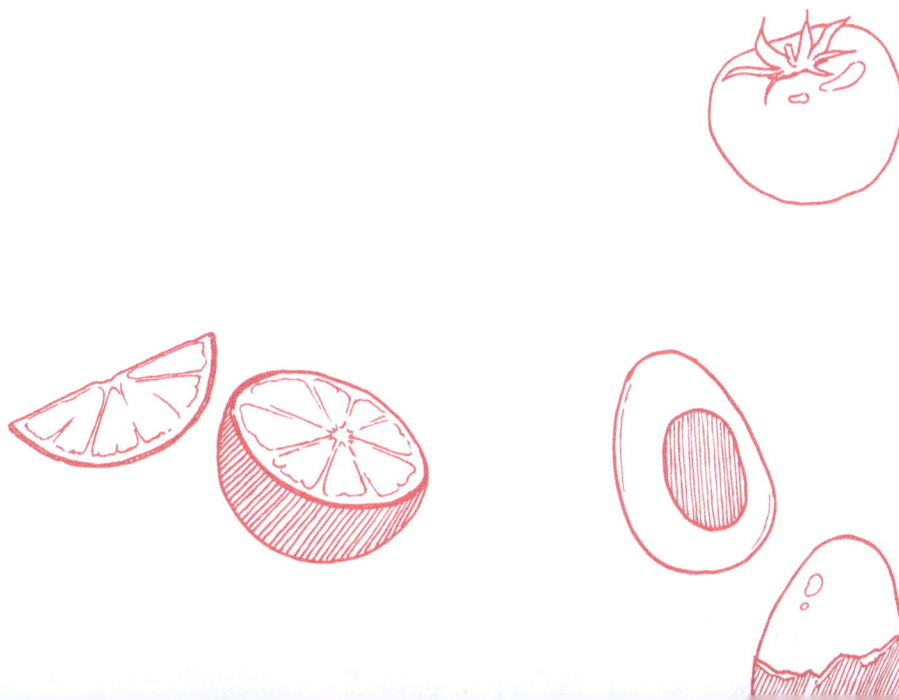

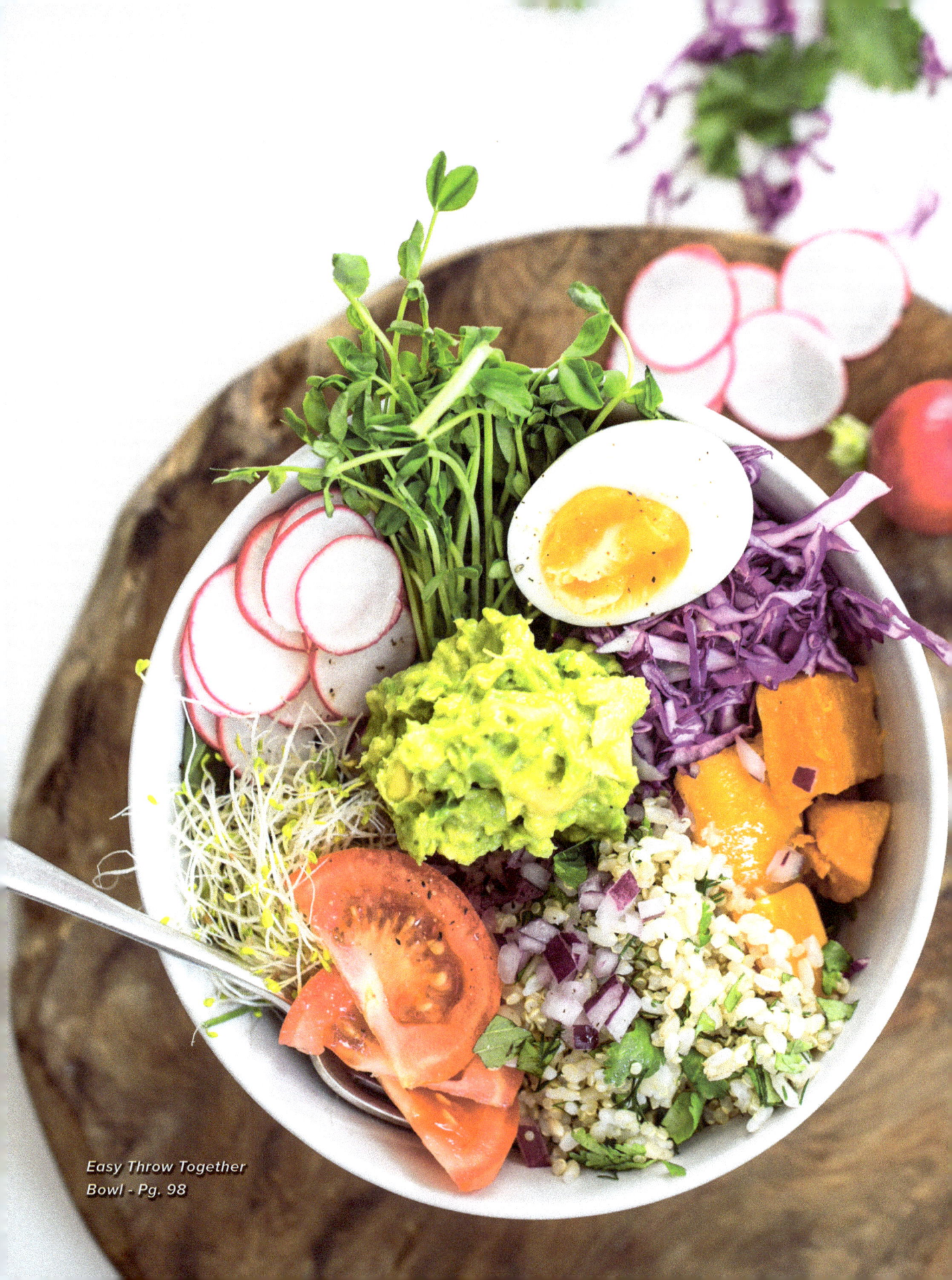

Easy Throw Together
Bowl - Pg. 98

Haloumi Salad with Quinoa and Avocado Salsa

Stephanie Geddes @nutritionist_stephgeddes

What do you think of when you hear the word "salad"? Limp lettuce leaves and some cold cherry tomatoes? Well forget everything you thought you knew about salads, because this salad by nutritionist, recipe developer and ambassador Steph Geddes is one you'll want to make friends with.

'Clients were coming to see me and telling me they ate salad leaves and tuna for lunch and that they were bored of eating healthily,' Steph says. 'So I decided to start creating salads like this, which are hearty, filling and so satisfying.'

Trust us, you'll never get sick of eating healthy food tucking into this dish!

Vegetarian, gluten-free, refined sugar-free

Ingredients

2 packets organic halloumi, cut in half and then into triangles

1 packet vine-ripened cherry tomatoes

2 cobs of corn

½ cup red quinoa (or any colour), rinsed well

¼ cup pumpkin seeds

4 large handfuls of rocket (arugula)

1 avocado, diced

1 long green chilli, diced

1 lime

Salt and pepper

Method

Preheat the oven to 200°C (400°F). Line a baking tray with baking paper, place the tomatoes on the tray and pop in the oven for 20-25minutes.

Meanwhile, place the rinsed quinoa in a saucepan with 1 cup of water. Bring to a boil then cover and turn to a low heat. Simmer until the water has absorbed then set aside for 5 minutes.

While the quinoa is cooking, prepare the avocado salsa by combining the avocado, chilli, zest of the lime, juice of ½ the lime and a sprinkle of salt and pepper and then set aside.

Lightly steam the corn. Using either a grill pan or BBQ, char the steamed corn and grill the halloumi slices for 1-2 minutes each side. Slice the corn kernels off the cob.

Combine the rocket, quinoa, corn, halloumi, tomatoes and pumpkin seeds and drizzle with olive oil. Top with the avocado salsa.

Serves 4

Soba Noodle Bowl with Creamy Chilli Peanut Sauce

Kat Nguyen-Thai @katnt

There's a lot to love about bowl food, says plant-based recipe developer Kat Nguyen-Thai. You start with a grain base, add whatever vegetables you like and before you know it you have a quick, delicious meal. The secret, however, to making them taste incredible lies in the sauce, she explains.

'Bowls are great because there are no rules to them - they're like the rebel of the food world,' she laughs. 'You just add whatever veggies you have on hand and as long as there's a great sauce it's always going to taste amazing.'

The rich, creamy dressing that accompanies this soba bowl is one of Kat's favourite. She regularly makes a big batch and stores it in her fridge to make midweek lunches and dinners all the more delicious. She recommends tossing any leftover sauce over noodle bowls, into stir fries and enjoying it with tofu.

Vegan, vegetarian, gluten-free, refined sugar-free

Ingredients

For the salad

180 grams (6 oz) 100% buckwheat soba noodles

2 carrots, julienned

2 cucumbers, julienned

1 capsicum, thinly sliced

Bunch of broccolini, roughly chopped

1 packed cup of parsley

Method

Preheat the oven to 175°C (350°F) and line a baking tray with baking paper.

To prepare the tempeh, cut the tempeh into 1⁄4 inch slices. In a small bowl, mix the tamari and sesame oil together and add the sliced tempeh.

Coat the tempeh in the sauces and place it in a single layer on the lined baking tray.

Cook tempeh in oven for 20 minutes until crispy and golden. Remove from the oven and set aside.

For the tempeh

1 x 225 grams (8 oz) packet of tempeh

2 tablespoons tamari

2 tablespoons sesame oil

For the chilli peanut sauce

½ cup peanut butter

Juice of ½ lime

2 tablespoons of tamari

2 tablespoons of maple syrup

1 tablespoons sesame oil

1 teaspoons chilli paste

½ cup water

1 tablespoon minced ginger

While the tempeh is cooking, in a small saucepan cook the soba noodles according to packet instructions. Set aside once cooked.

Blanch the broccolini in a pot of boiling salted water for 2 minutes. Drain immediately and run under cold water to stop from cooking further. Set aside.

Add the broccolini, carrots, cucumber, capsicum, baked tempeh and soba noodles into a large bowl. Using your hands, gently toss all ingredients together until the vegetables are evenly dispersed.

To make the sauce, add all ingredients in a small blender and blend until combined and creamy.

Pour the chilli peanut sauce into the bowl with noodles and vegetables and gently mix until the noodles, tempeh and vegetables are coated.

Serve immediately and share with friends!

Serves 2

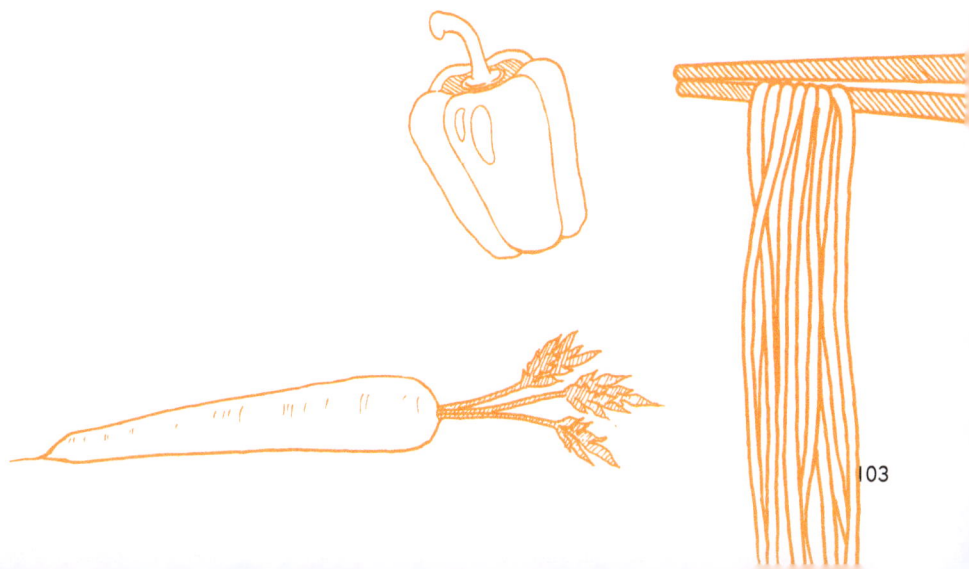

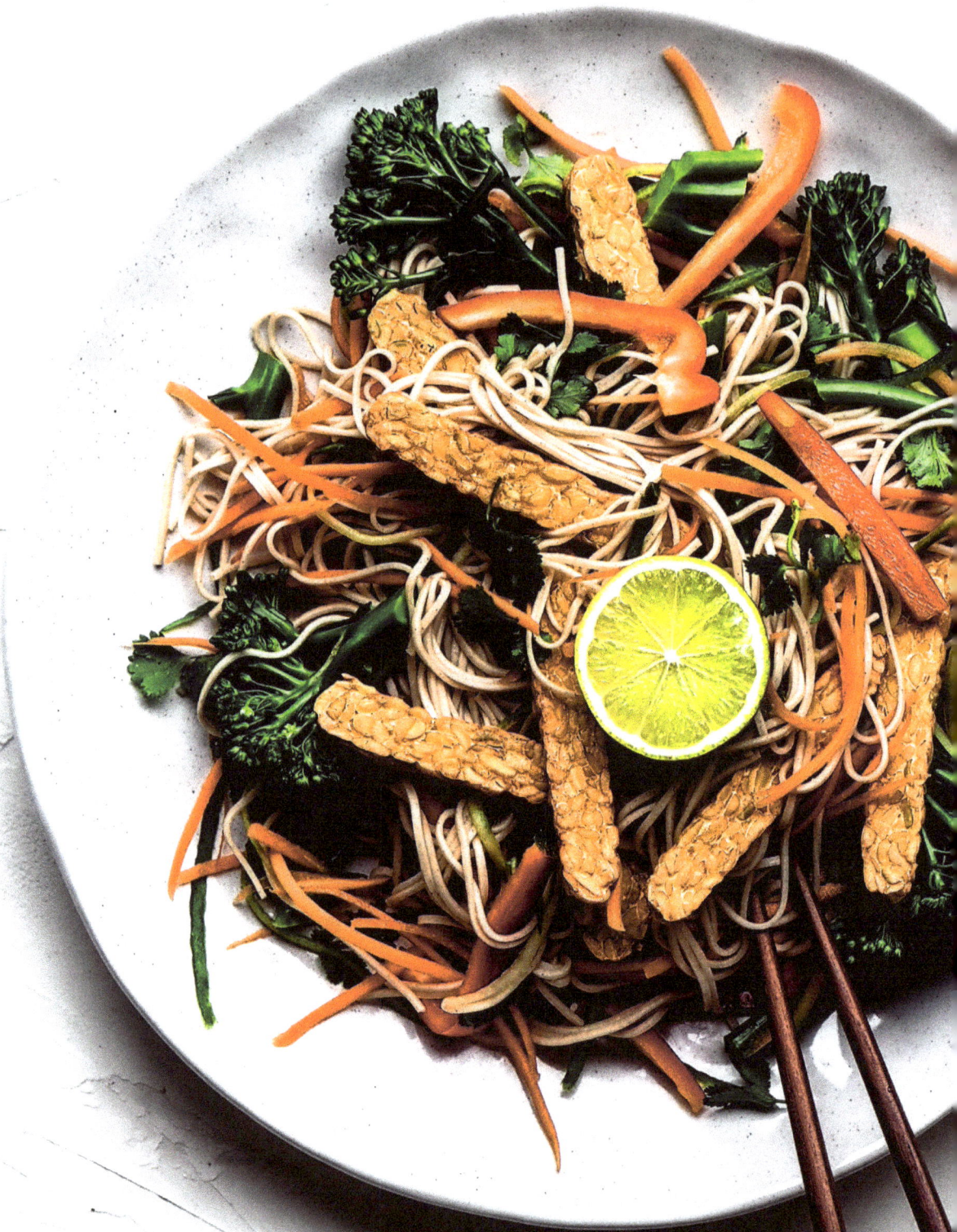

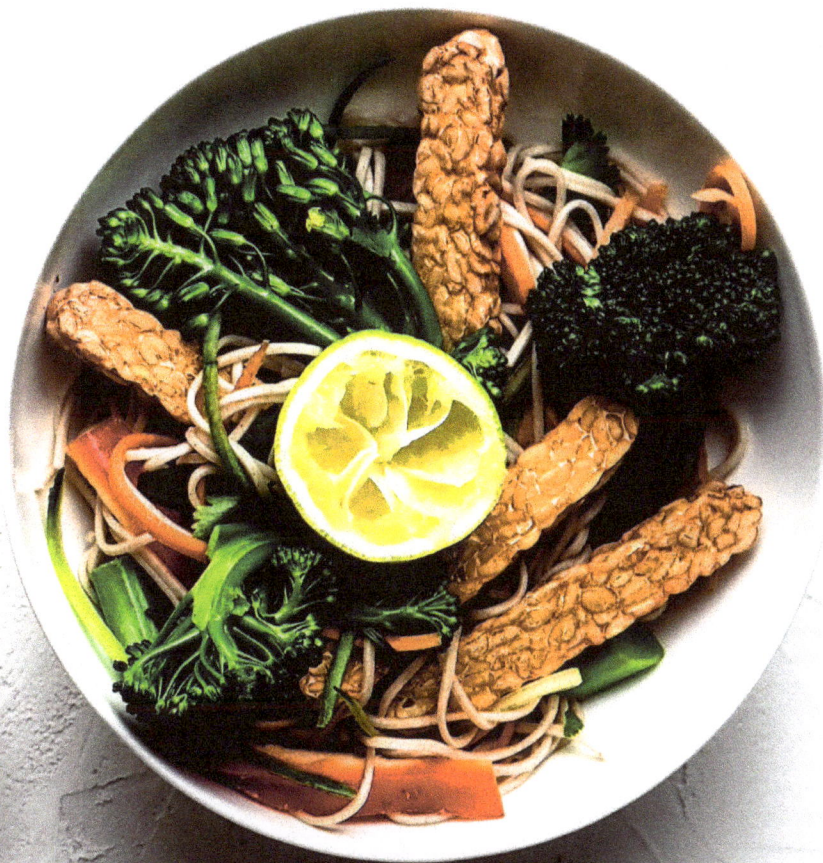

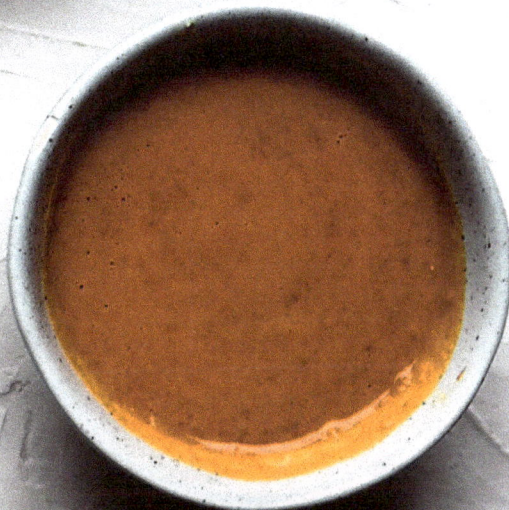

Soba Noodle Bowl with Creamy Chilli Peanut Sauce- Pg. 102

Golden Turmeric Cauliflower with Dukkah, Pomegranate & Pepitas

Sarah Cooper @scoopitup_

Having a few basic spices such as turmeric, cumin, chilli flakes and dukkah in your cupboard will significantly up your cooking game. Even the smallest amount will give your food serious cred, explains founder of Scoop it Up bliss balls, Sarah Cooper.

The combination of turmeric and cumin give this incredible salad a toasty, nutty flavour, that sets off the sweet bursts of pomegranate perfectly.

Serve this next to a portion of your favourite protein - salmon, chicken or tofu.

Vegan, gluten-free, dairy-free, refined sugar-free

Ingredients

1 head cauliflower

2-3 tablespoons olive oil

1 tablespoon turmeric

1 tablespoon cumin

1 teaspoon chilli flakes (optional)

3 tablespoons dukkah or sesame seeds

½ cup pomegranate seeds

¼ cup pepitas, toasted

salt and pepper

1 big handful fresh mint, chopped

2 cups fresh greens, rocket (arugula) and spinach work well

Method

Preheat oven to 180°C (350°F).

Cut your cauliflower into florets and place into a bowl with the olive oil, turmeric, cumin, chilli flakes and dukkah. Toss all together to make sure all the calufilower is covered in the oil and spices.

Place cauliflower on a baking tray lined with baking paper and bake for 45 minutes or until soft, golden and crispy

Arrange the fresh greens on a large serving plate and top with the roast cauliflower, pomegranate seeds, pepitas and fresh mint. Add extra olive oil, dukkah, salt and pepper if you wish

Serves 4 as a side

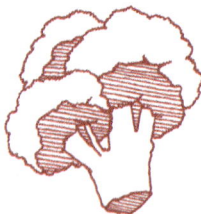

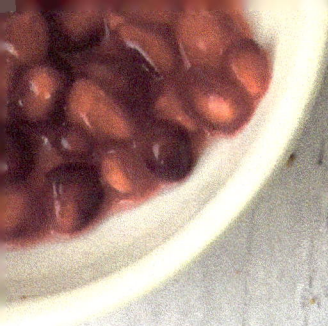

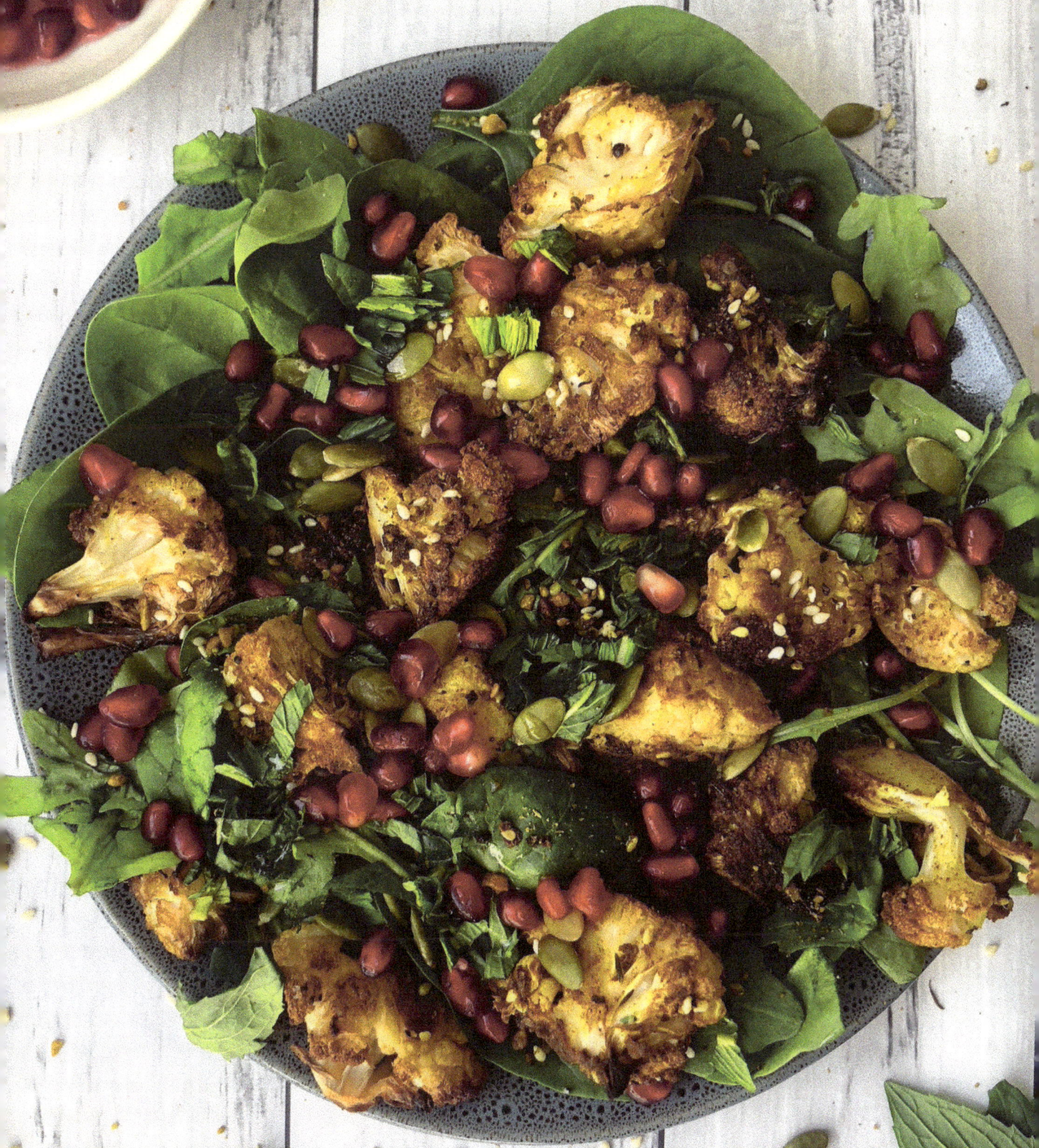

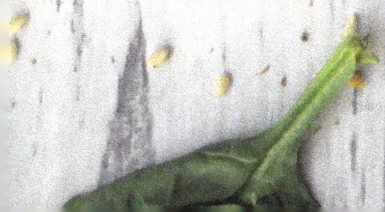

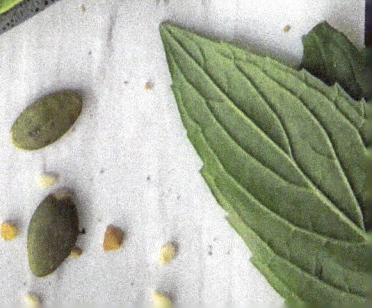

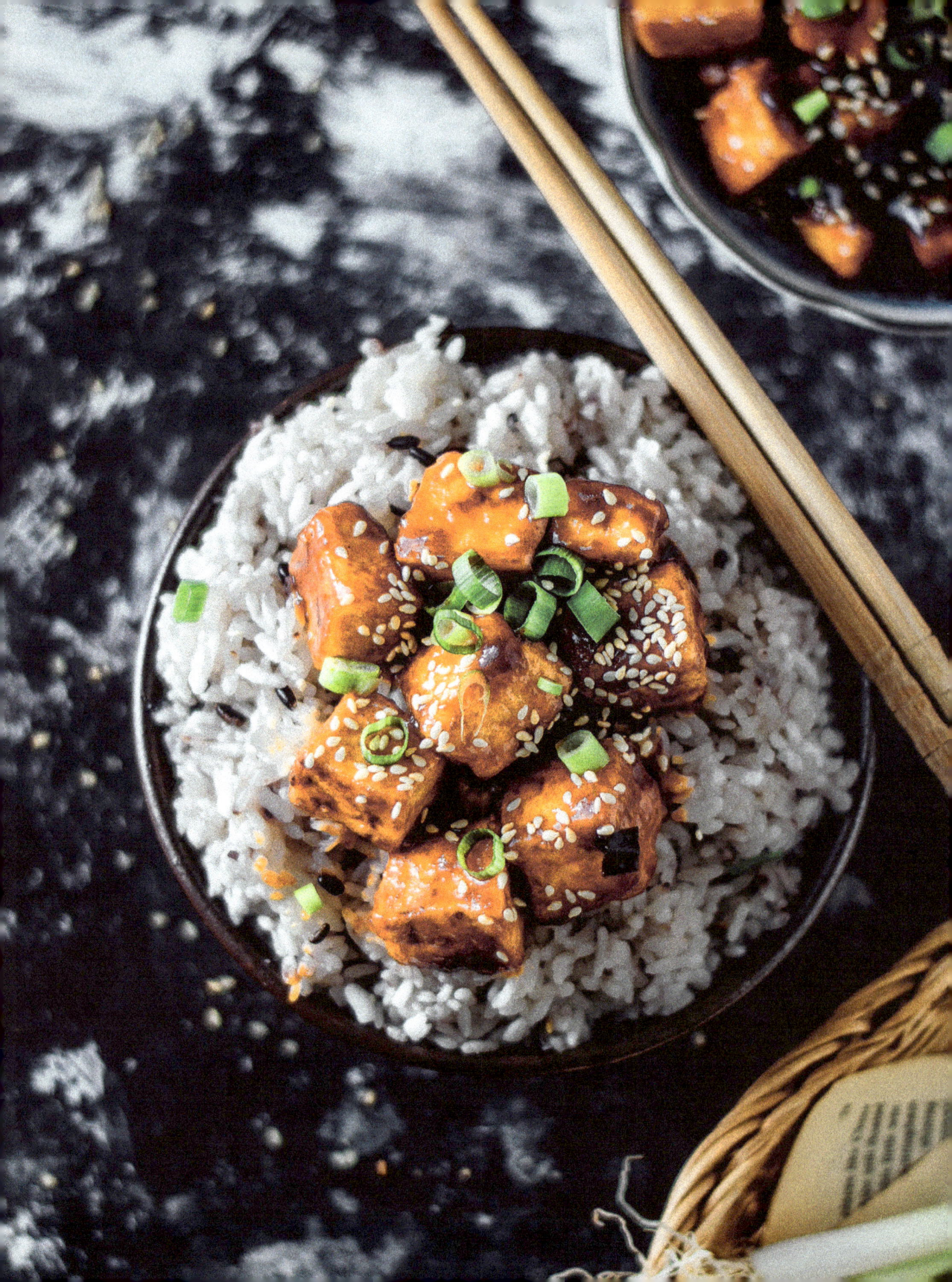

Sweet and Spicy Korean Tofu

Sasha Back @earthlingsasha

'When I first went vegan I didn't eat much of my traditional cuisine because I was branching out and trying new foods,' says food blogger Sasha Back, both of whose parents come from Korea. 'But I found I was growing a bit nostalgic for those flavours, so I'm moving back into cooking the dishes that I grew up eating.'

It was this desire for the taste of home that drove Sasha to create this dish, which echoes the rich, umami flavours often found in Korean cuisine.

Sasha explains that in Korean culture a bowl of plain white rice is usually accompanied by an assortment of dishes, such as this tofu, which is how she recommends serving it.

Vegan, dairy-free, refined sugar-free

Ingredients

For the tofu

330 grams (11½ oz) medium firm tofu

1 ½ tablespoon potato starch or cornstarch

1 tablespoon coconut oil

Cooked rice, sesame seeds and sliced spring onions, to serve

For the sauce

3 tablespoons maple syrup

2 tablespoons soy sauce

2 tablespoons gochujang (Korean red chilli paste)

1 tablespoon rice vinegar (or apple cider vinegar)

½ tablespoon sesame oil

½ teaspoon ground garlic

¼ teaspoon white pepper

½ tablespoon spring onion, chopped

Method

Start by pressing your tofu to release the moisture. To do this, place the block of tofu on a bench in between 2 clean tea towels. Place a heavy bowl or chopping board on top and leave for 5-10 minutes.

While tofu is pressing, make the sauce by combining all the ingredients in a bowl and mix well to combine.

Once the tofu has been pressed, cut it into cubes. Fill a shallow plate with the potato starch and coat your tofu cubes in the starch.

Heat a large pan with 1 tablespoon of oil and cook your coated tofu until all sides are nicely brown and crispy. This will take around 4-7 minutes.

Turn down the heat to low and add the sauce to the pan along with the tofu. Let this simmer and continue stirring for 5 minutes.

Turn off the heat from under the pan and let the contents cool for around 4 minutes, or until the mixture thickens slightly.

Serve over rice with spring onions and sesame. Enjoy!

Serves 3-4

Creamy Pumpkin Soup

Jen Murrant & Hannah Singleton @healthyluxe

There's something incredibly nostalgic about a steaming bowl of pumpkin soup on a cold winter evening. And this version from the mother daughter duo behind Healthy Luxe is no exception.

'Pumpkin soup has always been an old favourite and is something that mum always made for me when I was growing up,' says Hannah Singleton. 'It's so easy, nourishing and perfect for those nights when you want something really comforting.'

This soup gets its creamy consistency from homemade cashew milk, which Jen and Hannah create by simply blending one cup of raw cashews with three cups of filtered water. It might sound like a bit of work, but Jen guarantees it takes no time at all and is worth the extra effort.

Vegan, gluten-free, dairy-free, refined sugar-free

Ingredients

1 tablespoon coconut oil

1 leek, chopped

1 small brown onion, chopped

500 grams (1 lb) pumpkin

500 grams (1 lb) sweet potato

2 cups filtered water

1 tablespoon turmeric, grated

1½ tablespoon ginger, grated

¼ teaspoon Himalayan salt

½ cup cashew milk (homemade or store-bought)

Coconut yogurt, fresh herbs and toast to serve

Method

Braise the onion and leek in coconut oil in a large saucepan over low heat for 3-5 minutes.

Add chopped sweet potato, pumpkin and filtered water. Cover and leave to simmer for 10-15 minutes, or until vegetables are tender.

Add turmeric, ginger and salt to the pot and simmer for a further 5-10 minutes. Transfer the mixture to a blender, or use a handheld blender and blend until smooth.

Return the soup to your saucepan and reheat, slowly adding your cashew milk while stirring. Depending on how you like your soup you can add more if you prefer a thinner consistency.

Pour the soup into 4 bowls and top with a dollop of coconut yoghurt, fresh herbs, salt and pepper. Serve with a side of toast, if you like.

Serves 4 as a starter

Feel free to use store bought cashew milk if you're really pressed for time, or even coconut milk if that's what you have in your cupboard.

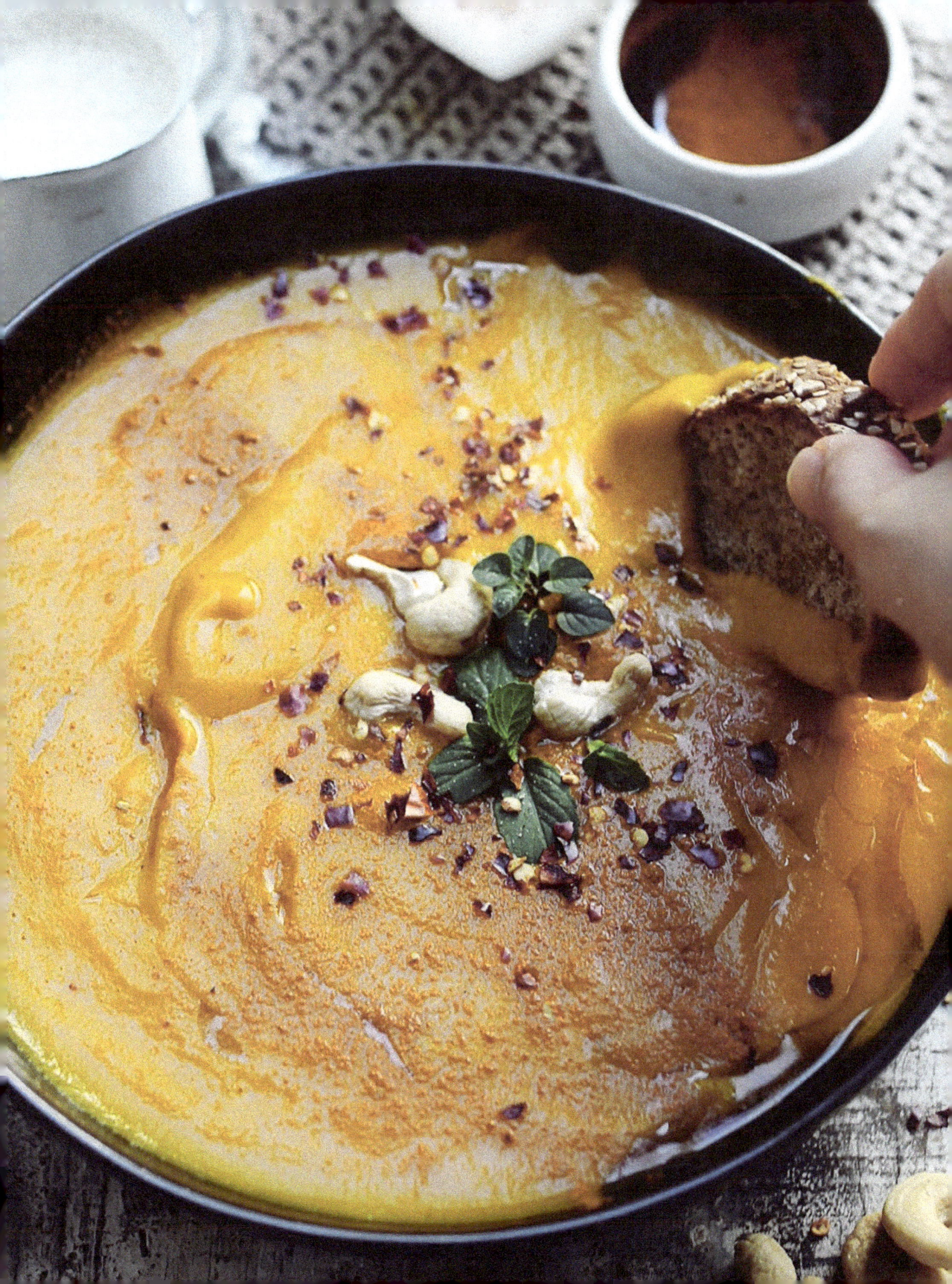

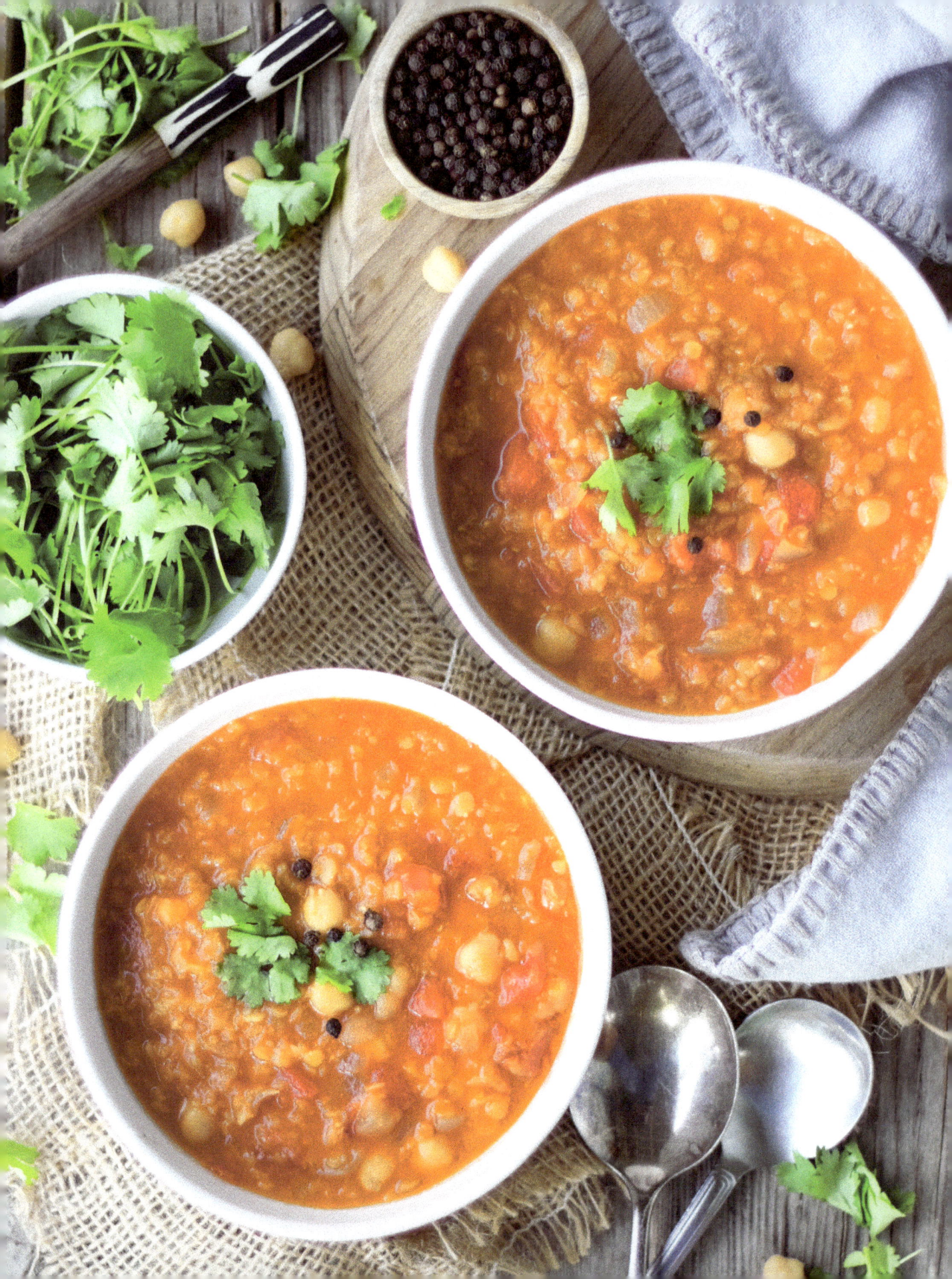

Smoky Lentil & Chickpea Soup

Chloe Munro @the_smallseed_

While winter on Victoria's Mornington Peninsula doesn't quite compare to the harsh, cold of England, where Chloe Munro grew up as a child, it can still get pretty darn cold. So when the frost starts to appear Chloe turns to this hearty, veggie-filled soup to warm her soul.

'This soup is one of my favourite winter dishes,' she says. 'It's filled with amazing plant protein, so is really satiating and so warm and nourishing. I brought it to a neighbourhood soup party one day and now everyone always asks me to cook it for them!'

This dish is a simple way to pack lots of nutrient-dense vegetables into your day with very little effort. And while Chloe's young son might pick out the chickpeas (kids, what can you do!), they provide a great dose of plant protein.

Vegan, gluten-free, dairy-free, refined sugar-free

Ingredients

200 grams (7 oz) red lentils

1 large red onion, diced

2-3 cloves garlic, crushed

1 teaspoon smoked paprika

½ teaspoon cumin

1 litre vegetable stock

1 x 400 gram (14 oz) tin tomatoes

¼ tin chickpeas, drained

¼ cup tomato purée

Pinch of cayenne pepper (optional)

Fresh coriander (cilantro) and crusty bread to serve, optional

Method

Gently fry the onion in a little olive oil in a large saucepan over a medium-high heat.

When the onion is translucent, add crushed garlic, lentils and spices. Cook for 1-2 minutes, stirring to ensure all the lentils are covered with the spices.

Add tinned tomatoes, vegetable stock, tomato purée and let simmer, half covered, on a low heat until the lentils are cooked through, approximately 15-20 minutes.

Add the chickpeas to the saucepan and remove from the heat.

Ladle into bowls and serve with a few sprigs of fresh coriander and a side of crusty bread.

Serves 5

Asian Broth with Chicken Meatballs

Phoebe Conway @pheebsfoods

A love of Asian food coupled with a busy schedule resulted in recipe developer Phoebe Conway buying ready-made dumplings from the supermarket on the reg. Eventually, she put her foot down and decided to create this more wholesome, nourishing alternative.

'This is such a beautifully aromatic dish and so full of nutrients,' she says. 'It's high in protein, low in fat and contains vegetables you might not eat as regularly, such as bok choy, giving you greater variety in your diet.'

The best part about this dish is you can really make it your own. Throw whatever vegetables you like into the mix and top it with your favourite garnishes; fresh chilli, coriander, spring onions, fried shallots, lime juice - whatever takes your fancy!

Gluten-free option, dairy-free, refined sugar-free

Ingredients

For the broth

4 cups chicken bone broth

2 spring onions

1 tablespoon ginger, grated

2 garlic cloves, crushed

1 lemongrass stalk, bruised and finely chopped

1 tablespoon tamari, to taste

1 teaspoon fish sauce. optional

1 teaspoon sesame oil

Juice of 1 lime

Sesame seeds, to garnish

Method

Preheat your oven to 200°C (400°F) fan forced, and line a baking tray with paper.

Combine all of the meatball ingredients into a bowl and mix until well combined. Roll into meatballs —around 16 balls.

Spread the meatballs out evenly on the tray and bake for 15-20 minutes or until just cooked through.

While the meatballs are baking, combine all of the broth ingredients in a pot and bring to the boil. Lower to a simmer until the meatballs have finished cooking - around 15 minutes.

Add your chosen vegetables into the broth and cook for 3-5 minutes until just tender.

For the meatballs

500 grams (1 lb) chicken mince

1 tablespoon ginger, grated

1 garlic clove

1 red onion, finely chopped

1 teaspoon sesame oil

1 tablespoon asian chilli garlic sauce

1 egg

½ cup panko bread crumbs (sub for almond meal to make gluten-free)

Zest of 1 lime

2 serves of rice noodles, prepared according to packet instructions

Vegetables of choice (E.g. bok choy, snow peas, mushrooms, sprouts)

Chilli oil, lime juice, fresh coriander (cilantro) and fried shallots, to serve

Divide the noodles, meatballs (you will most likely have meatballs left over -YES, lunch tomorrow!), vegetables and broth between two bowls. Top with desired condiments.

Serves 2

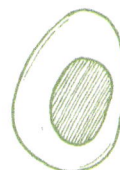

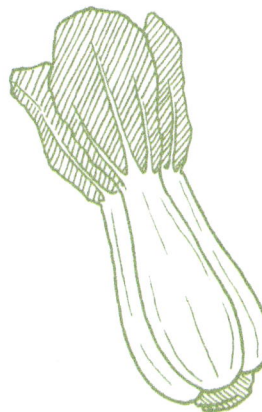

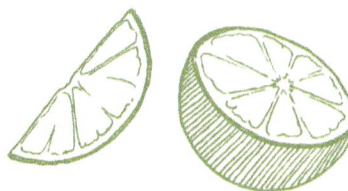

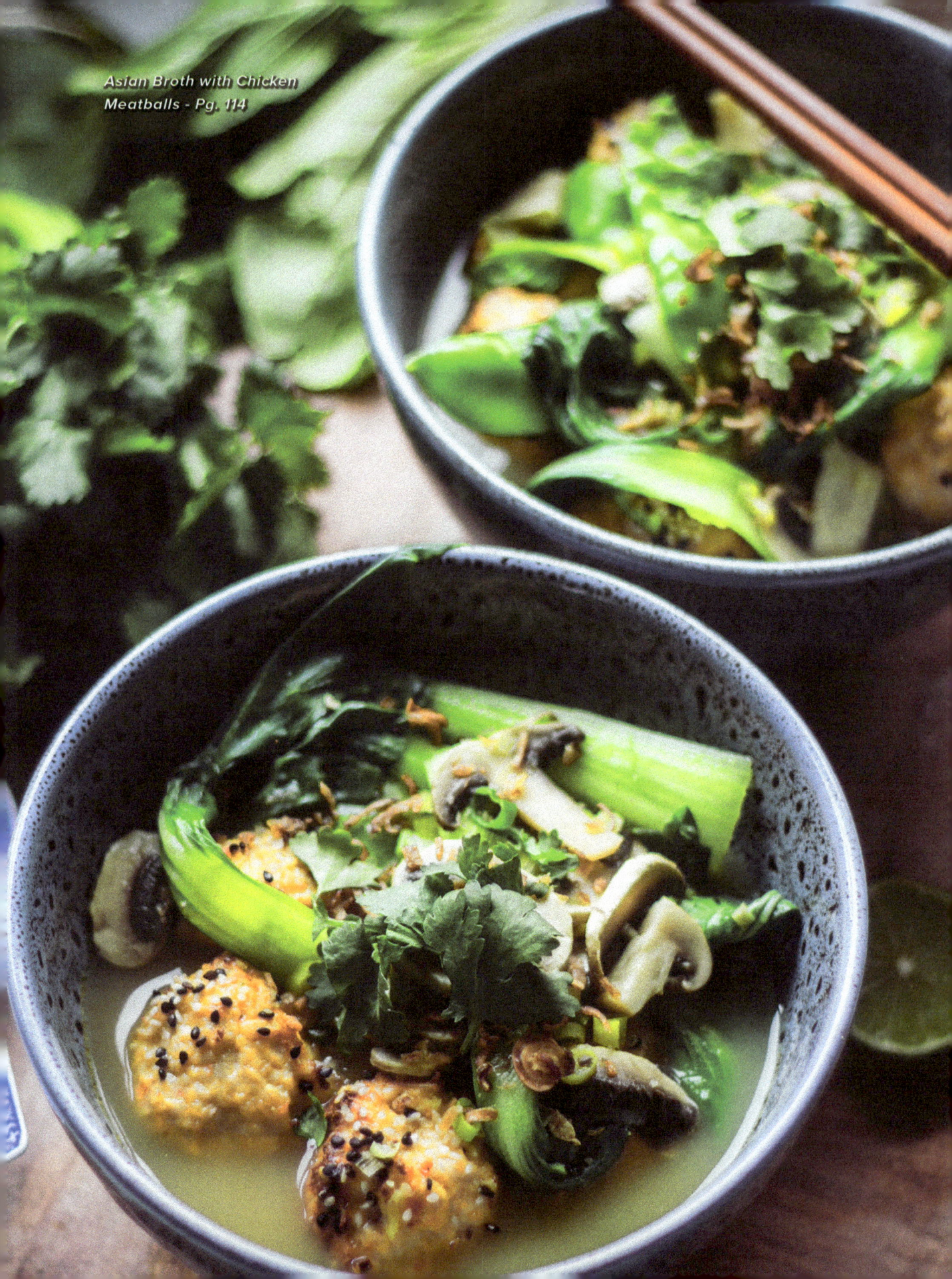

Asian Broth with Chicken
Meatballs - Pg. 114

Vegetarian Nut Loaf

Melanie Lionello @frommylittlekitchen

Christmas can be a challenging time for vegetarians when the rest of your family is tucking into a roast or seafood platter that you can't share. It was for this reason that Melbourne-based recipe developer Melanie Lionello decided to create a dish that celebrates the flavours of Christmas without the meat.

'I wanted to create a vegetarian dish that was festive and Christmassy, so people weren't missing out on those flavours,' Mel explains.

'The aged cheddar in this recipe adds a salty, umami richness that's so often missing in vegetables, so there's a depth of flavour here that would otherwise be hard to achieve.'

And while this dish is perfect at Christmas time, after one taste you'll definitely find yourself making it more than once a year.

Vegetarian, gluten-free, dairy-free, refined sugar-free

Ingredients

3 tablespoons extra virgin olive oil

1 large onion, finely chopped

2 sticks celery, sliced

2 garlic cloves, finely sliced

200 grams (7 oz) button mushrooms, sliced

1 capsicum, grated

1 large carrot, grated

1 tablespoon smoked paprika

100 grams (3½ oz) red lentils

2 tablespoon tomato paste

1 cup stock of choice

100 grams (3½ oz) breadcrumbs

150 grams (5 oz) hazelnuts

3 large eggs, lightly beaten

100 grams (3½ oz) mature cheddar, grated

Method

Heat the oven to 180°C (350°F) and line a loaf pan with baking paper.

Heat olive oil in a large fry pan and cook onion and celery for 5 or so minutes, until beginning to soften and turn translucent.

Stir in garlic and mushrooms and cook for a further 10 minutes.

Add capsicum and carrot and cook for 3 minutes, then add smoked paprika and cook for another minute.

Stir the lentils and tomato paste to pan and cook for around 1 minute, then add the stock and simmer over a medium heat until all the liquid has been absorbed and the mixture is pretty dry. Set aside to cool.

Place cooled mixture into a bowl and add breadcrumbs, hazelnuts, eggs, cheese and a pinch of salt and pepper to taste.

Stir to combine all the ingredients very well, then spoon the mixture into the loaf tin and press down firmly to evenly compact and smooth the top.

Continued over page.

Cover with foil and bake in the oven for 30 minutes. After 30 minutes, remove the foil and bake for a further 30 minutes until the loaf is quite firm when pressed and is nicely golden on top.

Allow the loaf to cool in the tin for about 10 minutes then turn out onto a serving board or plate to slice. The longer you leave the loaf to cool, the easier it'll be to slice, so you can bake it a day ahead then reheat the next day before serving.

Serves 6-8

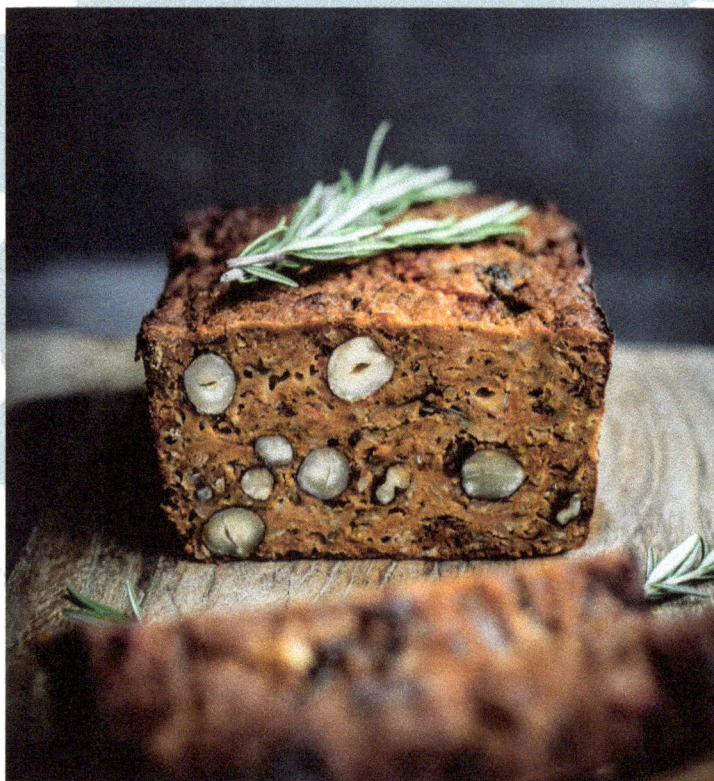

Spiced Quinoa and Lentil Veggie Burger

Phoebe Conway @pheebsfoods

Everyone loves a good veggie burger. And if you don't, you haven't tried this version from Adelaide-based nutritionist Phoebe Conway.

Filled with lentils, quinoa and oats, these patties are so packed with plant-based nutrients, one bite will basically turn you into Superwoman.

So load up your burger with whatever takes your fancy - tomato, cucumber, beetroot (ignore the haters) and get your Superwoman underpants on, because some serious burger business is about to go down.

Vegetarian, gluten-free option, dairy-free option, refined sugar-free

Ingredients

2 teaspoons olive oil

1 x tin brown lentils, drained

1 red onion, finely diced

2 garlic cloves, crushed

1 tablespoon ginger, finely grated

1 teaspoon fish sauce – optional

½ teaspoon cinnamon

½ teaspoon cumin

½ cup oats

1 egg

Juice of 1 lemon

⅓ cup parsley, chopped

½ cup cooked quinoa

4 wholegrain or gluten-free buns (halved), your favourite salad ingredients, natural yoghurt and chilli sauce, to serve

Method

Preheat oven to 200°C (400°F).

Heat 1 teaspoon of the olive oil in a frypan pan over a medium heat. Saute the onion, garlic and ginger until lightly browned. Add spices into pan and cook for a further 1 minute.

Place half of the lentils in a bowl and set aside. In a food processor combine the remaining lentils, cooked onion mixture, egg and oats and blend to combine.

Transfer the mixture from the food processor to the bowl with the other half of the lentils. Add the quinoa, parsley and lemon juice to the bowl and mix well.

Shape the lentil and quinoa mixture into 4 evenly sized patties. You can wet your hands slightly to avoid the mixture sticking too much.

Heat the remaining teaspoon of oil in the same frypan over a medium high heat. Fry each pattie for 3 minutes on each side or until browned. Transfer to a plate.

Place patties into the oven for 10-12 minutes until they have firmed up.

Remove patties from the oven and serve on burger buns with salad, yoghurt and chilli sauce.

Serves 4

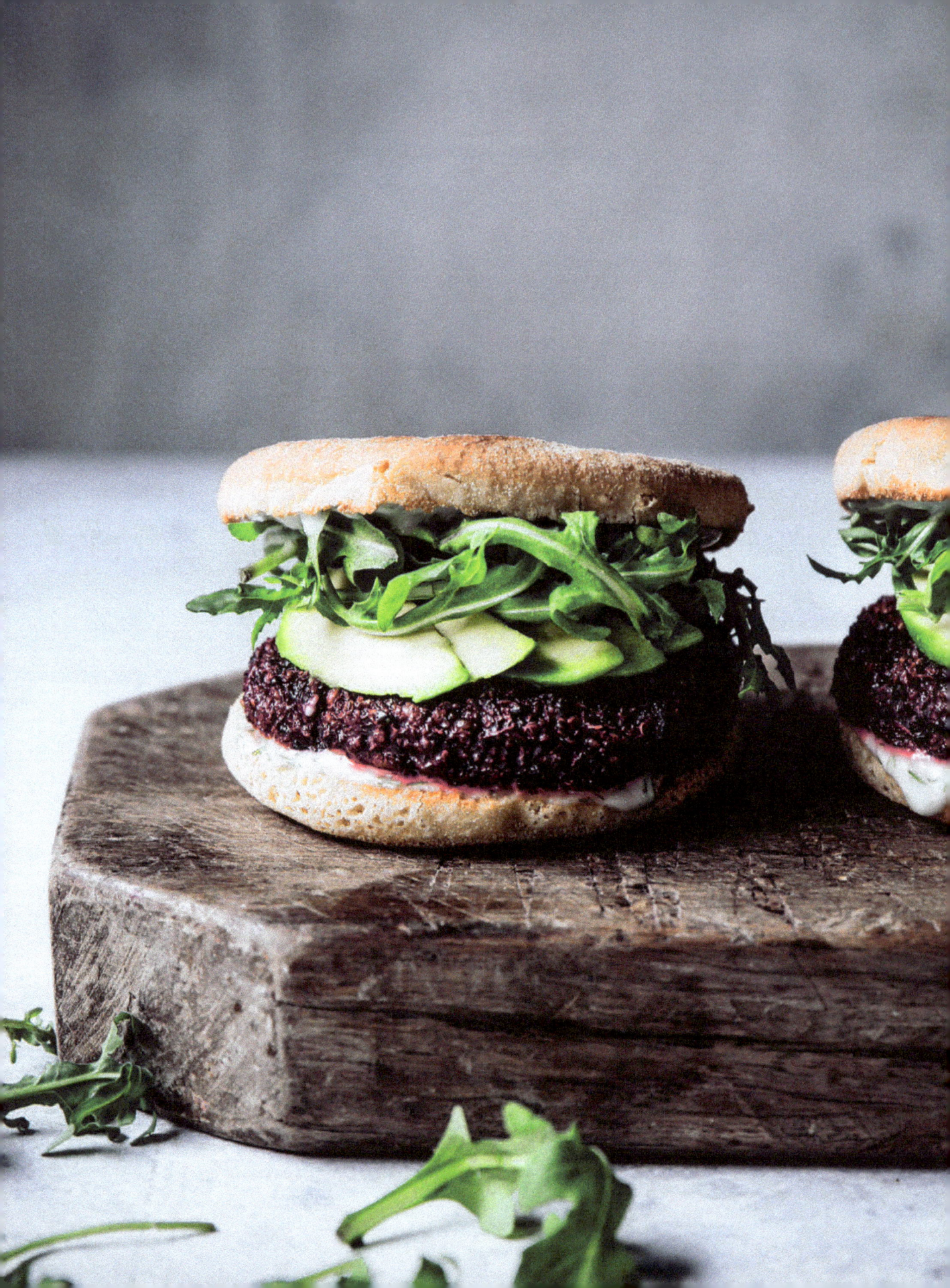

Beetroot & Blackbean Burgers with Herbed Yogurt

Sarah Bell @ournourishingtable

'I'm always experimenting in the kitchen to find ways to make plant-based dishes more appealing to my children,' says nutritionist and mother of three, Sarah Bell. 'This burger has exciting textures and different spices which gives it a meatier flavour that they love.'

If you're looking for a way to enjoy a plant-based burger, then look no further. With sweet beetroot and earthy black beans, these burgers won't just give you an excellent hit of protein and fibre, but also flavour.

If you have kids that are picky with their veggies, get them involved in the process by allowing them to build their own burger with whatever toppings they like. Do this and there won't be anything but smiles at your dinner table.

Vegan option, vegetarian, gluten-free option, dairy-free alternative, refined sugar-free

Ingredients

For the patties

2 cups grated beetroot

1 x 420 grams (15 oz) organic black beans, drained and rinsed

1 cup cooked quinoa

½ teaspoon cumin powder

1 teaspoon smoked paprika

Pinch of sea salt

For the herbed yogurt

½ cup natural yogurt (use coconut if dairy-free)

A small handful of fresh dill, finely chopped

Squeeze of lemon juice

Sea salt

To serve

Burger buns of choice (use gluten free if necessary), sliced in half

1 avocado, sliced

Rocket (arugula) leaves

Method

Preheat oven to 180°C (350°F).

To make the burger patties, add all the pattie ingredients to a food processor and pulse to combine the mixture until it sticks together well.

Divide the mixture into 6 portions and form into burger patties. Place each pattie onto a baking paper-lined oven tray for 25 minutes. Once cooked remove from the oven and set aside.

While patties are cooking, prepare the herbed yogurt. Add the yogurt, dill, lemon juice and salt to a small bowl and mix well to combine.

To make the burgers, spread the herbed yogurt onto the base of each burger bun, top with a beetroot and black bean pattie, sliced avocado and rocket leaves. Serve immediately.

Makes 6 large burger patties

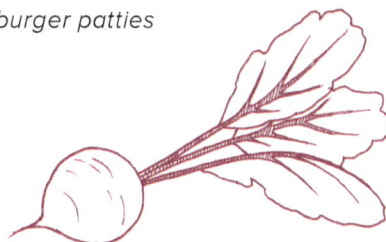

Grilled Mushroom Burger

Jessica Thomson @mindfullyjessica

Mushrooms have become ubiquitous in plant-based cooking for a reason. They're meaty, are a fantastic vehicle to carry flavour and are the perfect shape and size to stuff into a burger. Yup, when God was creating the portabello mushroom he certainly got a lot right.

Biting into this plant-based burger from recipe developer and yoga teacher Jess Thomson is a joy. One mouthful gives you a burst of flavours and textures that'll have you gobbling up every last bite, including licking the juice off your wrists!

Vegan, gluten-free alternative, dairy-free, refined sugar-free

Ingredients

2 large portobello mushrooms

3 tablespoons olive oil

1 tablespoons tamari or soy sauce

1 tablespoons maple syrup

1 teaspoon mixed herbs

To serve:

2 burger buns or rolls, cut in half (use gluten-free if necessary)

Red onion, sliced thinly

tomato, sliced

Kale, lettuce or spinach

Avocado, sliced

Tomato relish, hummus and/ or vegan mayonnaise

Method

In a bowl, mix together the olive oil, tamari or soy sauce, maple syrup and mixed herbs. Coat the mushrooms in this mixture and let them marinate for around 10 minutes.

While mushrooms are marinating, prepare your burger toppings and preheat your grill or grill pan.

If you're using a grill pan, drizzle with a bit of olive oil before adding the mushrooms. Cook the mushrooms on the grill over a medium-high heat for a few minutes before flipping over for an additional 3-5 minutes.

Once the mushrooms are cooked, place them on a paper towel to remove a little bit of the liquid, so they don't make your burger buns soggy.

Spread the halves of the burger buns with desired sauces, and pile the mushrooms along with the other toppings on top. Serve immediately.

Serves 2

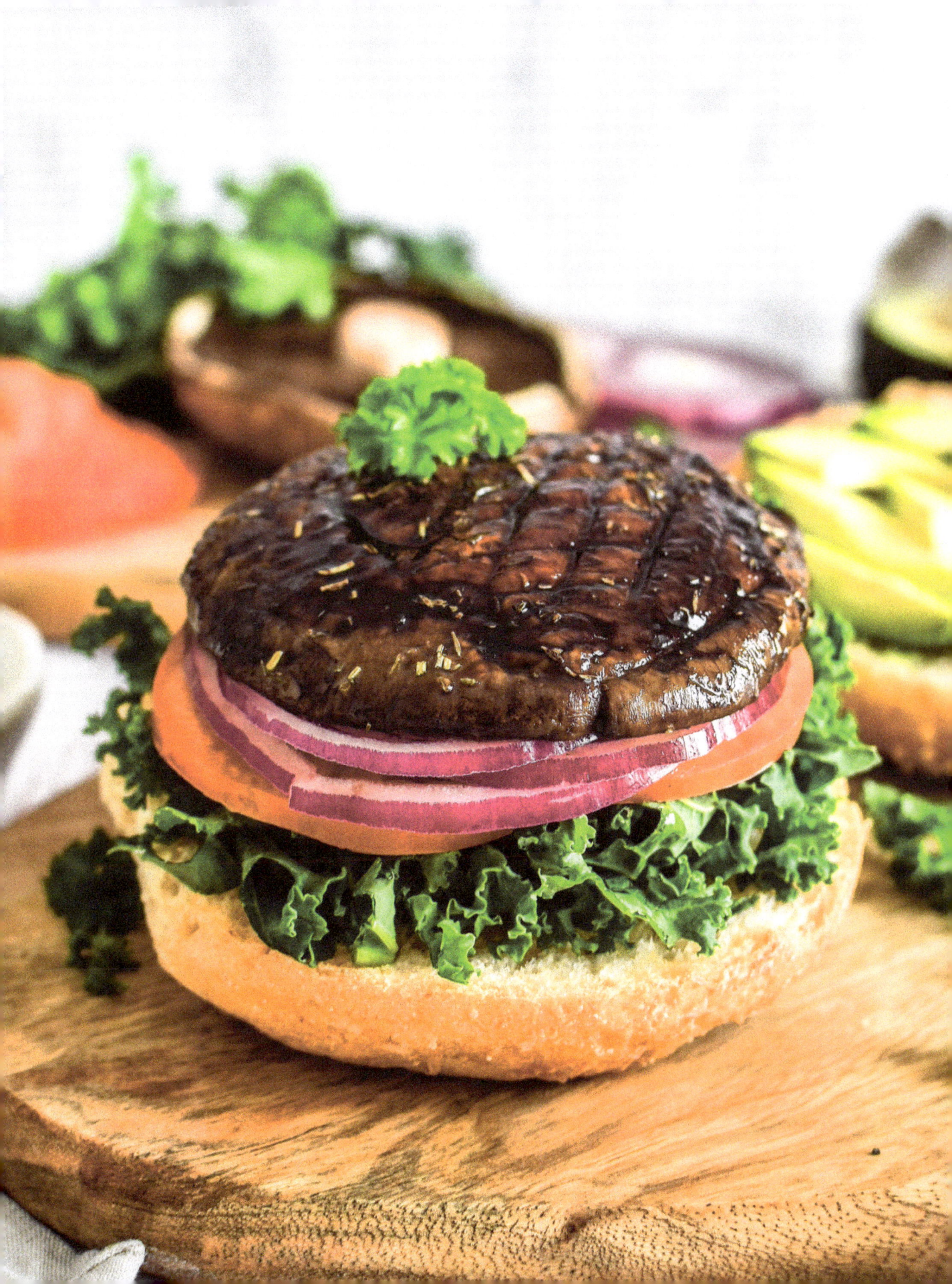

Mushroom Risotto

Melanie Lionello @frommylittlekitchen

10 years ago, nutritionist and recipe developer Melanie Lionello stayed with her Italian family in a picturesque town just outside of Venice. It was here, learning how to make risotto from her aunt, that she realised the incredible power of food.

'When I make this dish, I'm immediately transported back to Italy, chopping mushrooms with the snow falling outside the window,' says Melanie.

'For me, food ecompases so much more than just good, bad, healthy or unhealthy. It has the power to make you feel good beyond just a functional sense. It can make you feel nostalgic, connected, excited and comforted.'

So, if you're feeling a little nostalgic or in need of some comfort on a cold night, we recommend cooking up this creamy, oozy dish that's rich with the umami flavour of mushrooms. We guarantee you'll feel like you're being hugged from the inside out.

Vegan option, gluten-free, dairy-free, refined sugar-free

Ingredients

700 grams (1.8 lbs) portobello or field mushrooms, sliced

1½ - 2 litres chicken or vegetable stock*

2 very generous (Italian-style) slugs of extra virgin olive oil

1 brown onion, finely chopped

3 garlic cloves, minced

2 cups arborio or cannerolo rice

1 cup dry white wine

Salt and pepper to taste.

*You may need a little more or less depending on your cooking technique

Method

Heat one slug of olive oil in a non-stick fry pan over medium-high heat. Add mushrooms and cook until they are browned and beginning to crisp up, turning over every couple of minutes. Remove from the pan and set aside.

Heat the stock in a saucepan over medium heat until almost boiling, then reduce heat to very low, just to keep warm.

In a large heavy-based pot, add the remaining slug of olive oil and add onion and garlic, cook on a medium heat until onions are translucent. Add cooked mushrooms to the pot.

If you have some caramelised, brown bits left on the mushroom pan, you'll want to add this into your risotto, because there's so much flavour there! To do this, simply add a little stock to the fry pan pan to deglaze it, then pour it back into your stock pot.

Add the rice to the pot with the onions and mushrooms and cook on a low heat for 2 to 3 minutes until the ends of the grains of rice are beginning to look translucent.

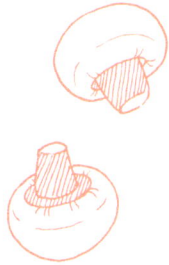

Add the wine and cook until it has evaporated, around 2 minutes.

Add 1 ladleful of stock to the rice and gently stir until stock is absorbed. You'll want to stir pretty consistently, which is tedious but so worth the effort. (Here, Melanie recommend getting a glass of wine and chatting with whoever is home about your day while you do this).

Continue adding the stock into the rice ladle by ladle and letting it cook away until the rice is tender with just a slight bite, like 'al dente' pasta.

Season with salt and pepper to taste then pour into bowls and serve with parmesan cheese. Buon Appetito!

Serves 4

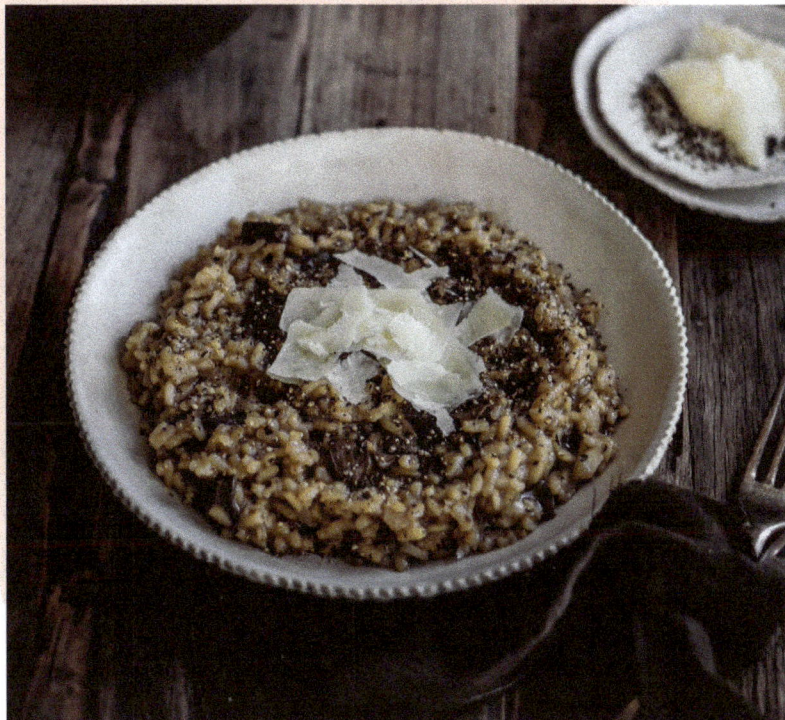

Creamy Carbonara

Courtenay Perks @wholeremedy

Whenever Courtenay's parents took her out for Italian when she was little, she vividly remembers always ordering the carbonara - a token comfort food for many of us.

Now a recipe developer, health coach and yoga teacher, Courtenay found herself nostalgic for the creamy, comforting bowls of carbonara from her youth, so she tasked herself with creating this vegan, nutrient-dense alternative.

The coconut yogurt and Japanese pumpkin give this dish a rich, creamy texture, while the addition of sage takes this humble bowl of pasta to the next level, giving it a depth of flavour that will make you look super chef-y to all your friends and family.

Vegan, dairy-free, refined sugar-free

Ingredients

1 small Japanese pumpkin skinned and diced into 1cm (4") dice

2 tablespoons cold pressed organic olive oil

1 onion, diced

2 garlic cloves, finely sliced

1 handful sage leaves

2 cups almond milk

¼ cup natural coconut yoghurt

1 tablespoon savoury yeast flakes

¼ teaspoon red chilli flakes (optional)

Cracked Himalayan sea salt and pepper

300 grams (11 oz) rigatoni pasta

Method

In a deep saucepan set over a medium-high heat, sauté sage in olive oil until crispy. Remove and set aside.

Keeping the saucepan over the heat, add the onion and garlic and sauté until soft and golden, around 3-4 minutes. Add pumpkin and almond milk to the pan and simmer uncovered for 30 minutes until the pumpkin is soft. Add chilli flakes, cracked pepper and Himalayan sea salt.

Cook rigatoni pasta following instructions. Drain and set aside in a saucepan.

Transfer pumpkin mixture to a blender or use a stick blender to purée until smooth. Add coconut yogurt and savoury yeast flakes and blend to combine well.

Stir the sauce through the pasta over low to medium heat until well combined and heated through.

Serve topped with crispy sage leaves, cracked pepper and salt. This is also delicious with a sprinkle of cashew parmesan cheeze if you have some on hand!

Serves 4

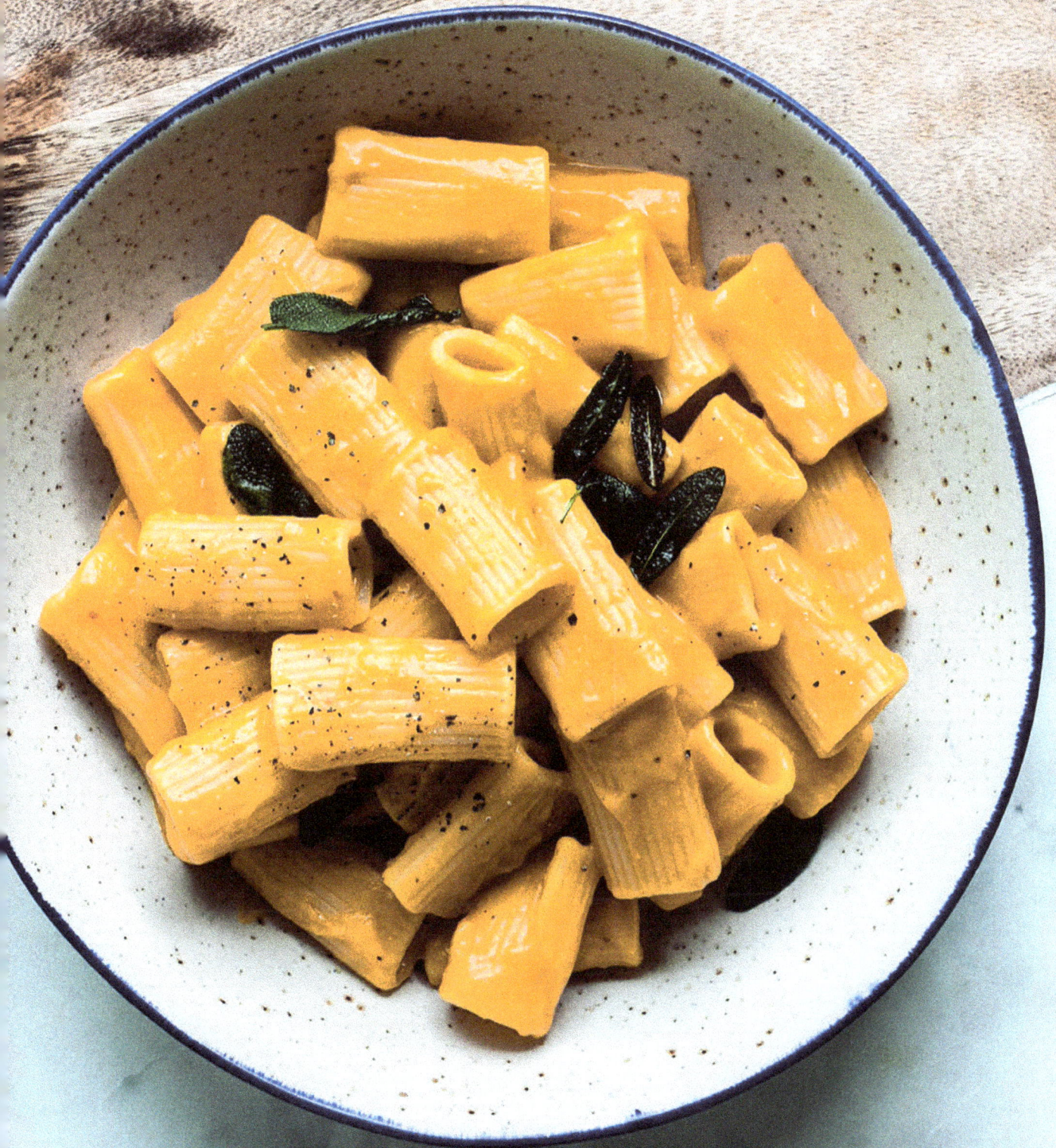

Spaghetti Bolognese with Lentil & Walnut Meatballs

Talida Voinea @Hazel_and_cacao

This recipe packs an incredible nutritional punch, with heaps of vegetables as well as legumes and wholegrains. And while it might not be quite like nonna used to make, damn it tastes just as good!

Talida recommends making this dish for anyone who might be hesitant about trying more plant-based foods. Her husband, a big meat lover, actually had a dream about this dish. Yes, really.

Vegan, gluten-free option, dairy-free, refined sugar-free

Ingredients

300 grams (11 oz) of wholewheat spaghetti (use buckwheat or quinoa pasta for a gluten-free alternative)

For the vegan meatballs

1 x 400 gram (14 oz) tin brown lentils, drained and rinsed

½ cup rolled oats

¼ cup walnuts

¼ teaspoon garlic powder

½ teaspoon mixed herbs

2 tablespoons tamari

2 tablespoons barbeque sauce

2 tablespoons bread crumbs

For Bolognese sauce

10 button mushrooms

1 large carrot, diced

1 zucchini, diced

3 celery sticks, diced

1 tablespoon extra virgin olive oil

1 brown onion, diced

Method

Preheat your oven to 180°C (350°F).

Begin by making the vegan meatballs. Add walnuts and oats to a food processor and blend until a fine crumble forms.

Add drained lentils and remaining spices, barbecue sauce and breadcrumbs to the food processor and blend until combined. The mixture should be sticky. Add some water if the mixture is too dry, one tablespoon at a time.

Roll mixture into meatball-sized balls. Place balls onto an oven tray lined with baking paper and into the oven for 20-25 minutes.

Meanwhile, cook pasta according to packet instructions. For the Bolognese sauce, in a food processor, process mushrooms until fine. Attach the grater attachment and process the carrot, zucchini, and celery and set aside. If you don't want to use a food processor for this step, simply finely dice the vegetables.

In a saucepan over a medium heat, fry the diced onion in olive oil. Once lightly browned (3-4 minutes), add crushed garlic ensuring not to burn.

Add the chopped mushrooms, zucchini, carrot and celery to the pan and cook until soft. The vegetables will release their water and you should continue cooking until the water has evaporated.

1-2 cloves garlic, crushed

1 cup organic tomato passata (pure tomato sauce/puree)

Himalayan salt and pepper to taste

½ teaspoon paprika

2 teaspoons Italian herbs

1 teaspoon maple syrup (optional)

Additional fresh herbs of choice and vegan parmesan, to serve (optional)

Add tomato passata sauce and tomato paste and mix well. Reduce heat and allow to simmer, covered, for about 20 minutes or more. The longer it cooks, the more flavour it'll have, but you still want it to be saucy.

Add salt and pepper to taste, paprika, Italian herbs and cook for a few more minutes. Add in maple syrup (if using) and stir well.

Portion spaghetti into bowls and top with Bolognese sauce. Top with vegan meatballs and garnish with additional herbs and vegan parmesan, if you like.

Serves 4

Use as many meatballs as you like for the Bolognese, the rest can be frozen and used in different dishes!

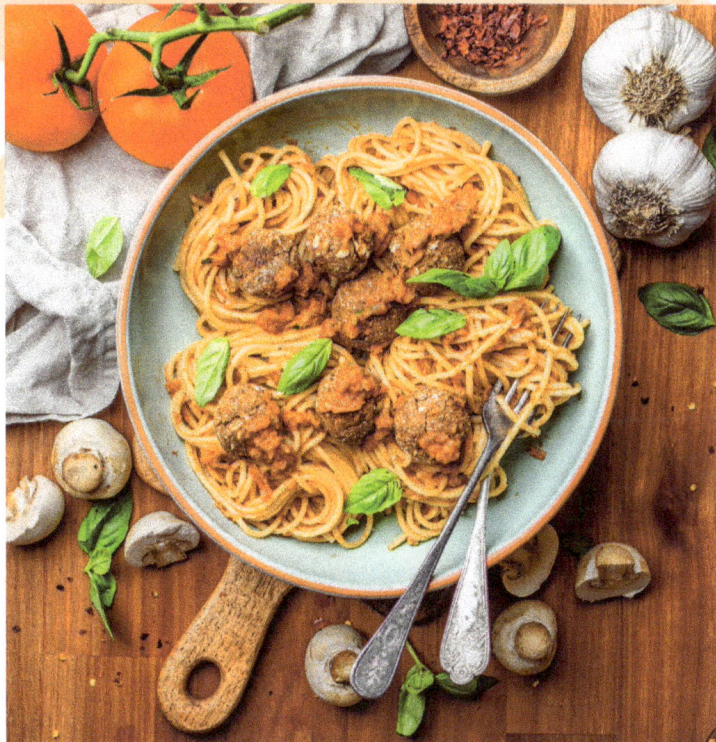

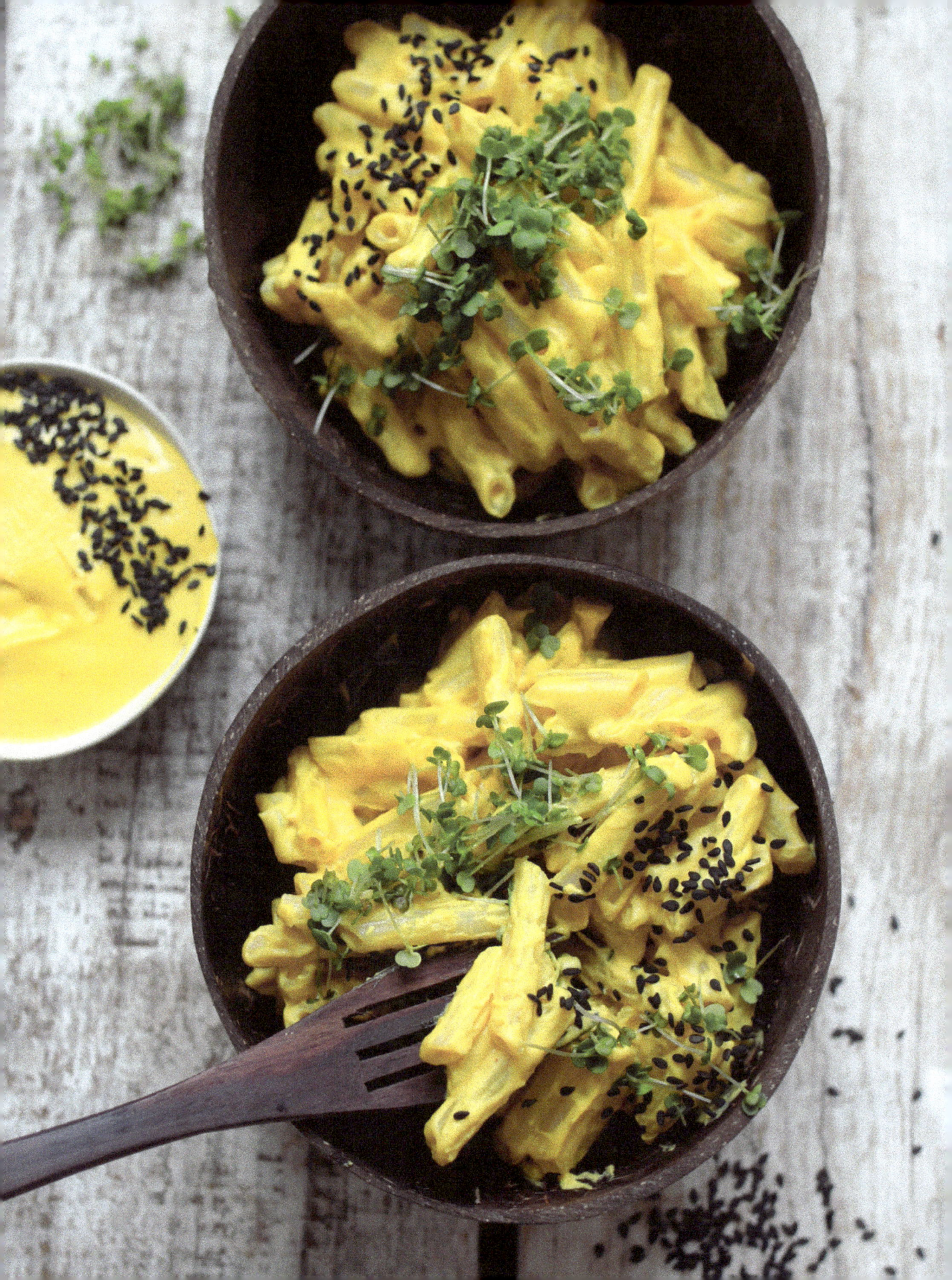

Vegan Mac & Cheese

Jen Murrant & Hannah Singleton @healthyluxe

This rich and creamy mac and cheese is just like the real deal, but somehow, miraculously, contains no dairy, gluten or unnecessary additives. The combination of cashews and pumpkin creates the soft, creamy texture, while nutritional yeast adds the cheesy taste and is also high in vitamin B12.

'This dish is lovely and indulgent, but because we don't use dairy and we choose a gluten-free pasta it won't leave you with a heavy, weighed down feeling,' says nutritionist Jen Murrant from Healthy Luxe. 'Quite a lot of people find themselves deficient in vitamin B12, which is crucial for blood formation and neurological function, so it's something we should all try to eat more of!'

Vegan, gluten-free, dairy-free, refined sugar-free

Ingredients

1 tablespoon coconut oil

1 small brown onion, finely chopped

150 grams (5 oz) pumpkin, roughly chopped

¼ cup water (+ additional ¼ cup)

1 cup cashews (soaked for 2-3 hours)

1 tablespoon nutritional yeast

2 tablespoon lemon juice

1 teaspoon turmeric

¼ teaspoon paprika

1 teaspoon Dijon mustard

½ tablespoon coconut oil

1 pinch salt and pepper

3 cups pasta (we use gluten free amaranth/rice pasta)

Method

In a fry pan over a medium heat braise the onion in 1 tablespoon of coconut oil for around 5 minutes.

Add pumpkin and ¼ cup water to the pan and cook for 10 minutes, or until soft.

Add remaining water to the pan if it gets too dry to stop the pumpkin from sticking.

Meanwhile, cook the pasta as per packet instructions.

Place the cooked pumpkin mixture and all the other ingredients (except pasta) in a high speed blender and blend until smooth and creamy*. That's your "cheese" sauce done!

Tip your pasta into serving bowls and mix through your sauce. Garnish with sprouts.

* The mixture will be hot and does not need to be reheated (unless pumpkin was pre-cooked and allowed to cool).

Serves 4

Basa & Cashew Stir Fry

Sally O'Neil @thefitfoodieblog

When Sally O'Neil first moved to Australia from the UK she admits her diet was far from healthy, having spent most of her student life living off chocolate and microwave meals.

When she moved to Sydney she realised she'd have to learn to cook for herself (boiling an egg was first) and that's when her passion for creating nutritious, soul-satisfying recipes began. This tasty and incredibly easy stir fry pays homage to those first years in Australia, when she was looking for uncomplicated yet nourishing dishes to fuel her busy life.

Gluten-free option, dairy-free, refined sugar-free

Ingredients

2 teaspoons sesame oil

130 grams (4½ oz) basa fillet

¼ cup cashews

2 bok choi, leaves separated

½ fresh red chilli, sliced, plus extra to garnish

½ lemon

½ tablespoon tamari or soy sauce

Black sesame seeds, to garnish

Method

Set a fry pan or wok over a medium heat and add 1 teaspoon of the sesame oil. Add the basa fillet, cooking for 5-8 minutes until cooked through. Remove the fish from the pan and set aside.

Keep the fry pan over the heat and add the remaining teaspoon of sesame oil, bok choi, red chilli and cashews. Sautee these for 3-5 minutes, or until the greens have started to wilt but still have some bite to them.

Squeeze the lemon juice into the pan and add the soy sauce, then toss it all together and remove from the heat. Add the greens to a bowl and top with the basa fillet. Finish with a sprinkle of black sesame seeds and fresh chilli.

Serves 1

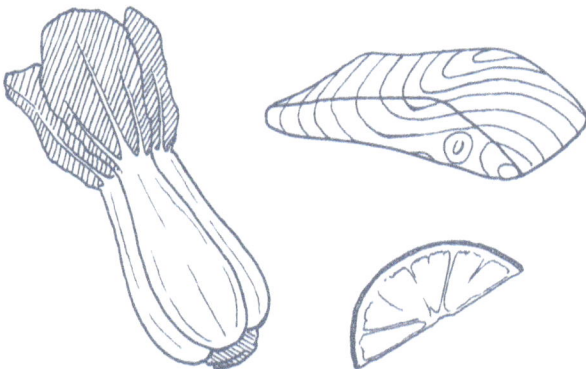

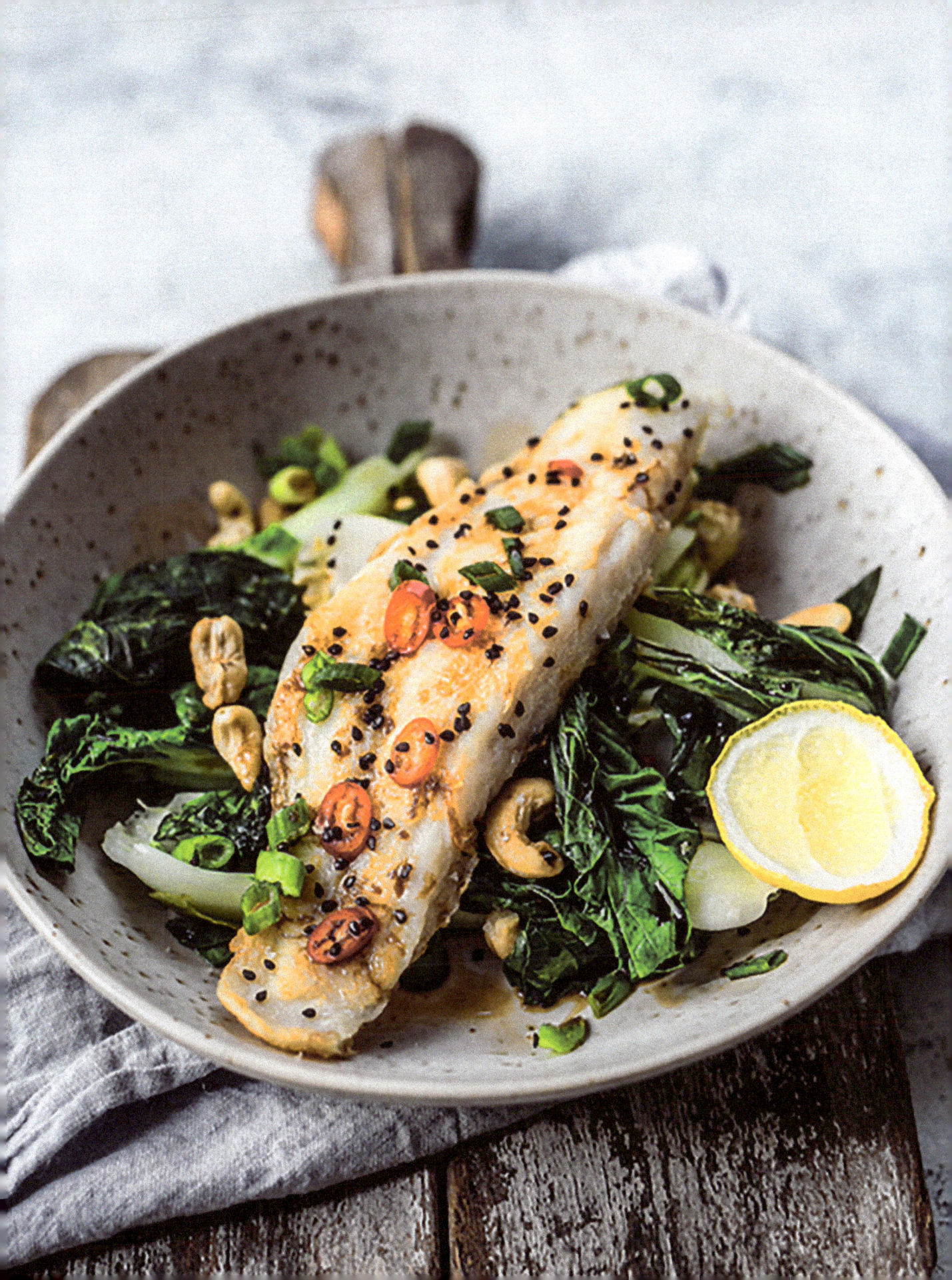

Crispy Skin Salmon with Mashed Sweet Potato & Greens

Sarah Bell @ournourishingtable

There's something incredibly comforting about having a go-to dish. No matter how little time you have or how few ingredients you have in your fridge, you can always manage to cobble it together when you're in a pinch.

This crispy skin salmon dish is one such go-to meal for recipe developer and food photographer Sarah Bell. She affectionately refers to this as her "fish and three veg" dinner, and is her fall back when she needs to get a nutritious meal on the table for her and her family.

'This is the easiest thing to make and is a staple in my house,' says the Brisbane-based nutritionist. 'You know you're getting a healthy dose of vegetables, high quality protein and a good source of fibre and quality carbohydrates.'

Sarah serves her salmon with sweet potato mash (her daughters' favourite), kale, broccoli and green beans, but she suggests using whatever veggies you have on hand in your fridge.

Gluten-free, dairy-free option, refined sugar-free

Ingredients

4 x Atlantic salmon fillets

Extra virgin olive oil

Salt and pepper, to season

500 grams (1 lb) sweet potato, skin removed and diced

1 tablespoon butter (or vegan butter)

¼ cup plant-based milk of choice

Small handful of fresh dill, roughly chopped

Method

Remove salmon fillets from the fridge at least 15 minutes before cooking.

Place sweet potato in a saucepan of a double boiler. Top with water and place steamer on top. Cover with lid and bring to a boil. Alternatively, steam sweet potato using your preferred method.

While the sweet potato is boiling, drizzle a generous amount of olive oil in a large frypan and bring to a medium-high heat. Once the pan is hot, add the salmon fillets to the pan, skin side down. Make sure to leave at least a couple of centimeters between each fillet. Season fillets with salt and pepper.

6-7 kale leaves, stems removed and roughly chopped

1 large head of broccoli

Handful of green beans, topped and tailed

The colour of the salmon will start to change to deep pink while cooking. Once the salmon is light pink to around ¾ of the way up the fillet, it's time to flip it onto the other side. Pro-tip: use a metal egg-flip to help prevent the skin from sticking to the pan.

At the time of flipping the salmon, place the broccoli, beans and kale into the steamer with the sweet potato and replace the lid.

Cook both the salmon and greens for a further 2-3 minutes. Once the salmon is cooked to your liking, turn off the heat and allow to rest. Once the greens are cooked through, but still bright green, remove them from the steamer and set aside.

Strain the sweet potato and return to the pan. Add the butter and milk to the pan and mash with the sweet potato with a potato masher until creamy and smooth. Add dill and season with salt and pepper, stirring to combine.

To serve, divide the potato mash between each serving plate and place a salmon fillet on top. Then divide green amongst the plates and serve immediately.

Serves 4

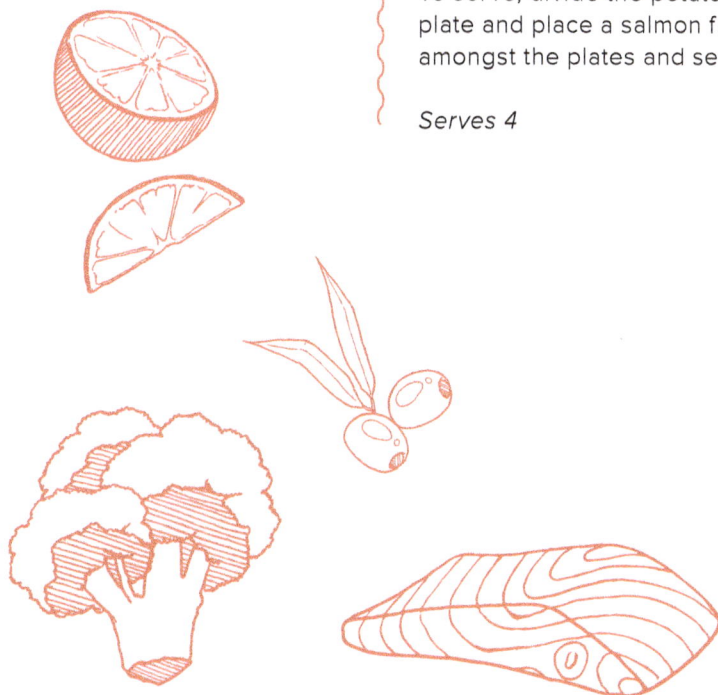

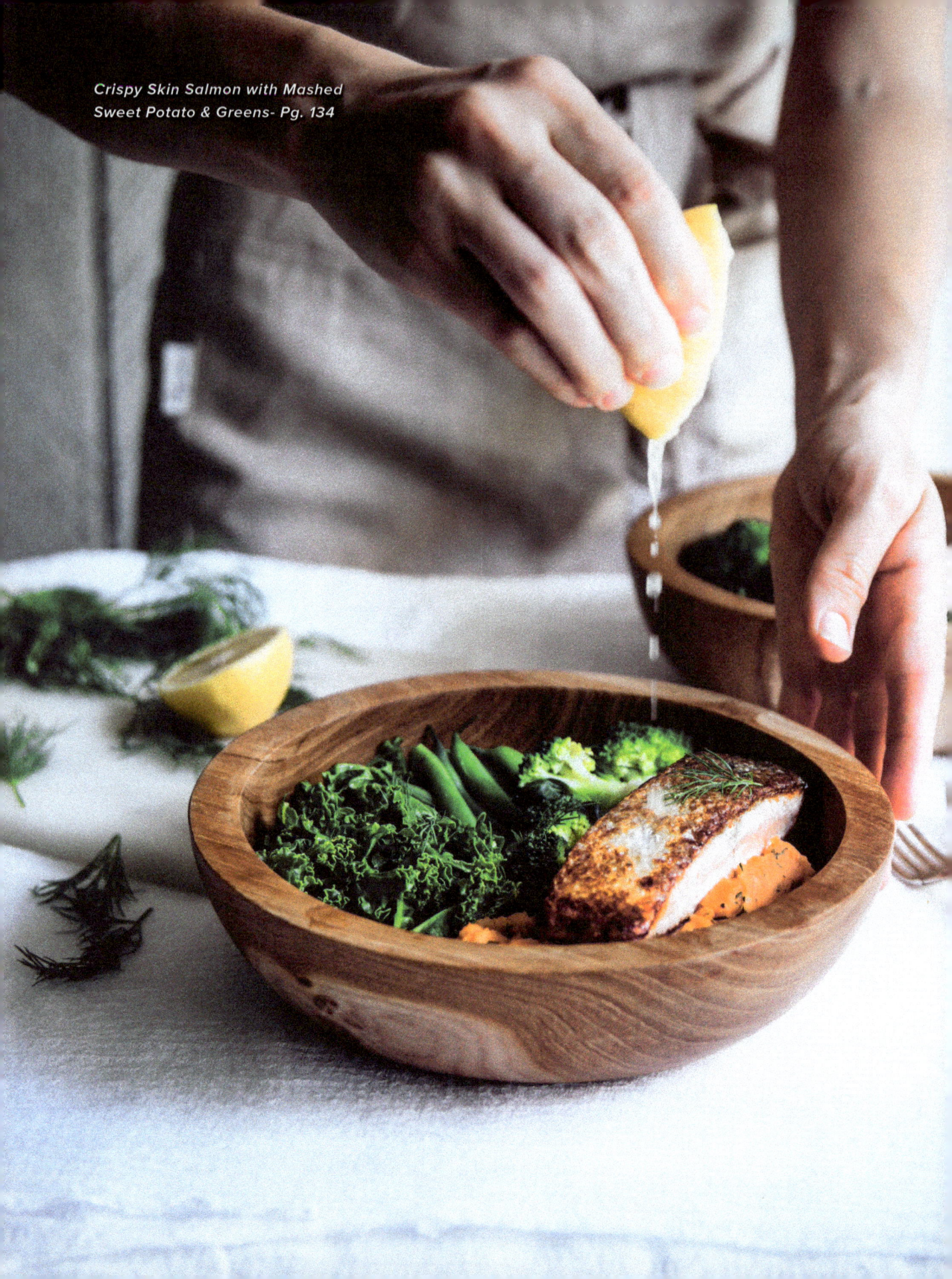

Crispy Skin Salmon with Mashed Sweet Potato & Greens- Pg. 134

Tasty Lamb Meatballs

Nadia Felsch @nadiafelsch

Growing up, Sydney nutritionist Nadia Felsch loved watching her Hungarian grandmother, or Nagymama, cook for her and her family. She believes it was here that her passion for food and cooking began.

While this hearty dish is slanted towards Greek cuisine, Nadia says it's nourishing, nostalgic food that reminds her of her Nagymama's cooking - with extra veggies thrown in for good measure!

'I'm actually a bit fussy when it comes to food, so I add in vegetables wherever I can,' Nadia laughs. 'The carrot adds sweetness and interest to the meatballs, and the almond meal also gives them a lovely nutty flavour. My favourite way to eat these meatballs is in a rice or quinoa bowl with roast veggies. Then I top it with greek yogurt, feta and tomato for freshness.'

Gluten-free, dairy-free, refined sugar-free

Ingredients

400 grams (14 oz) lamb mince

¼ heaped cup carrot, grated

1 small garlic clove, crushed

2 tablespoons red onion, finely diced

2 tablespoons mint leaves, finely chopped

2 tablespoons coriander leaves, finely chopped

3 tablespoons almond meal

Salt and pepper, to taste

2 tablespoons extra virgin olive oil, to cook

Method

Add all ingredients, except the oil, together in a mixing bowl and use your hands to mix it together well.

Roll the mince mixture into small balls using 1-2 tablespoons-worth of mixture per ball. Wet your hands slightly if the mixture starts to stick to them.

Heat the oil in a large frying pan on medium-high heat and once hot, add the meatballs to the pan. Use a spoon to turn the meatballs carefully and once firmer, you can shake the pan. Cook for 10 minutes or until browned on the outside and cooked through.

Remove the meatballs from the hot pan and drain on paper towel before adding to a rice or quinoa bowl and topping with your favourite toppings.

Makes 21 small meatballs

Enjoy alone or make a meal of these meatballs by adding to a quinoa or rice bowl with cherry tomatoes, cucumber, fetta, mixed leaves, avocado and a simple yoghurt and lime dressing.

Ridiculously Good Moong Dal Tadka

Sasha Back @earthlingsasha

It's easy to get into a cooking rut when you're stressed out and busy, which is exactly where Sydney-based food blogger Sasha found herself while in the throws of studying.

'I knew I needed to branch out and get creative in the kitchen again, so I used a recipe I'd seen in a magazine and worked out a way to make it vegan,' she explains. 'Moong Dal Tadka normally has quite subtle flavours, so I created a temper to really enhance these so you're left with something really delicious and wholesome.'

Vegan, gluten-free, dairy-free, refined sugar-free

Ingredients

¾ cup moong dal (split yellow lentils), washed and rinsed well

3 cups water

½ teaspoon ground turmeric

1 teaspoon salt

Crispy kale chips to top (optional)

For tempering

1 tablespoon coconut oil or vegan ghee

1 teaspoon ginger, finely chopped

2 garlic cloves, finely chopped

1 teaspoon cumin seeds

½ teaspoon chilli powder

1 small onion, finely chopped

1 medium tomato, chopped

½ teaspoon garam masala

1-2 lime leaves (can substitute for curry leaves)

Method

Add the lentils, water, turmeric and salt to a pot and bring this to a boil. Lower the heat and simmer for 20-30 minutes or until the lentils have broken down considerably and the mixture has thickened.

If you prefer your dal to be a smoother consistency you can use a stick blender to puree lentils, however the mixture is nice with a little bit of texture. This can be achieved by just allowing the lentils to naturally break down.

Meanwhile, in a small pan, heat coconut oil or vegan ghee. Add the ginger, garlic and cumin seeds and fry until aromatic - around 30 seconds.

Add the onion, tomato ground cumin, garam masala, chilli powder and lime leaf to the spices and cook until onions are transparent and tomatoes have broken down. Be careful here not to burn the spices.

Once the dal is cooked, add the tempered mixture into the dal and stir well to combine.

Serve the dal over hot rice and top with kale chips

Serves 2-4

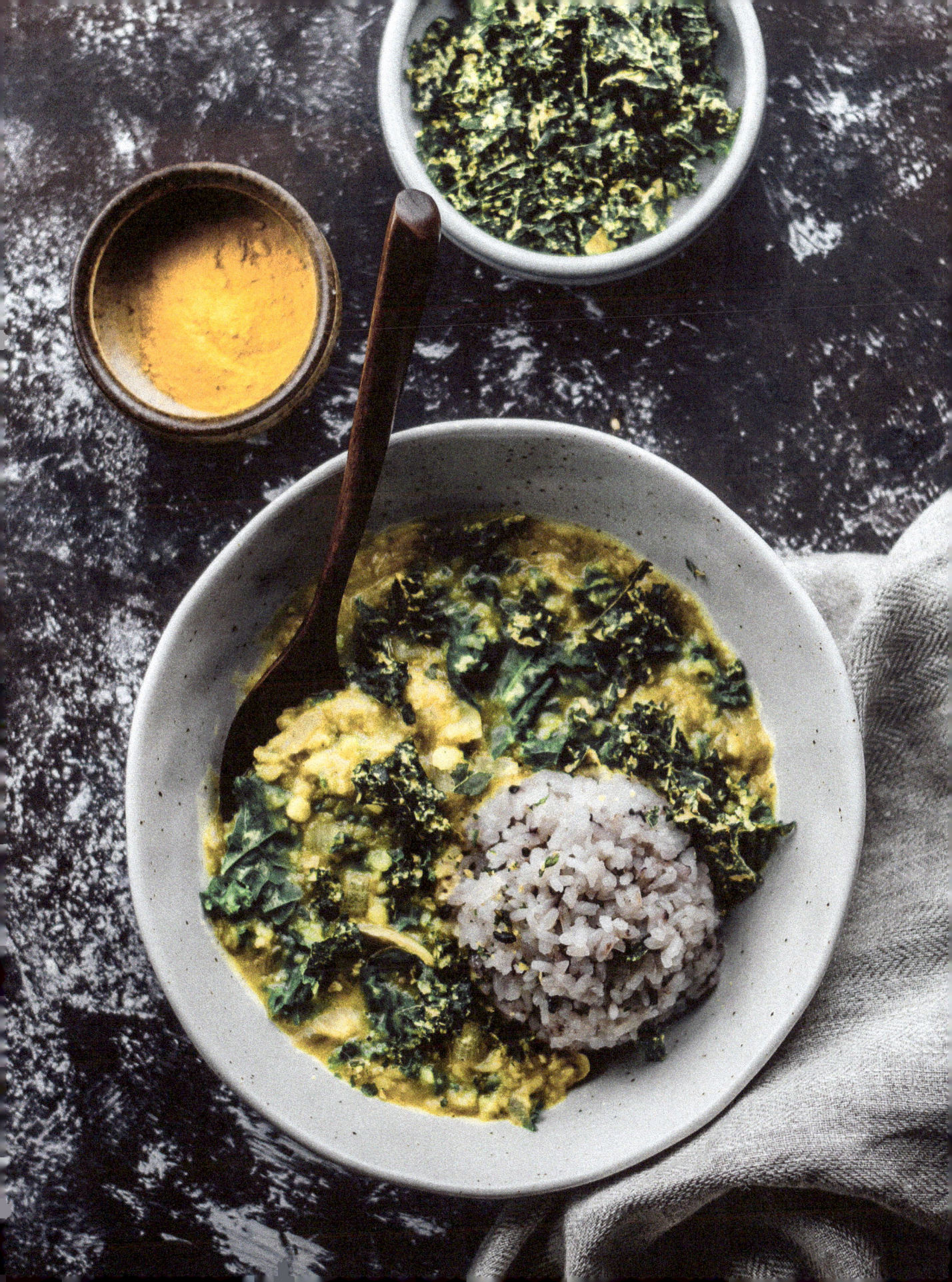

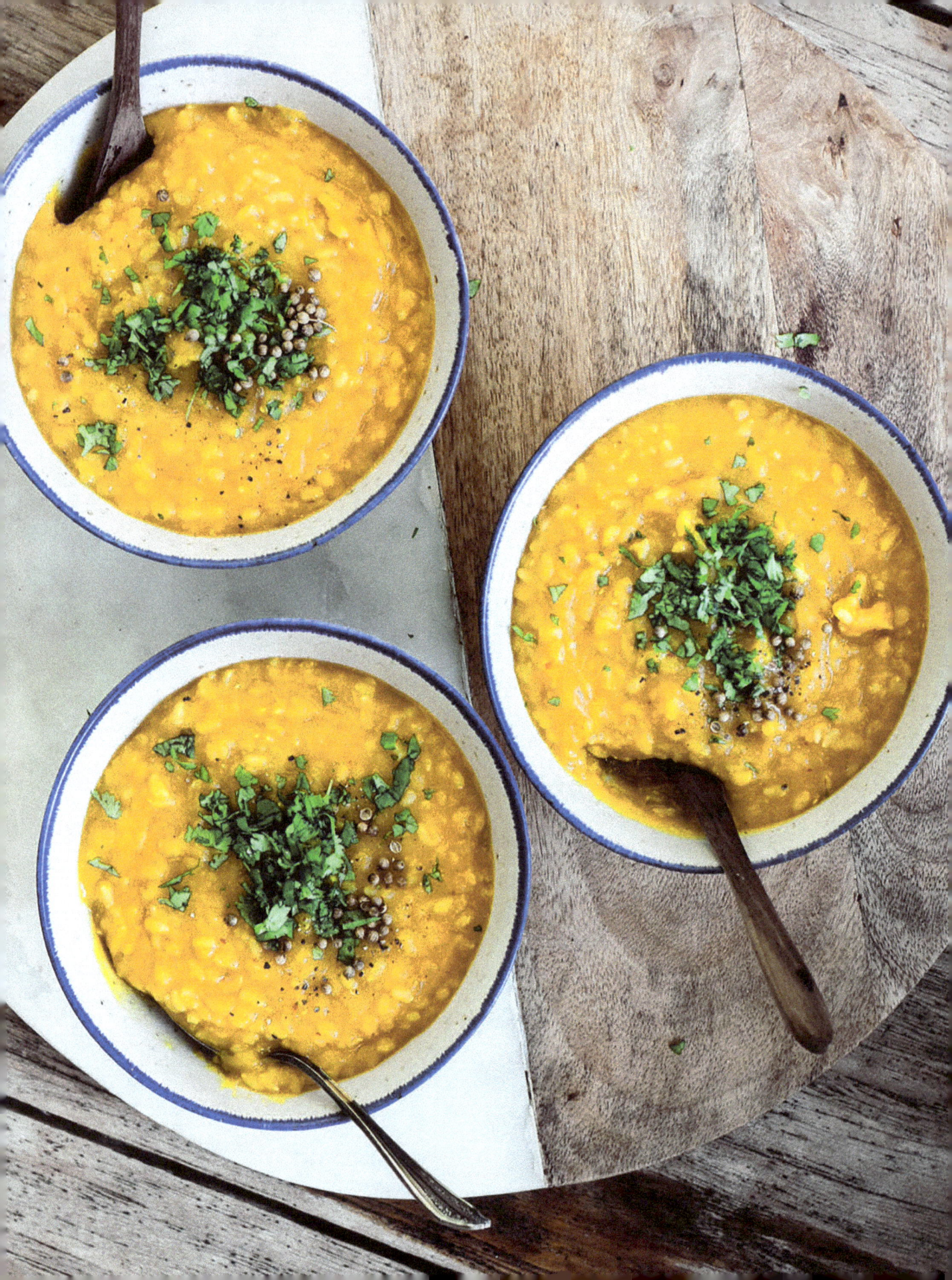

Ayurvedic Kitchari

Courtenay Perks @wholeremedy

While difficult to encapsulate the principles of an Ayurvedic diet in a few sentences, we'll try our best. Ayurvedic is basically a health modality that is based on the belief that health and wellness depend on a delicate balance between the mind, body, and spirit.

It is a way of eating that yoga teacher and vegan recipe developer Courtenay Perks thrives on, allowing her to balance out her "flighty" Vata tendencies with the more grounding elements of Kapha foods (see note).

'Kitchari is the traditional cleansing food of Ayurveda, and provides a grounding dinner filled with nourishing ingredients that come from the earth,' explains Courtenay. 'This dish is easy to digest, allowing your body to put its energy towards recovery and rest, rather than adding stress to the digestive system.'

Vegan, gluten-free, dairy-free, refined sugar-free

Ingredients

1 large organic pumpkin, skinned and diced in 1cm (½") dice

1½ teaspoons coconut oil

1 thumb-size piece of fresh ginger, skinned and grated

1 teaspoon ground cumin

1 teaspoon ground coriander

1 cup organic brown rice

½ cup red lentils

8 cups filtered water combined with 2 tablespoons low-sodium vegetable bouillon powder

1 teaspoon ground turmeric

½ teaspoon ground Himalayan sea salt

Cracked black pepper

Finely chopped organic fresh coriander (cilantro)

Method

Steam pumpkin using your preferred method until completely soft. Place pumpkin in a food processor and purée until smooth.

Add coconut oil to a large, deep saucepan. Add the ginger, cumin, ground coriander and sauté for 1-2 minutes.

Add rice and lentils to the pot and stir to ensure the spices are mixed through. Add the bouillon water and simmer uncovered for 30 minutes.

Stir the pumpkin puree, turmeric, and sea salt into the saucepan and allow the flavours to combine for 3 minutes.

Serve warm with cracked black pepper and coriander.

Serves 4

Vata and Kapha are two of the three 'doshas', which Ayurvedic medicine believes are biological energies found throughout the human body and mind.

Nourishing Chicken & Tumeric Curry

Leanne Ward @the_fitness_dietitian

When Sydney dietitian Leanne Ward spoke to clients in her Love Living Lean program, she realised many of them thought a healthy diet consisted of two things; limp salad, or the exceedingly boring meal of chicken, rice and broccoli.

This led her to create this nourishing chicken curry, to prove that healthy food can still be hearty and satiating.

'Many people think that healthy eating means they have to miss out on the comforting meals they used to love, but that's just not true,' says Leanne.

'Takeaway curries are often laden with excess fat and contain hardly any vegetables, so I wanted to make something that was worlds away from that, but that still tasted amazing.'

This dish is perfect for leftovers or you can portion it into individual containers and freeze it for quick midweek dinners!

Vegan option, gluten-free, dairy-free, refined sugar-free

Ingredients

300 grams (11 oz) raw chicken

100 grams (3½ oz) raw brown rice (250g cooked)

2 tablespoons extra virgin olive oil

3 tablespoons curry powder

3 teaspoons turmeric powder

2 x 400 millilitre (13½ fl oz) cans of light coconut milk

Chilli flakes (optional)

2 large carrots, diced

2 large zucchini, diced

Method

Heat a large fry pan over a medium heat and add 1 tablespoon of oil. Add the onion, 1 tablespoon of curry powder and 1 teaspoon of turmeric and stir for a few minutes until fragrant and the onion is translucent.

Add the chicken and 1 can of coconut milk. Bring to a simmer and allow the chicken to cook for 15-20 minutes. Once cooked through, remove pan from heat and put to the side.

Meanwhile, cook the rice according to the packet instructions.

Next, heat a large clean fry pan over medium heat and add the rest of the oil, turmeric and curry powder. Add the chilli flakes here if you like it spicy! Stir the spices until fragrant.

½ (300 grams/11 oz) small cauliflower, chopped into medium-sized florets

½ (300 grams/11 oz) small broccoli, chopped into medium-sized florets

8 medium button mushrooms, diced

250 grams (8½ oz) green beans, diced

1 medium brown onion, diced

Add all the chopped veggies to your pan and stir to combine, allowing to soak up the flavours of the spices for a 2 minutes.

Pour the second can of coconut milk over the veggies and allow the milk to come to a simmer. Turn the heat to low, put a lid on the fry pan and allow the veggies to cook in the coconut milk until they are cooked through, approximately 10 minutes.

Once cooked to your liking, remove the pan from the heat. Divide the chicken and rice into 4 portions and add ¼ of the veggies to each portion. Stir and enjoy!

Serves 4

To make this dish vegan, simply substitute the chicken for firm tofu.

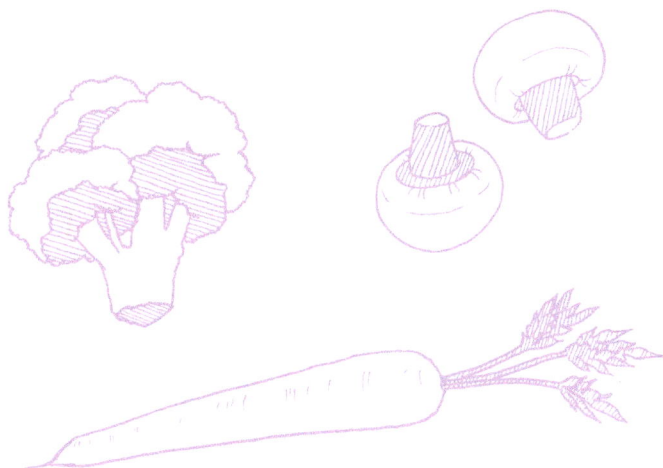

Vegan Jackfruit Ragu

Kitch Catterall @soybabie_

If you live in or have ever visited Melbourne, hopefully you've been lucky enough to visit one of the city's most renowned vegan restaurants, Smith & Daughters. If not, then go there ASAP. It was here that vegan food blogger Kitch Catterall tried a mushroom-based ragu that made her determined to create her own version at home.

'After eating the ragu at Smith & Daughters I really started to crave the warm, hearty flavours of osso bucco, so I started thinking about how I could create an easier version of the dish at home,' Kitch says.

The result was this jackfruit ragu, which contains all the rich, deep flavours Kitch was hoping to capture.

Kitch says you can pick up tinned jackfruit in brine or springwater from Asian grocers for a couple of bucks. 'It does look a bit anemic when you take it out of the tin,' she laughs. 'But once you pan fry it and add your spices it tastes like the real deal!'

Vegan, dairy-free, refined sugar-free option

Ingredients

1 onion, diced

2 x cans of jackfruit in brine (drained)

Olive oil

3 garlic cloves, finely diced

1 teaspoon paprika

1 teaspoon garlic powder

½ teaspoon cayenne pepper (optional, for spice)

1 teaspoon thyme

⅓ cup red wine

Worcester sauce, to taste

½ tablespoon soy sauce

BBQ Sauce, to taste (optional)

Method

Add a splash of olive oil to a large pan set over medium heat. Cook the onion and jackfruit until it's slightly browned. Add paprika, cayenne pepper, garlic powder to the pan and continue to pan fry for 3 minutes.

Add Worcester sauce to taste, soy sauce and the red wine and reduce the heat under the pan.

Add the water and pink salt to the pan and then cover and allow the mixture to reduce for 15 minutes.

Depending on how saucy you want your ragu, you can add some more water, red wine and Worcester sauce at this point, along with the chopped garlic.

Add a squeeze of BBQ sauce and coconut sugar here if using, this will make it nice and sticky and a little sweet.

Stir and cover again for another 10 minutes.
Once the jackfruit has become tender, you can start pulling it apart in the pan with a fork.

2 teaspoons coconut sugar (optional)

3 tablespoons tomato paste

Black pepper

Pink salt

Water

1 teaspoon dried sage

Favourite kind of pasta or soft polenta, to serve

Nutritional yeast and fresh basil, to serve

Add tomato paste, 1 cup of water, another splash of wine, thyme, sage and pepper to the pan and stir together.

Cover the pan, reduce the heat to a simmer and allow the mixture to cook until it's a thick, rich ragu! The longer you leave it, the better the flavour becomes.

Meanwhile, cook pasta according to packet instructions. Once cooked, stir through a little vegan butter and place into serving bowls.

Taste your ragyu and add any last minute touches as per your tastes.

Pour ragu over the top of your pasta and serve with a sprinkle of nutritional yeast, cracked pepper and fresh basil.

Serves 4-6

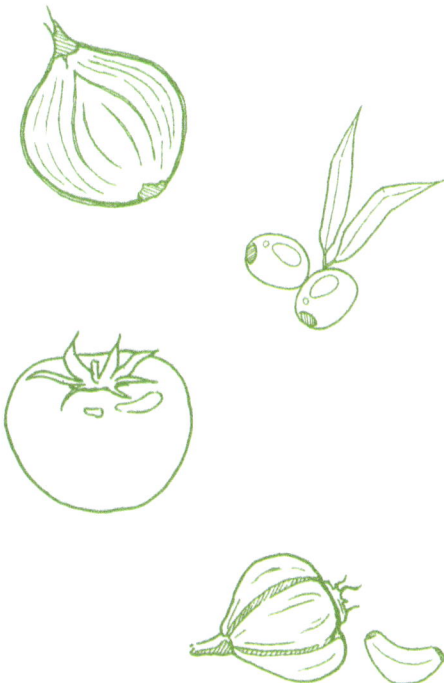

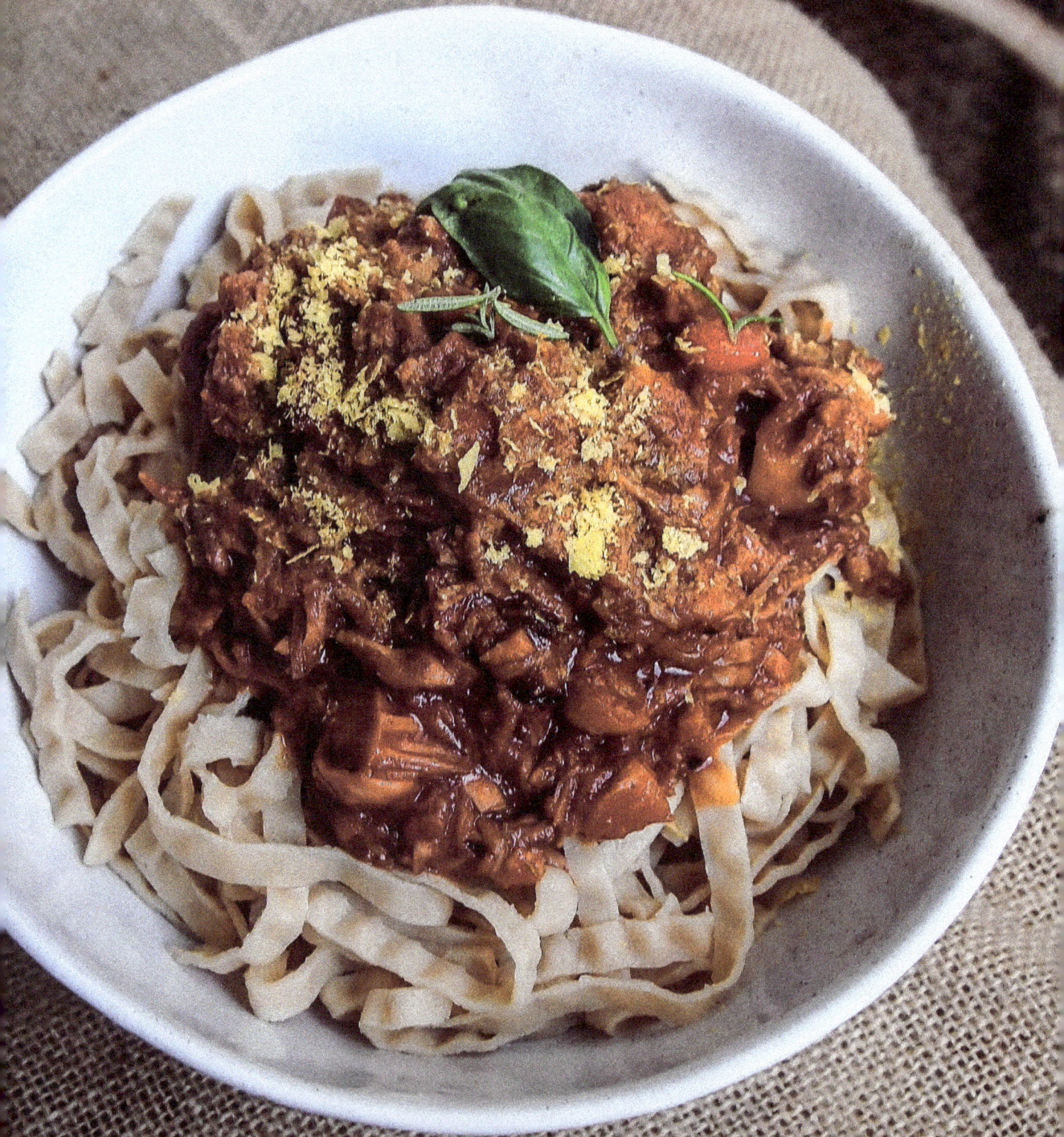

Eggplant Parmigiana

Sami Bloom @samibloom

Many people will have fond childhood memories of the classic parmigiana, traditionally made with chicken and plenty of cheese. So when Sydney-based nutritionist Sami Bloom wanted to include a mediterranean-inspired recipe in her eBook, she tasked herself with recreating a plant-based version of this nostalgic dish.

The various textures - the meaty eggplant, crumbly quinoa, and smooth sauce spiked with herbs - makes this an extremely satisfying dinner that will make you wish you'd been served this healthified adaptation as a child.

Vegan, gluten-free, dairy-free, refined sugar-free

Ingredients

1 eggplant

1 cup cooked quinoa

⅓ cup, plus 2 tablespoon ground flax seeds

½ cup nutritional yeast

⅓ cup brazil nuts

¼ bunch parsley

1 large roma or heirloom tomato, diced

½ onion, diced

2 cloves garlic, minced

2 x 400 gram (11 oz) tins tomatoes

1–2 teaspoons dried italian herbs

Salt and pepper, to taste

Method

Preheat the oven to 200°C (400°F). Slice eggplant into 1.5cm (½") rounds or sliced vertically along the full length of the eggplant. If you have time, allow each sliced eggplant to sweat by sprinkling it with a pinch of sea salt and letting it sit for 15-30 minutes. Rinse and pat dry with a clean kitchen towel.

Meanwhile, in a medium bowl soak ⅓ cup ground flax seeds in approximately ⅓ cup water for around 5-10 minutes until gluggy. Set aside.

Pulse the nutritional yeast, the additional 2 tablespoons of ground flax seeds, brazil nuts and parsley together until they form a chunky powder. This is your herb-parmesan! Set aside.

Place a deep pan or small pot over a medium heat and add the diced roma tomato, onion, garlic, dried herbs, salt and pepper and simmer for around 10 minutes, stirring occasionally.

Pour one tin of the tinned tomatoes into the base of a medium baking dish, using a spatula to spread it evenly over the dish.

Once eggplant is ready, set-up the soaked flax and a bowl of cooked quinoa next to each other.

Continued over page.

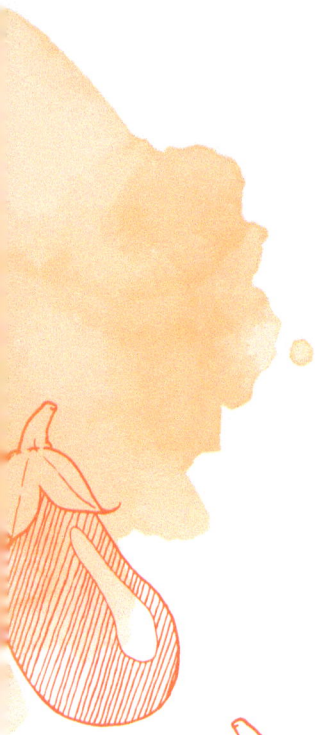

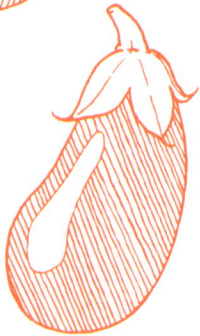

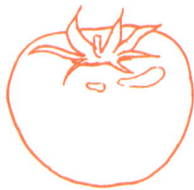

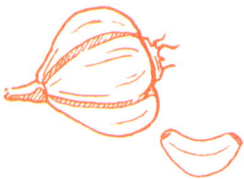

Dip a slice of eggplant into the ground flaxseed to wet it first, and then into the quinoa to bread it. This won't be perfect, just cover the piece as much as possible, then place the eggplant in the dish. Repeat this with all the eggplant slices, layering them on top of the sauce in the baking dish as you go.

Once you've layered all your eggplant, cover with the remaining sauce. Sprinkle the herb-parmesan over the top of the eggplant, patting down evenly. Cover the dish in aluminum foil and bake for 30 minutes until the top is brown and golden.

Allow to stand for 20 minutes before slicing and serving.

Serves 6

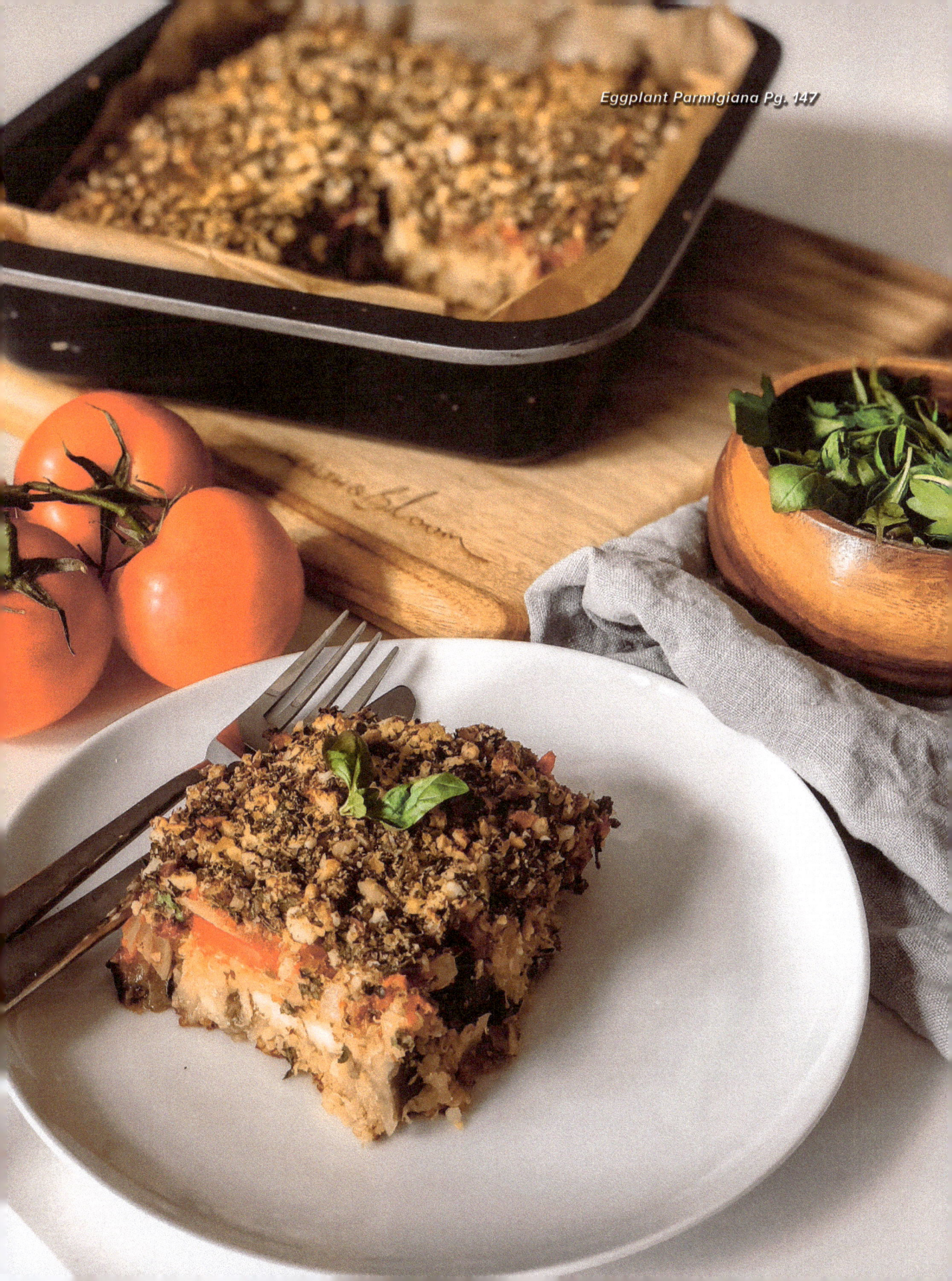

Eggplant Parmigiana Pg. 147

Tully Humphrey on Conquering Mental Illness Through Movement

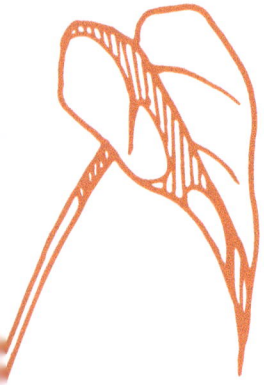

"Yoga became an escape from the voice that told me I wasn't enough. I would get on my mat and it was my escape from the world - from those negative thoughts inside my head. In those classes, I learnt to be so present with my body and to love myself again."

This is how Tully Humphrey, founder of activewear label Tully Lou, feels after a session on her yoga mat: filled with a sense of inner euphoria and quiet peace that she finds difficult to cultivate in any other way.

But despite her positive relationship with exercise and her body now, it wasn't always this way.

Tully's story begins in the Victorian country town of Kyneton, where she was raised in a loving, supportive family comprised of her parents and younger sister. Living in the country, a love for being active and outdoors was instilled in her from a young age.

'I was always outside running around, exercising and being very physical on a daily basis,' Tully says, playing with one of the chunky gold rings that adorns her index finger. 'Mum was always very

health focused and would cook a lot of our food from scratch. I was always that weird kid at school who got rye instead of white bread, and was only allowed coco pops on my birthday,' she laughs.

Looking back on this wholesome upbringing, Tully says she's grateful that her parents adopted this healthy way of living. But at that point in her life, she wasn't to know how those views might manifest themselves in her teenage years to become unhealthy obsessions.

Too Much of a 'Good' Thing

Team sports had always been an important part of Tully's childhood. She played netball, basketball and was always running around her family's property. But what started out as harmless activity became a fully-fledged dependence on exercise around the age of 13.

'I soon realised that if I exercised between my usual sporting and recreational activities that I could lose weight, and I became obsessed with the idea of that,' she admits.

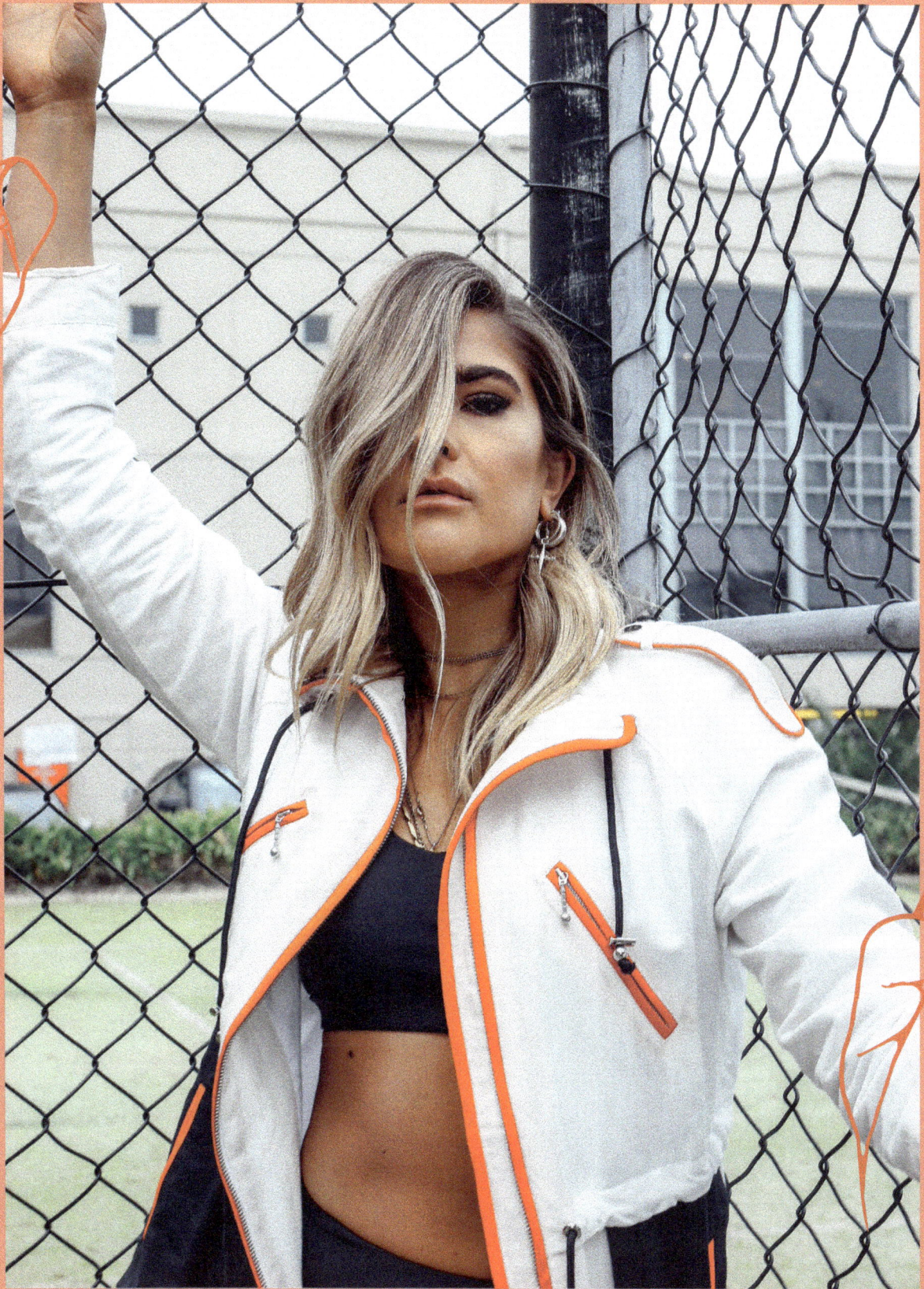

Tully says that by the time she was 14 the joy had been sucked out of exercise entirely, with her sole focus being on losing weight rather than simply moving her body for the innocent pleasure that it once was.

'I would count how many calories I ate each day and knew how far I had to run to burn them off,' she admits. 'I was doing crazy shit, like setting my alarm at 1am to get out of bed and do 50 squats. Then I would go back to sleep and get up again at 4am to do another 50 squats.'

It was at this point in her life when Tully realised that what had previously been a passion for moving her body had become something much more sinister. There was an obsessive compulsive intention behind how she exercised and ate, which she began to realise wasn't normal. In her pursuit of "health", she had, in fact, fallen into a routine that was so mentally and physically destructive that she hardly recognised herself.

Eventually Tully's parents, who had grown increasingly worried about her behaviour, asked her to visit a psychologist. After her first visit she was diagnosed with Anorexia Nervosa, a serious mental illness that is defined by low body weight and body image distortion, with an obsessive fear of gaining weight. Coupled with her exercise addiction, it was a potentially life-threatening combination for young Tully.

Even after the diagnosis, Tully wasn't ready for the internal battle that was to ensue between her and her eating disorder for years to come. They would be the hardest years of her life.

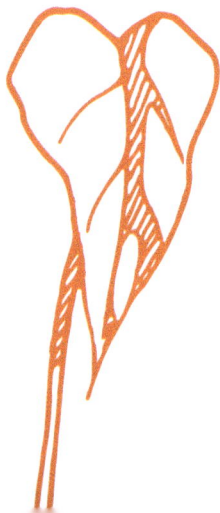

The debilitating mental illness completely dictated her every waking move and thought. It was a loud, persistent voice in her head that forced her to act against the most basic human instincts: rest, nourishment and survival.

'Anorexia has a terrible way of connecting all your self worth to how much you weigh, what you eat and how much you exercise. I used to believe that if I didn't engage in the exercise it told me to, I wouldn't be successful, happy or achieve anything significant. I associated so much of who I was with one tiny, relatively insignificant part of myself; my body.'

'At this time of my life I hated my body,' Tully says, pushing a strand of golden blond hair behind her ear. 'I was never happy when I looked in the mirror and there would always be some part of myself that I would pick at and criticise. I would stand there and think 'I'm fat, I'm fat, I'm fat', over and over again - it was a thought that I lived and breathed. For most of my day my whole mind would be consumed by these thoughts. It was relentless and never ending.'

Movement as Medicine

In her early adult years, Tully became interested in the practice of yoga as an alternative form of exercise, though she admits that her intentions were stilled marred by her disorder.

'Initially when I started yoga I was 100 percent doing it to burn off calories, which was still my main reason for exercising at that time of my life,' she says. 'But after engaging in the practice for a while, I began to realise that after every time I did yoga, I was happier. And not just happier because I had satisfied a need to burn calories or obey my eating disorder, but because it helped me find a kind of peace and acceptance with my body that I hadn't been able to achieve before.'

'I found that the more I did yoga, the more the voices in my head began to quieten, until eventually they almost completely disappeared. And don't get me wrong, those voices sometimes still pop up, I think they do for most people, but yoga has helped me get to a place where if I ever do have those thoughts, I can turn them around straight away.

If I ever start to get stuck in that rut again I know I can turn to yoga because of how powerful it is. It connects my body to my mind and allows me to get out of my own head and listen to what's really happening inside my soul, which I think so many of us struggle with these days.'

Tully explains that it isn't just yoga that can help create this mind-body connection, and what works will vary from person to person. Any form of movement, whether it be walking, pilates, swimming or a sweaty HIIT class, that gives you a sense of inner strength, empowerment and acceptance of yourself is beneficial.

As women, we are so often taught that we should place the needs of others above our own, but putting aside time for you to move your body in a way you love is a sign that you respect yourself.

You're giving yourself permission to spend time within yourself and your own body, not to criticise and judge, but to simply be.

If you don't have time to do this every day, aim to carve out just a few times in your week when you engage in some kind of fulfilling movement that allows you to disengage from the noise of society, social media and work emails.

Use this time to escape from any judgmental thoughts, whether they be about yourself or others, and find a place of fierce, beautiful peace within yourself.

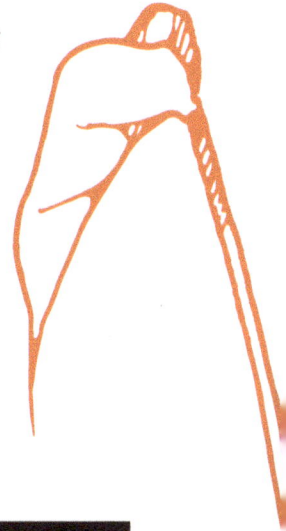

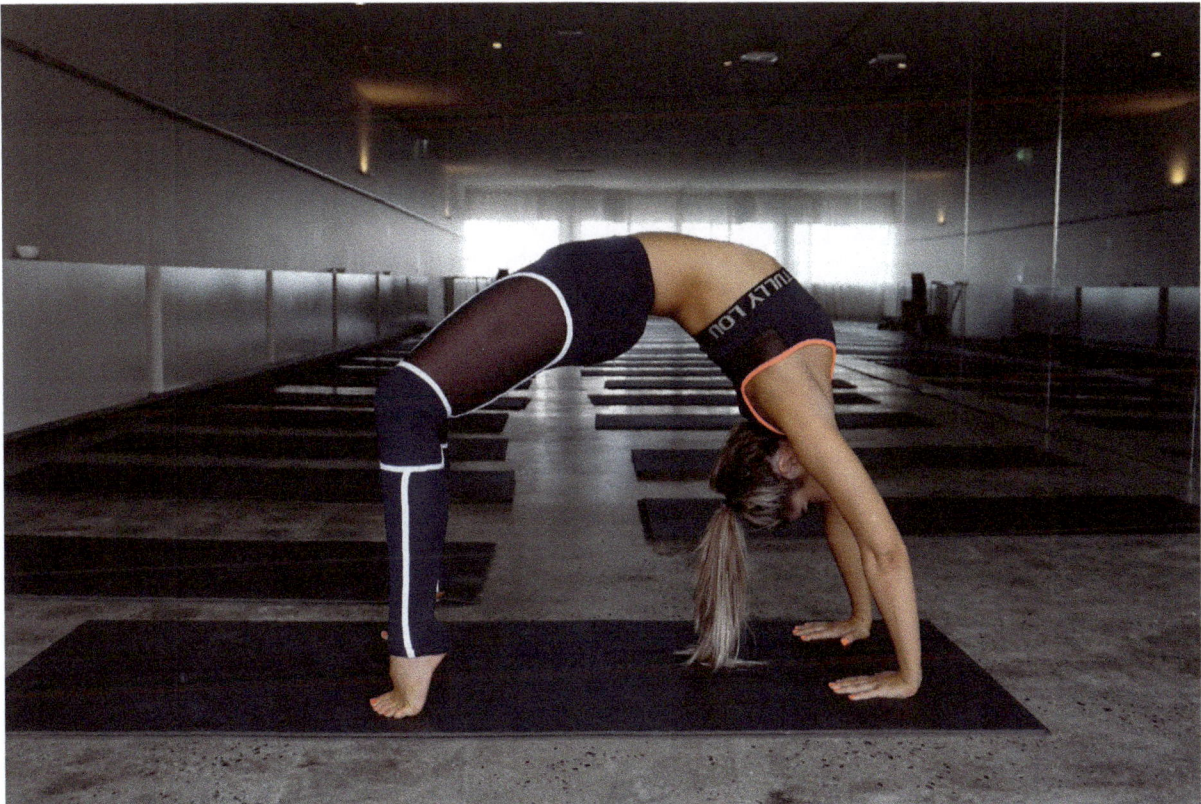

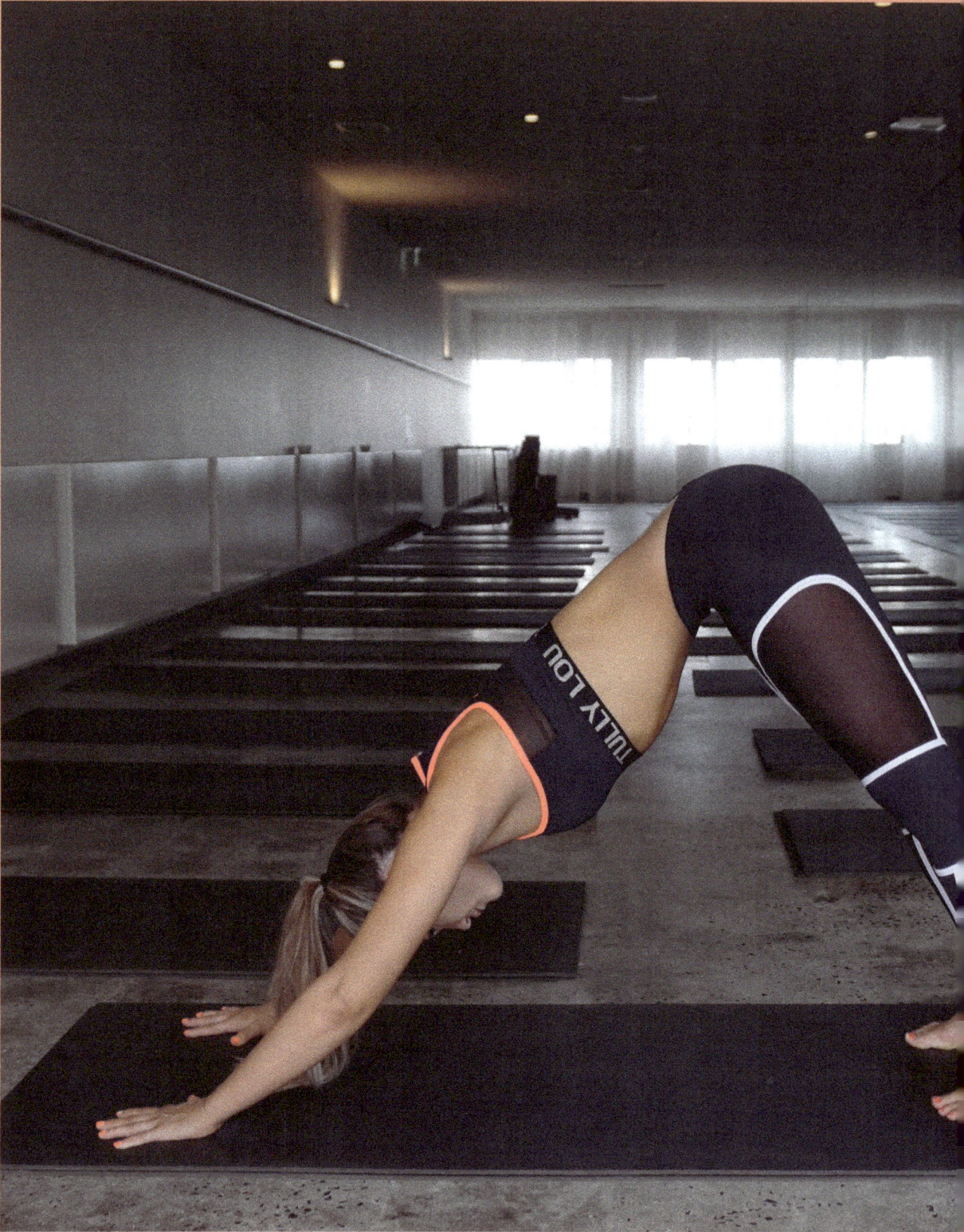

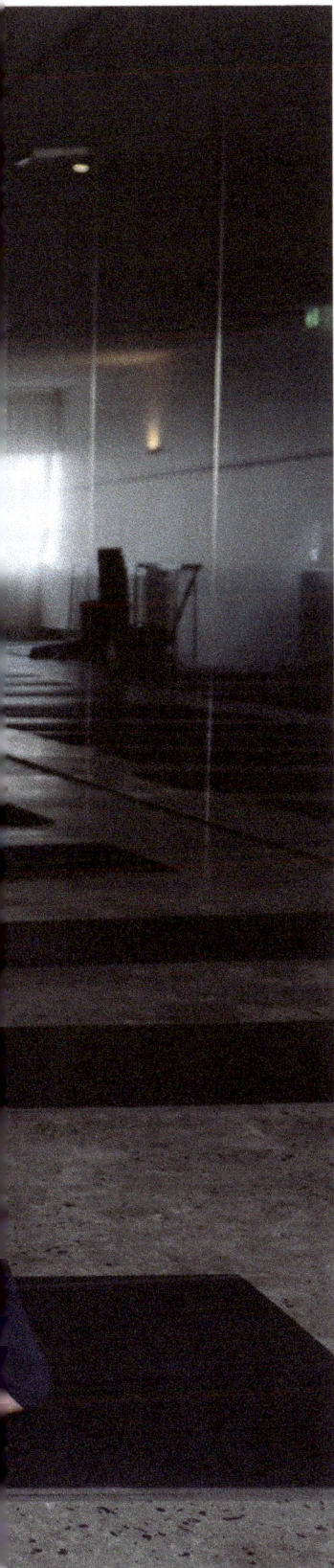

Knowing When to Stop

'I've spent years using exercise as a punishment,' Tully admits. 'It was really difficult, but I had to become self-aware and know when I was turning to exercise to deal with issues that were happening around me, or thoughts I was having about myself.'

While she says it's fine to go for a run when you're emotional or sign up for a boxing class to let off steam, Tully's experience has taught her that exercise should never be used as a coping mechanism.

If it becomes the way you deal with negative thoughts or external stressors - such as exams, your terrible job or dysfunctional relationships - that's when it can turn into a form of self-abuse.

The key here, Tully says, is identifying your main reasons for exercising. If you feel as though you might be abusing exercise, you need to ask yourself the purpose behind it. How does your body and mind feel at that point in time? Are there other stressors in your life that are contributing to your need to exercise? And, perhaps most importantly, is exercise really the healthiest thing for you in that moment? Maybe instead of exercising you should be sitting down to talk to someone, confronting something you're putting off, or surrounding yourself with loved ones. Maybe instead of moving, you actually just need to be still and show yourself some self care after a busy, stressful week.

'Listen to your body and don't let that controlling, judgmental voice take over,' Tully says. 'If the voice in your head says you "have" to exercise and you don't want to, then don't do it. Exercise should always be a choice, and if it feels like it isn't, then you should question your motives.'

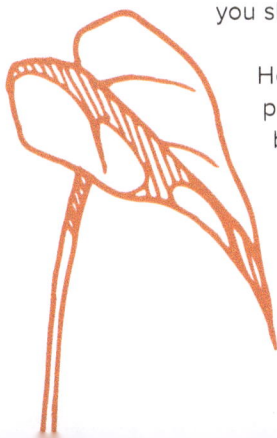

Healthy exercise is done when it's performed purely for the enjoyment of moving your body. It's time for you, and you alone. That's when movement is a truly beautiful, empowering thing.

The Birth of Tully Lou

Now 31 and living in Melbourne, Tully's remarkable journey has seen her become a passionate yoga instructor and founder of the sportluxe activewear label Tully Lou, which blends the lines between high-quality performance activewear and fashion forward streetwear. With a collection comprised of bold, fierce pieces, Tully says she launched her brand back in 2013 as a way to motivate and empower women to move their bodies and live healthier, happier lives.

'My eating disorder played a huge part in why I created my brand,' she explains, sipping on her strong soy latte. 'Having an eating disorder throughout my teenage years was the worst and most debilitating thing in the world. But it's a time in my life that has really shaped me and made me who I am today. It's made me want to help other women to feel strong and empowered within themselves and their own bodies.'

'So often when I was in my yoga class I would look around the room and see that all the women there were wearing dark, black baggy clothing. Athleisure wasn't a thing back then, and I realised there was nothing on the market that made women feel special or embraced their feminine form - it was like they were trying to hide themselves from the world, like they were ashamed.'

'So that's how Tully Lou was born,' she says. 'I wanted to inspire women to embrace their bodies, to workout and live healthier lives. I hope that my label can help women respect themselves and find the joy in the movement that they deserve.'

Tully's Tips for Healthy Movement

Here are some tips from Tully Humphrey that we hope you can adopt into your routine to help you motivate yourself to move your body in a truly healthy way that works for you.

1. Find What Works for You

Find out whether you're someone who likes to workout in the morning, afternoon or evening. Chances are, if you choose a time to exercise that suits when you have the most energy you won't just be more likely to do it, but you'll also have a more productive workout.

Tully is a self-confessed early riser, so sets her alarm bright and early to get her workout in. This is how she sets herself up for a positive and energised day ahead. But if you're not a morning person - don't sweat it! You shouldn't try to force yourself to the gym in the morning just because it feels like everyone on social media is doing it. If you're going to hate every second of it then you've already lost the purpose of movement - enjoyment. So choose a time that works for you and own it.

2. Become a Scheduler

If you're someone who finds it difficult to stick to an exercise routine once the businesses of your week kicks in, don't think it's just you. We all have times when we feel overwhelmed, and exercise is often the first thing to slip off our To Do lists.

If this is something you find regularly occurring, Tully suggests writing down the kind of movement you'd like to do that week. 'Schedule in any classes or gym time and see this as non-negotiable self-care time,' she says. 'It's an opportunity for you to respect yourself and value what makes you feel good.'

3. You Gotta Get With Your Friends

Exercising with friends is something that not only holds you accountable, but will also add more enjoyment to your workouts. Furthermore, if you find yourself becoming a bit obsessive about your workout routine, exercising with friends is a great way to take the focus off the calories your burning and helps you instead focus on connecting with others and having fun!

4. If You Hate It, Don't Do It

Find what exercise you enjoy doing. If you hate running so much that it makes you want to punch someone, then don't do it! If the idea of F45 makes you die a little bit inside, don't sign up! Essentially, if you try and make yourself do exercise that you don't enjoy, no matter how "trendy" it is, it will always be a struggle.

Moving your body should be a joy, never a chore. So, if you don't enjoy it then find something else. Tully suggests trying out a few things to see what you really love, because this will improve motivation and help you be consistent in your workout.

5. Mix It Up

'Incorporating diversity into your fitness routine is a great way to not only challenge your body, but also help reduce the risk of becoming overly obsessive about your exercise routine,' says Tully. 'If you do the movement over and over again, you can easily become disengaged from your workout and find yourself simply going through the motions.'
Diversity in your workouts adds fun and play to your routine. It helps to push you mentally as well as physically and let's you explore all the fantastic movements your body can perform. Think dance classes, rock climbing or mountain bike riding - anything that keeps your body guessing and your motivation high.

6. Hit Unfollow

Tully says that one of the most helpful things she did to heal her relationship with her body and exercise was to unfollow exercise and fitness accounts on social media that she found triggering.

'If looking at certain content makes you compare yourself to others or makes you feel less than anything but awesome in your own skin, then unfollow them,' she says resolutely.

And if you feel like you can't unfollow the account, Tully recommends using the mute function on Instagram, so you don't have to see their content. Genius.

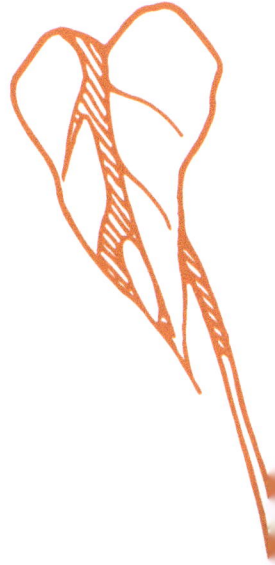

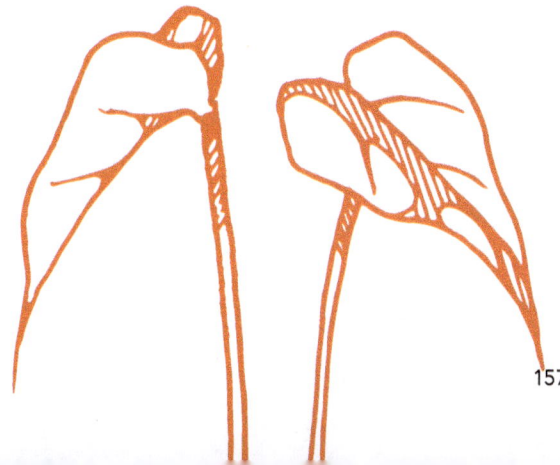

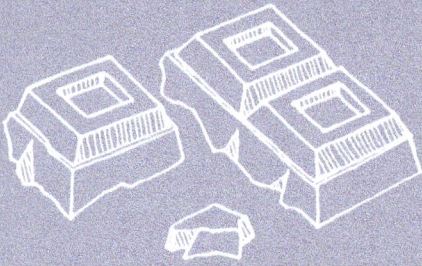

Snacks

While we may debate over which peanut butter is best (are you team smooth or crunchy?), one thing we can all agree on is that snacks are life.

Packed with energy-boosting ingredients, this selection of recipes was created to help you get through those energy slumps that hit you between meals. They'll quieten a rumbling tummy, satisfy a sweet tooth and help you get 100 percent out of your day.

Some people may still refer to "snacking" as a dirty word. We say ignore them, you don't need that kind of negativity in your life when you've got tasty bliss balls and beetroot-flecked hummus to eat and share with your friends.

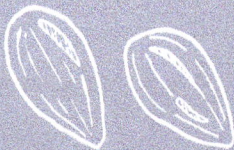

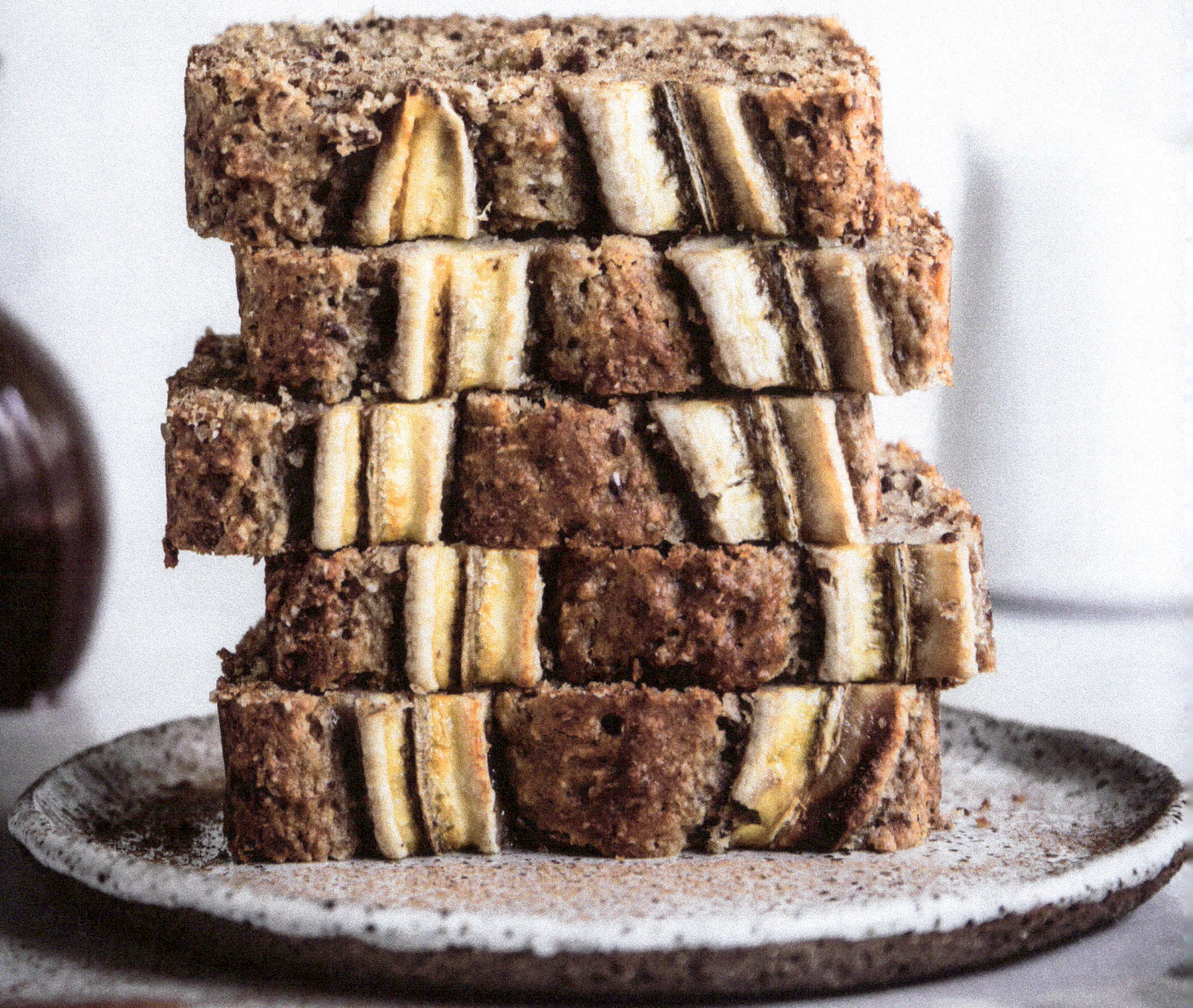

Salted Sesame Swirl Bark

Olivia Kaplan @livinbondi

How good is it when you put minimal effort into something and it's still manages to impress your friends? That pretty much sums up this incredibly quick and tasty snack from Bondi-based nutritionist, Olivia Kaplan.

In this creation, Olivia uses tahini, a paste made from sesame seeds that's high in calcium and healthy fats, to make a sophisticated treat that's not too sweet.

'Sesame is one of my favourite flavours in all its forms — sesame oil, sesame seeds, and sesame paste, AKA tahini,' Olivia says.

'Just like olive oil, tahini has a distinctive savoury and slightly bitter flavour that you can't get from anything else. This makes it perfect for desserts to counteract the sweetness and gives it a unique and surprisingly sophisticated flavour.'

Vegan, gluten-free, dairy-free, refined sugar-free

Ingredients

¼ cup tahini

2 tablespoons coconut oil, melted

15 drops liquid stevia, or to taste

200 grams (7 oz) dark chocolate (70–90%)

2 tablespoon toasted sesame seeds

Pinch of sea salt

Method

In a small bowl combine the tahini, melted coconut oil and stevia. Set aside.

Melt the chocolate either in the microwave or in a small bowl over a pot of simmering water. Remove from the heat and add in the stevia. If you like sweeter chocolate, add more liquid stevia until you reach your desired sweetness.

Line a large baking tray with baking paper.

Pour the melted chocolate over the baking paper in a large slab. Next, pour over the tahini mixture and swirl gently into the chocolate using a knife until you get a pretty marble pattern.

Sprinkle over sesame seeds and sea salt.

Place in the fridge or freezer until set completely, around 1-2 hours.

Break up into shards and store in the fridge.

Serves 10-15

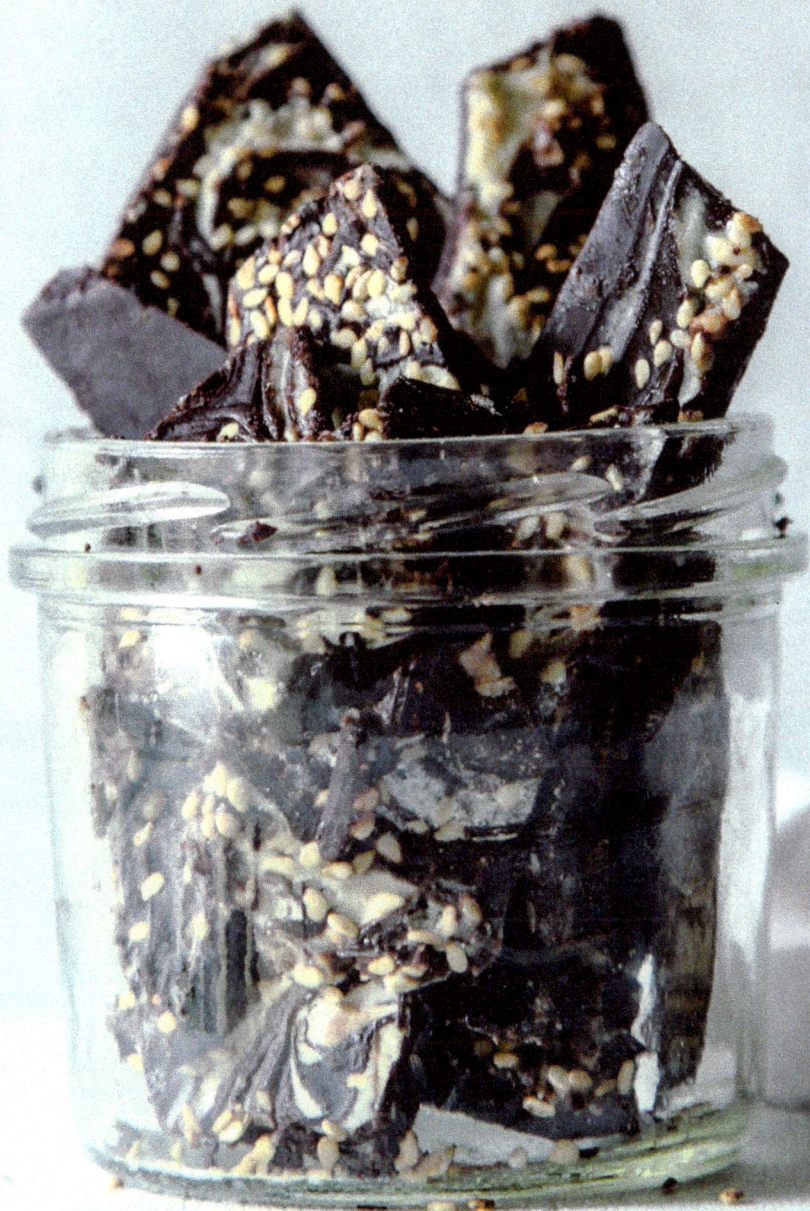

Strawberry Pitaya Almond Thumbprints

Leah Boston @simplyleahboston

Growing up in Pennsylvania, Leah Boston has been cooking since she could reach the kitchen counter-top. It was a family tradition to bake Christmas cookies, hand make Easter candy and decorate extravagant birthday cakes.

Now based in Australia, the plant-based recipe developer and yoga teacher keeps these customs alive through her delicious creations, like these healthi-fied thumbprint cookies.

'These cookies were a Christmas tradition in my house, except they were rich butter cookies filled with blackberry jam,' Leah says. 'When I overhauled my diet I didn't want to miss out on my favorite festive treat, so I decided to recreate them with this recipe.'

'Because they're full of all the good things, they're perfect for a morning snack, afternoon tea or a little something sweet before bed without feeling as though you've over indulged. Even after Christmas dinner!'

Vegan, gluten-free, dairy-free, refined sugar-free

Ingredients

For the cookie

1¼ cups almond meal

⅓ cups almond butter

3 tablespoons maple syrup

For the strawberry pitaya jam

1 cup frozen strawberries

1 packet Pitaya Plus frozen pitaya

1-2 tablespoons maple syrup

1-2 tablespoons freshly squeezed lemon juice

2 tablespoons chia seeds

Method

Preheat oven to 190°C (375°F).

For the jam, combine the strawberries, pitaya, maple syrup and lemon juice in a small saucepan over medium heat. Cook for 8-12 minutes until the fruit breaks down and becomes syrupy. Throughout this process use a fork to mash the strawberries.

Take the mixture off the heat and stir in chia seeds. Set aside and allow to stand for 5 minutes. As the mixture cools it will thicken to a jam-like consistency. If you want a thicker jam, simply add more chia seeds.

Transfer to a jar and allow jam to cool completely.

For the cookies, add all ingredients into a medium bowl and use a spatula or your hands fold together until dough forms.

Cover bowl with glad wrap and place in fridge for 30 minutes, allowing dough to chill making it easier to handle.

Once dough is chilled, portion into tablespoon-full amounts and roll into balls, placing on a tray lines with baking paper.

Using your thumb, press down into the center of each ball creating a little crater for the jam.

Fill each crater with a teaspoon of the cooled strawberry pitaya jam. Be careful not to overfill them or jam will spill over edges.

Place in the oven and cook for 8 to 10 minutes until slightly golden. Remove from oven, cool on a wire rack and serve.

Makes 10 cookies

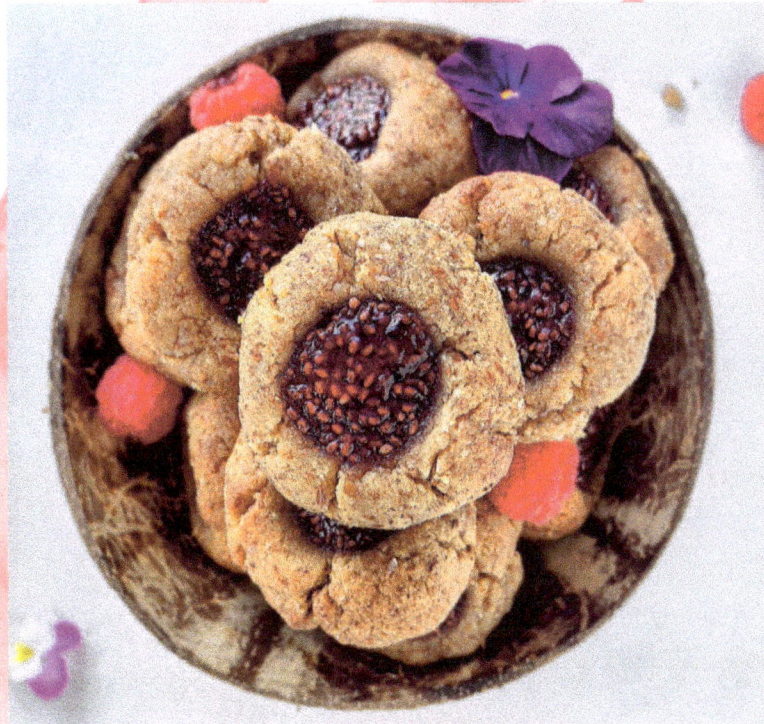

Gut Healthy Chocolate, Coconut & Chickpea Cookies

Leanne Ward @the_fitness_dietitian

We love chickpeas. And we love cookies. But together? Surely this is a joke, right?

We may be funny, but we would definitely not joke about cookies, especially these delicious, gut-loving morsels from Sydney-based dietitian Leanne Ward.

'I'm obsessed with gut health,' Leanne confesses enthusiastically. 'And the greater diversity of plant-based food you have in your diet, the better it is for your gut. I wanted to create a cookie that included some kind of legume - which are one of the best sources of plant fibre available.'

These cookies are also extremely allergy friendly, being nut free, gluten free, egg free and dairy free. The only thing they're not free from is deliciousness!

Vegan, gluten-free, dairy-free, refined sugar-free

Ingredients

1 x 400 gram (11 oz) tin of chickpeas, drained

½ cup tahini

¼ cup maple syrup

1 teaspoon vanilla bean paste

1 teaspoon baking powder

½ teaspoon salt

¼ cup psyllium husk

¼ cup shredded coconut

¼ cup dark chocolate chips

Method

Preheat oven to 190°C (375°F) and line a baking tray with baking paper.

In a food processor add the chickpeas, tahini, maple syrup, vanilla, baking powder and salt. Process all together until a smooth batter forms.

Pour batter into a large bowl and fold in the psyllium husk, coconut and chocolate chips.

Using a tablespoon, drop spoonfuls of the batter onto your tray. Allow enough space between the cookies as they'll expand when they cook. Shape the batter into balls.

Place the tray in the oven to bake for 25 minutes until lightly browned.

Allow to cool and store in an airtight container.

Makes 14 cookies

Coconut, Spiced Apple & Blueberry Breakfast Cookies

Sami Bloom @samibloom

Nutritionist Sami Bloom dreaded the 6:45am starts during her dietitian clinical placement and, understandably, she found it difficult to fit in her usual bowl of porridge before rushing out the door. This lead to her creation of what she now affectionately calls her 'portable porridge cookies', which made sure she was fueled for her busy days.

'These cookies are packed with fibre, healthy fats and high-quality carbohydrates making them a great on-the-go breakfast if you're running out the door in the morning,' she says.

These cookies aren't just great for breakfast though. They'll help you power through any mid-afternoon energy slump.

Vegan, dairy-free, refined sugar-free

Ingredients

Dry ingredients

1 ½ cup rolled oats

½ cup ground flaxseeds

½ cup shredded coconut

½ teaspoon baking soda

1 teaspoon cinnamon

Pinch of sea salt

Wet ingredients

½ cup unsweetened apple sauce

3-4 tablespoons maple syrup

2 teaspoon vanilla extract

1 teaspoon lemon juice

1 small green apple, shredded

⅓ cup blueberries

Method

Preheat your oven to 180°C (350°F).

Pulse all your dry ingredients in a food processor until around ¾ of the mixture is floury and the rest is still a bit chunky.

Transfer mixture to a medium bowl and add the apple sauce, maple syrup, lemon juice and vanilla. Stir well to combine. Fold in the blueberries and shredded apple.

Line a large baking tray with baking paper. Take 2 tablespoons-worth of the cookie batter and roll into balls. Gently flatten them onto the tray with a spatula.

Place in the oven and bake 25 minutes, or until slightly golden and cooked through.

Allow the cookies to cool for 15-20 minutes then store in an airtight container and refrigerate. These will keep for around 5 days.

Makes 10 cookies

Nut Butter-filled Dates

Laura Ford @laurafordnutrition

'I was surprised how delicious these turned out when I first made them,' laughs dietitian Laura Ford. 'My husband's a building surveyor and he's always hesitant to try my healthy snacks, but he loves these so much he takes them to work to share with his mates!'

These stuffed dates are the perfect 3pm pick me up if you're craving something sweet and delicious to see you through the afternoon. They have a rich, caramel flavour and just one or two are enough to satisfy your sweet tooth. We wouldn't judge you if you had more though - they're that good!

Vegan, gluten-free, dairy-free, refined sugar-free

Ingredients

10 Medjool dates, pits removed

10 teaspoons natural peanut butter (can sub with any nut butter you like)

¾ cup dry roasted peanuts, roughly chopped

150 grams (5 oz) vegan mylk chocolate

½ teaspoon coconut oil

Method

Gently open the dates in half and place one teaspoon of peanut butter in each.

Press ½ teaspoon (or more if it fits) of chopped peanuts into each date on top of the nut butter and set aside. Repeat with remaining dates.

Once all the dates are stuffed, melt the chocolate and coconut oil together in a microwave and stir to combine. Dip the stuffed dates in the chocolate then place on a tray lined with greaseproof paper.

Place the chocolate-dipped dates in the fridge until the chocolate is set.

Makes 10 dates

You will need to use medjool dates for this recipe, not the dried kind.

Lemon Bliss Balls

Tarni Deutsher @healthywholefood

When it comes to raw treats, once you know the ratio of dry to wet mixture, it's often simply a matter of choosing your favourite flavours, throwing them together and voila! You have your own perfect portable snack.

These fresh, zingy bliss balls from plant-based blogger Tarni Deutsher came to life during one of her creative sessions in the kitchen when she was developing a snack she could take to university that would satisfy her sweet tooth. As she puts it, 'these are the ideal snack if you want something fruity that's a little more delicious than fruit.' Amen.

Vegan, dairy-free, refined sugar-free

Ingredients

2 ¼ cup oats

7 dates, pits removed

3 tablespoons coconut oil, melted

Juice and zest of one lemon

1 teaspoon vanilla essence

2 tablespoons maple syrup or honey

3 tablespoons chia seeds

¼ cup desiccated coconut, plus extra for rolling

2 tablespoons pitaya powder (optional)

Method

Firstly, soak dates in warm water for 30 minutes. In a high-speed blender, add the oats and quickly pulse until a fine, flour-like consistency is achieved. Place the oats in a large mixing bowl and set aside.

Drain the soaked dates and add them to the blender with melted coconut oil, lemon juice, vanilla essence and maple syrup. Blend until it becomes a smooth "date paste".

Add the date paste into the bowl with the oats along with the lemon zest, chia seeds, desiccated coconut and pitaya powder (if using) and mix until well combined. Go with your gut here, and if the mixture feels a little too wet, add more oats. If it seems too dry, then add a splash of plant-based milk.

Roll the mixture into desired sized balls and then into desiccated coconut. You can also roll them into some additional lemon zest for an extra lemony kick!

Store in the fridge for 3-5 days or in the freezer for around a month if you want to keep them longer.

Makes 12-14 balls

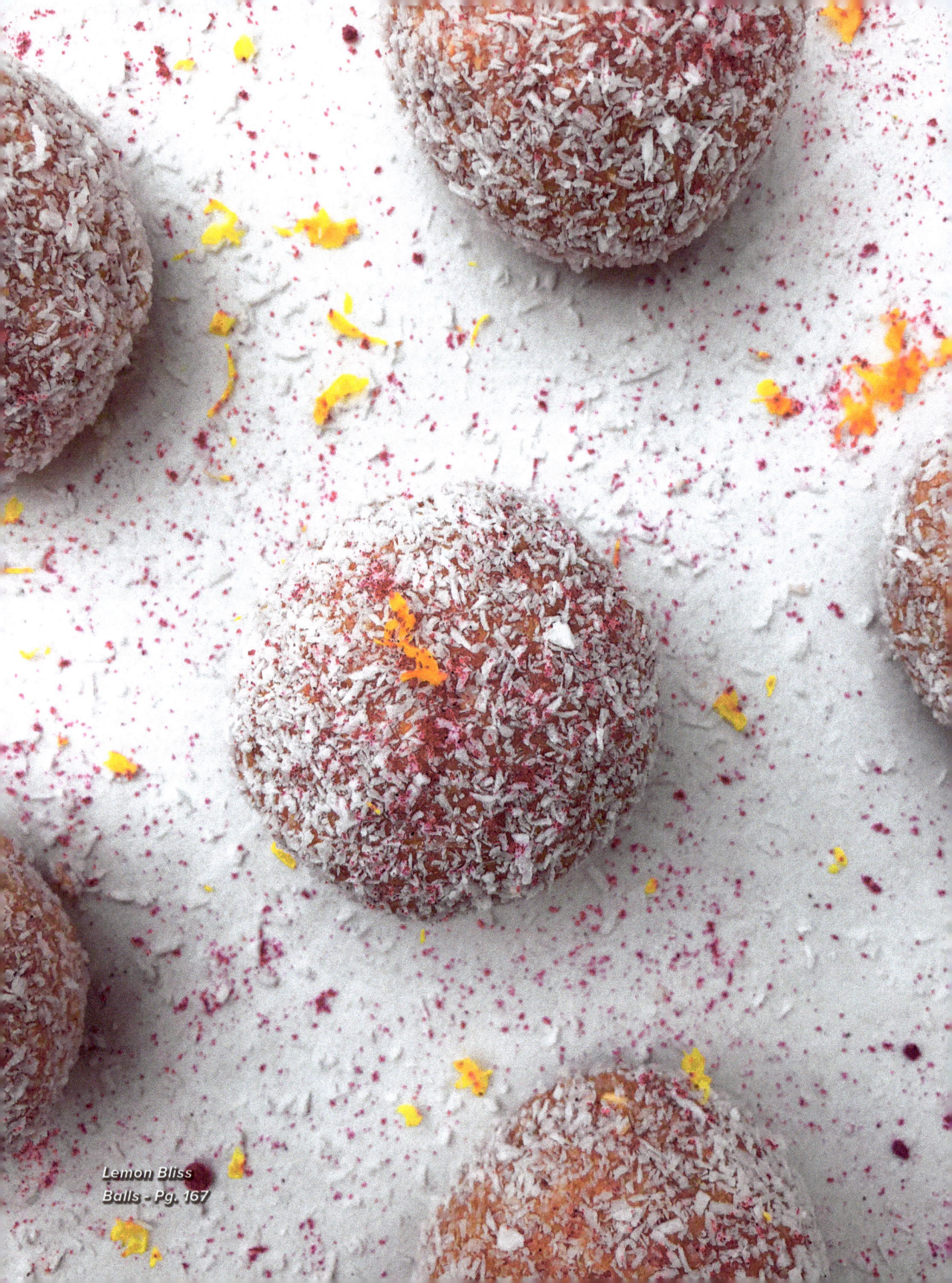

*Lemon Bliss
Balls - Pg. 167*

Peanut Butter Choc-Chip Cookie Dough Protein Balls

Michelle Chen @run2food

There's something wonderfully nostalgic about the act of baking cookies and eating the dough along the way, which we all know is obviously the best bit.

'Once you bake the cookies you always wish you'd eaten more of the dough,' laughs vegan food blogger Michelle Chen. 'That's why I wanted to make a snack that let people eat the dough without any regrets!'

Vegan, gluten-free, dairy-free, refined sugar-free

Ingredients

1 cup almond meal

¼ cup coconut flour

1 scoop (40 grams/1 serve) vegan protein powder

¼ cup almond milk

¼ cup smooth peanut butter

¼ cup maple syrup

¼ cup vegan chocolate chips

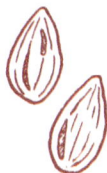

Method

In a large bowl, mix the almond meal, coconut flour and protein powder together.

In a separate bowl, combine the almond milk, peanut butter and maple syrup and mix well until smooth.

Transfer the wet mixture to the bowl with the dry ingredients and stir until a cookie dough-like consistency forms. Fold in the chocolate chips and mix until well distributed.

Divide the dough into 8 portions and roll into balls. Store in the freezer and allow to thaw for 5 minutes at room temperature before eating.

Makes 8 balls

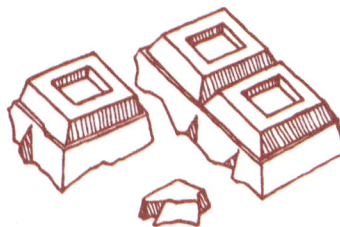

Gluten-Free Banana Bread

Sarah Bell @ournourishingtable

Nutritionist and recipe developer Sarah Bell has always been a foodie to the core. Growing up in Queensland's little bushland town of Mount Crosby, she fondly remembers baking cakes and biscuits with her Nana and mum.

Many years on, she uses cooking as a creative outlet and particularly finds comfort in baking, except, she jokes, when her three children are in the kitchen with her.

Sarah uses buckwheat flour in her banana bread to give it a fluffier texture that she often finds is missing from healthier, gluten-free baking. And once drizzled in the caramel sauce, there's no way you'd think this is banana bread is anything but decadent.

Gluten-free, dairy-free,

Ingredients

1 cup almond meal

1 cup buckwheat flour

¼ cup tapioca starch

2 teaspoons baking powder

½ cup coconut sugar

1 teaspoon ground cinnamon

½ teaspoon ground nutmeg

2 eggs

2 ripe bananas

¾ cup extra virgin olive oil

Buckwheat flour can be substituted for brown rice flour if preferred.

Method

Preheat oven to 180°C (350°F) and line a tin loaf with baking paper.

In a large mixing bowl, all the almond meal, buckwheat flour, tapioca starch, baking powder, cinnamon, nutmeg and coconut sugar. Stir to combine.

In a separate bowl, mash the bananas with a fork. Add the extra virgin olive oil and eggs and whisk well.

Pour the wet ingredients into the dry ingredients and stir well to combine, until the mixture is smooth and doesn't have any lumps of flour in it.

Pour the mixture into the lined baking loaf tin and place in the oven for 50 minutes or until a skewer comes out clean when tested.

Once cooked, remove the loaf from the oven and allow to cool before serving.

Makes 1 loaf

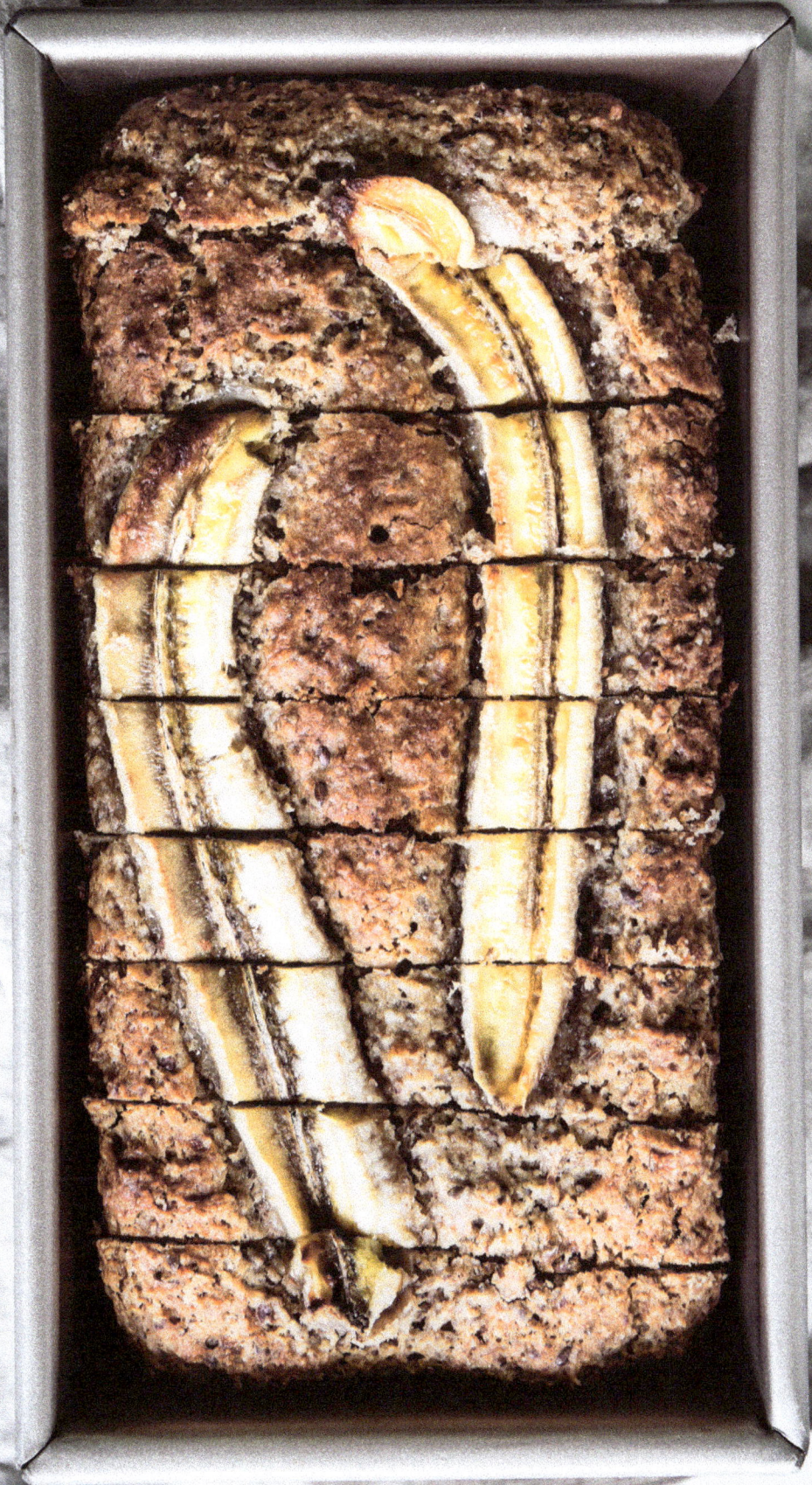

Almond, Banana Chocolate Chunk Loaf

Leah Boston @simplyleahboston

'If there's one thing I can't live without, it's bananas,' admits plant-based recipe developer and yogi Leah Boston. 'And nothing makes me happier than consuming them in a freshly baked loaf of banana bread!'

Her happiness might be due to bananas natural level of tryptophan (a chemical that feeds the serotonin pathway in the brain that makes us happy), but we think that even without the science-y stuff, the taste alone is enough to put a smile on your face.

Vegan, gluten-free, dairy-free

Ingredients

1 chia egg (3 tablespoons water + 1 tablespoon chia seed)

2 ½ medium ripe bananas, mashed

¾ cup full fat coconut milk

3 tablespoon almond butter

½ cup coconut sugar

2 tablespoon maple syrup

⅔ cup almond flour

⅔ cup + 2 tablespoons tapioca (cassava) flour

1 cup oat flour

3 ½ teaspoons baking powder

1 teaspoon cinnamon

½ teaspoon each nutmeg, ginger, sea salt

⅓ cup chopped almonds

⅓ cup vegan dark chocolate chunks

Method

Preheat oven to 180°C (350°F). Line a 9x5 loaf pan with baking paper and set aside.

In a small cup mix up your chia egg and set aside.

In a large bowl mash your bananas until you reach a smooth consistency with no chunks.

Add your chia egg, almond butter, coconut sugar, maple syrup, baking powder and coconut milk to the bowl with the banana and mix until well combined.

In a medium bowl, combine the almond flour, tapioca flour, oat flour, cinnamon, nutmeg, ginger and sea salt.

Add your dry ingredients to the bowl with the wet ingredients, mixing until well combined.

Fold in chopped almonds and chocolate chunks and pour the batter into lined loaf pan. Place pan in the oven and bake for 45 minutes. At this point, remove the banana bread from the oven and pierce with a skewer. If the skewer comes out clean, the loaf is cooked through. If not, place banana bread back in the oven and check every 5-10 minutes until cooked through.

Once cooked, remove the bread from the pan and cool completely on a wire rack before slicing. Store banana bread in the fridge for one week or freeze for up to two months.

Makes 1 loaf

Spinach and Zucchini Loaf

Stephanie Geddes @nutritionist_stephgeddes

Delicious served warm with almond butter, or toasted and topped with avocado, it's no wonder why this healthful loaf is nutritionist Steph Geddes' most popular recipe in her 21 Day Detox Program.

Apart from being delicious, it's also incredibly convenient, with Steph suggesting freezing it and tossing it straight in the toaster for a quick snack when you're in a hurry.

Top it with your favourite toppings, such as ricotta, tahini or nut butters. And if you're in a pinch for lunch or dinner turn it into a meal by adding poached eggs and sauteed greens. However you choose to eat it, you'll get a boost of iron, calcium and folate from the spinach and some vitamin C and potassium from the zucchini.

Gluten-free option, dairy-free, refined sugar-free

Ingredients

1 cup almond meal

1 cup oats (sub quinoa flakes for gluten-free option)

½ cup buckwheat flour

1 tablespoon psyllium husk

¼ teaspoon salt

1 teaspoon baking powder

¼ teaspoon baking soda

¼ teaspoon ground nutmeg

4 eggs

½ cup coconut oil, melted

1 tablespoon honey

1 tablespoon apple cider vinegar

1 cup spinach, chopped finely

1 cup zucchini, grated

¼ walnuts, coarsely chopped

2 tablespoons pumpkin seeds

Method

Preheat the oven to 180°C (350°F). Grease a loaf pan and line it with baking paper.

Combine the almond meal, oats, buckwheat flour, psyllium, salt, baking powder, baking soda and nutmeg in a bowl.

In a separate bowl beat the eggs until pale and fluffy. Add the eggs, oil, honey and apple cider vinegar to the dry mixture and mix thoroughly. Add the spinach, zucchini and walnuts and stir until well combined.

Spoon the mixture into the loaf tin and smooth with the back of a spoon. Top with pumpkin seeds and bake for 30-35 minutes or until a skewer inserted into the middle comes out clean.

Remove the loaf from the oven, cool and slice.

Makes 10 slices

This loaf will keep in the fridge for 1 week or in the freezer for 1 month, simply toast before serving. If storing in the freezer, slice and place baking paper between each piece.

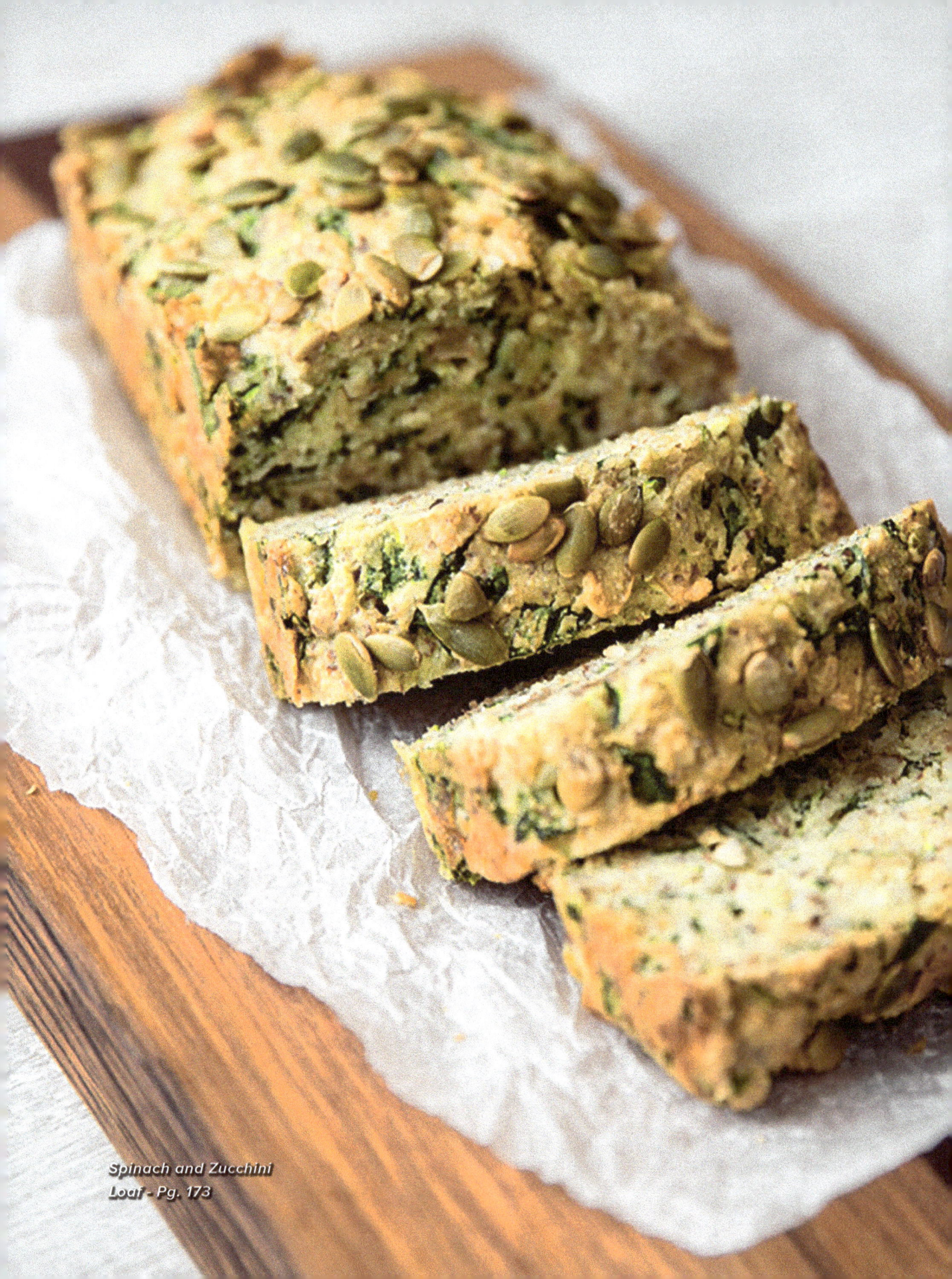

Spinach and Zucchini
Loaf - Pg. 173

Peanut Butter-Stuffed Raspberry Muffins

Miriam Haug @mealsbymiri

'I love peanut butter, I love berries and I love stuffing things,' laughs vegan recipe developer Miriam Haug. And thus, with those wise words, these oozy, peanut butter-filled muffins were born.

While baking was never her strong suit in the kitchen, Miriam admits that muffins were always something she could get right. That makes this recipe perfect for the novice cook who's just beginning to experiment in the kitchen.

Miri suggests having these on hand as a grab and go snack, or else topping them with some vanilla coconut yoghurt and raspberries for an after dinner treat.

Vegan

Ingredients

1 tablespoon flaxseed

210 millilitres (7 fl oz) almond milk

100 grams (3½ oz) banana

10 grams (0.3 oz) lemon juice

100 grams (3½ oz) whole wheat flour

150 grams (5 oz) plain flour

1 teaspoon baking powder

1 teaspoon baking soda

1 teaspoon cinnamon

1 teaspoon cardamom

¼ teaspoon salt

1 teaspoon vanilla extract

50 grams (1½ oz) raw sugar

100 grams (3½ oz) frozen raspberries

9 teaspoon salted peanut butter

You can use fresh or frozen berries for this recipe, just be mindful that if they're thawed they'll colour the batter as you mix them in!

Method

Preheat your oven to 200°C (400°F). Start by making your flax egg. Mix your flaxseed with 2 tablespoons of water in a small bowl and leave to set until it forms a thick paste.

Mash your banana in a bowl until smooth, then add in your flax egg, almond milk, lemon juice and vanilla extract and whisk to combine.

In another bowl, sift in your plain flour, whole wheat flour, baking powder, baking soda, cinnamon and cardamom. Add in your salt and sugar and mix to combine.

Pour the banana mixture into your flour. Add your raspberries and gently fold until no large dry lumps of flour are visible. Try not to crush up the raspberries too much in this process, otherwise they will colour the batter.

Line a muffin tray with squares of baking powder, or spray lightly with oil.

Spoon a tablespoon of muffin batter into each lined muffin tin and make a well in the centre. Add 1 teaspoon of salted peanut butter into the centre and cover with another 2-3 tablespoons of muffin batter. Repeat until all the batter has been used.

Bake in the oven for about 20 minutes, until cooked through and slightly golden.

Leave to cool before serving.

Makes 9 muffins

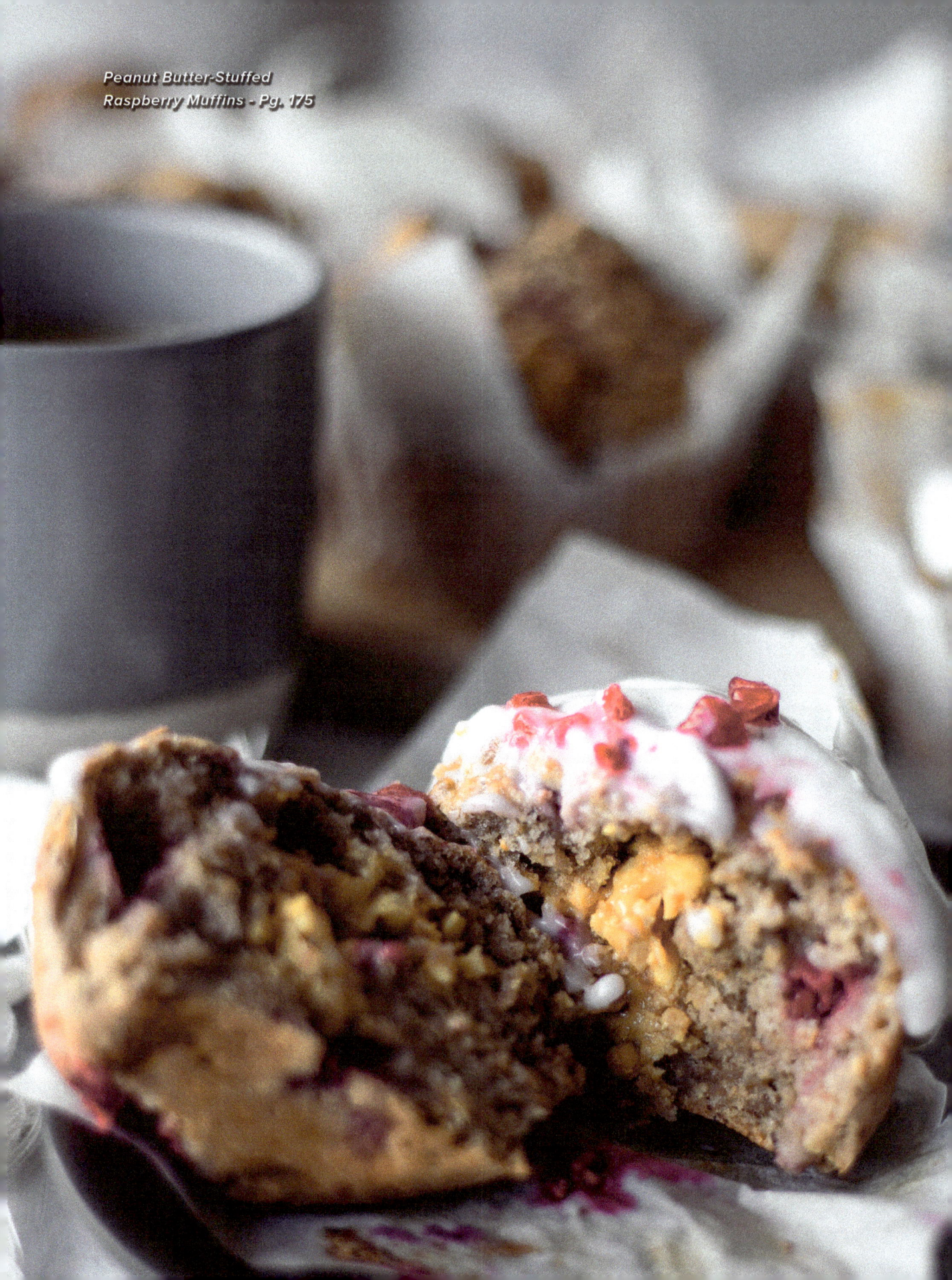

Gluten Free PB & J Muffins

Aliza Strock @shaktifresh

If you suffer from a gluten intolerance and thought we'd forgotten about you, don't worry, we've got the perfect PB & J muffin combo just for you.

After moving from Boston to Australia, personal chef Aliza Strock missed the American flavours she had grown up with as a child; most noticeably, Peanut Butter and Jelly.

'I had PB & J sandwiches most days for lunch, even into my teenage years,' says Aliza. 'But I don't think I really appreciated it as a flavour combination until adulthood when I was experimenting with food a lot more.'

There's something about the combination of salty peanut butter with the sweet homemade jam that's just addictively good. 'I love to slice one of these muffins in half when it's still a little warm and slather a bit of extra peanut butter or vegan butter on them,' Aliza admits with a sly grin.

She uses almond meal and gluten-free baking soda in this dish to make it coeliac-friendly. This makes them a little denser than your traditional muffin, but adds more fibre and protein along with a delicious nutty flavour.

Vegan, gluten-free, dairy-free

Ingredients

For the jam

300 grams (11 oz) frozen raspberries

½ cup black or white chia seeds

¼ cup maple syrup

For the muffins

1 cup gluten free baking flour (Aliza recommends Bob's Red Mill)

1 cup almond flour

½ cup coconut sugar

1 teaspoon baking soda

1 teaspoon cinnamon

¼ teaspoon sea salt

Method

Preheat your oven to 180°C (350°F).

To make the jam, place frozen berries in a container and let thaw completely. Once thawed, place in a bowl and stir through maple syrup.

Slowly add chia seeds to the berries and syrup, whisking the mixture to prevent clumps. Let this mixture sit for 10 minutes, then whisk again. Set aside.

In a large mixing bowl, combine all the dry ingredients with a wooden spoon.

In a smaller mixing bowl, peel and mash bananas before adding in the rest of the wet ingredients, including your chia or flax egg, and mix well to combine.

Add wet ingredients to the dry, and use a wooden spoon or silicone spatula to mix until well combined.

Continued over page.

3 very ripe bananas

¼ soy or unsweetened almond milk

2 tablespoons creamy peanut butter

2 tablespoons maple syrup

1 teaspoon vanilla extract

1 chia or flax egg (1 tablespoon of chia or flax + 2 ½ tablespoons water, left to sit for 5 minutes)

You may need to add more liquid at this stage, in which case just add a little bit at a time until you have a sticky batter.

Stir ½ cup of your raspberry jam through your batter. You can store the remainder in a container for up to 2 weeks in the fridge.

Transfer the batter into a non-stick muffin tin, or a tin lightly greased with vegetable oil.

Bake in the oven for 30 minutes or until a toothpick comes out of the centre of a muffin cleanly.

Once cooked, remove from the oven and let the muffins cool slightly before serving.

You can keep muffins in a container in the fridge for up to 5 days, or freeze them for the perfect on-the-go snack.

Makes 12 muffins

Substitutes

If you have a peanut allergy but tolerate tree nuts, you can easily substitute the PB for almond, cashew or walnut butter. If nuts aren't your thing, sunflower seed or pumpkin seed butter will do the trick!

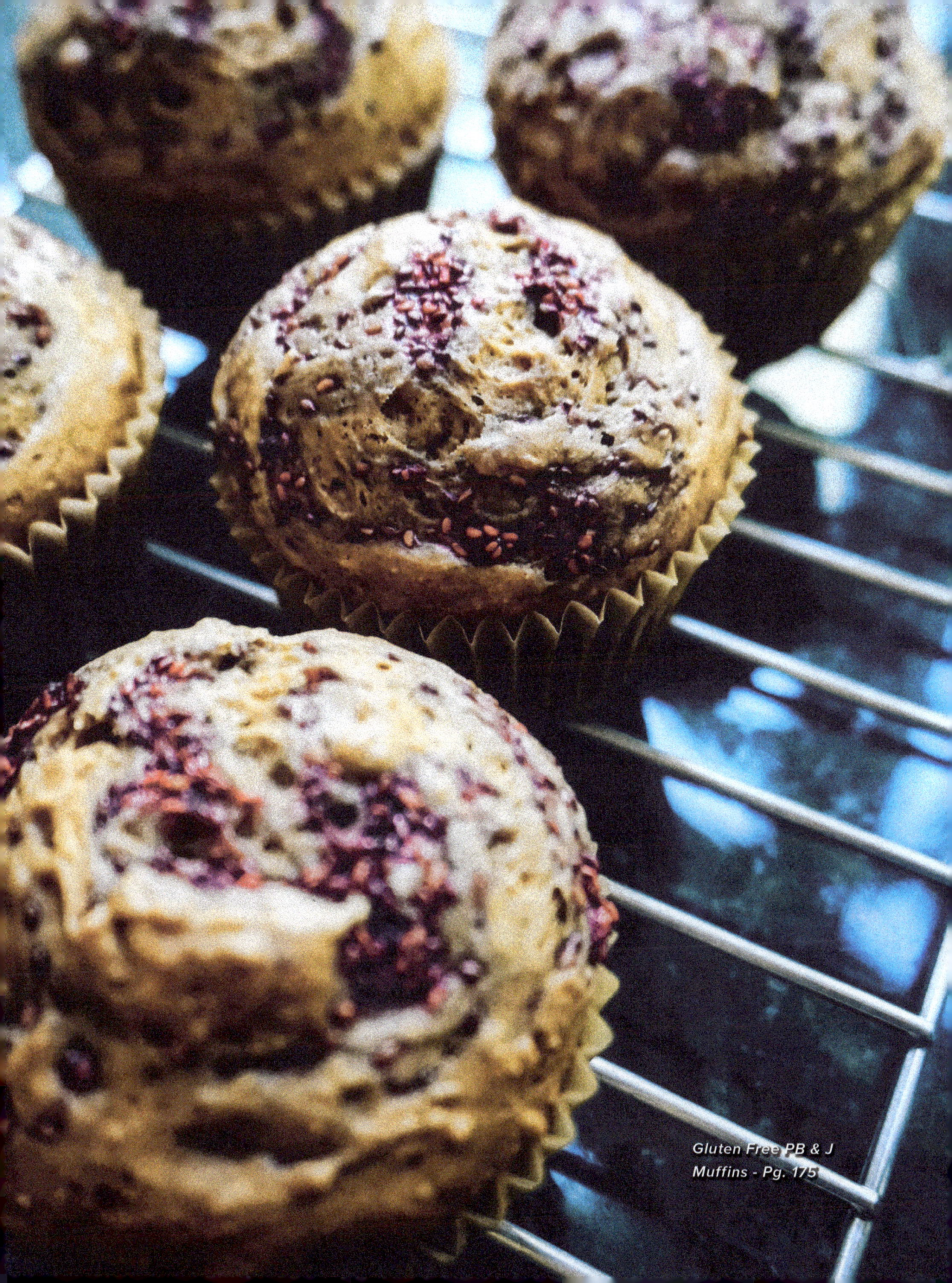

Gluten Free PB & J
Muffins - Pg. 175

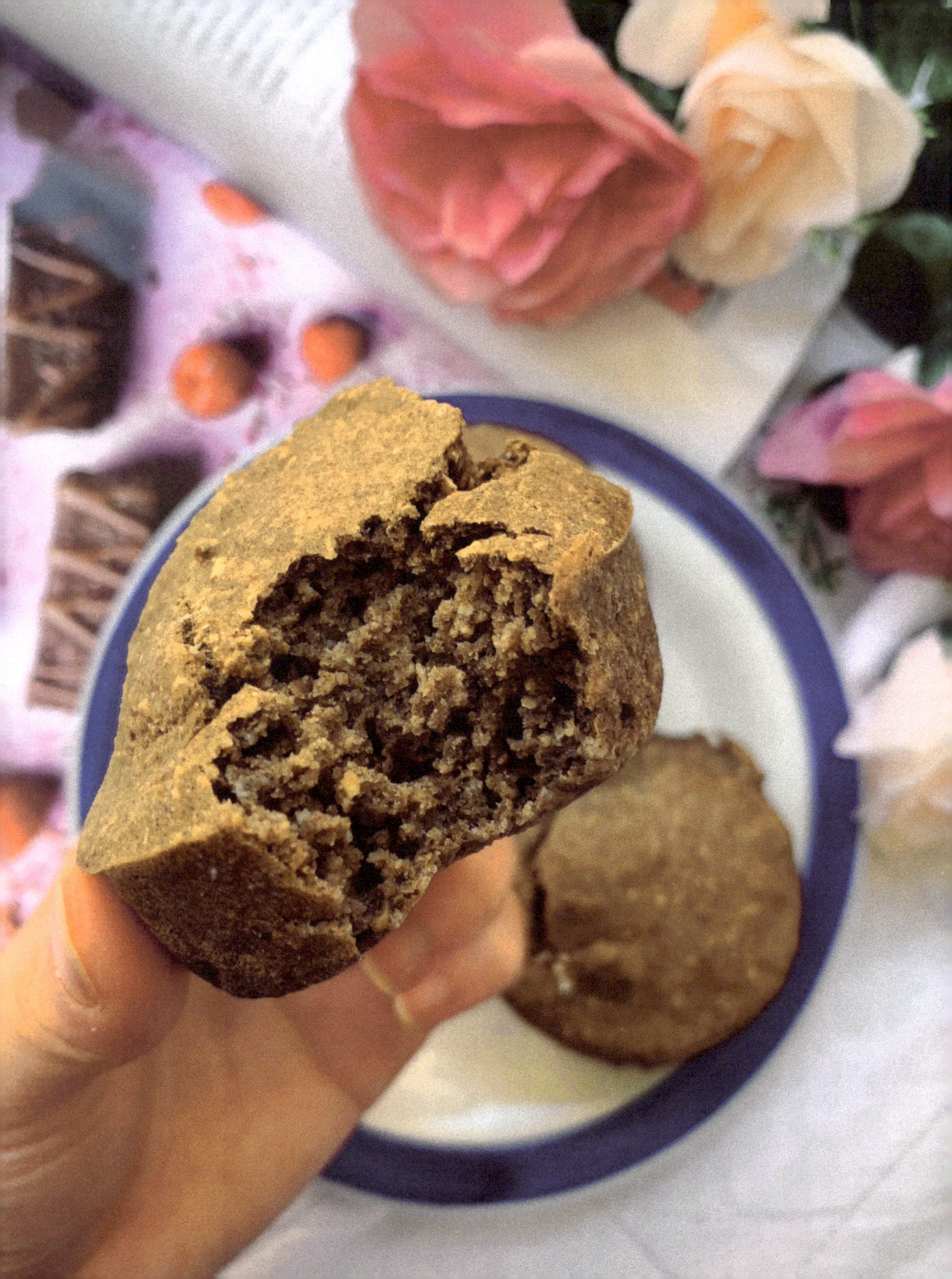

Chocolate Protein Muffins

Sabrina Lu @nourishfulsabrina

Having healthy homemade snacks on hand is a great way to keep energy levels up during the day and is also a good way to save yourself some money.

'I always have snacks with me when I go out', says Melbourne food blogger Sabrina Lu. 'I can't think clearly when I'm hungry, I get easily annoyed and I wind up spending so much money on food!'

Sabrina has created a muffin recipe which is incredibly adaptable, so she recommends adding whatever flavours you love most to the base ingredients and making it your own.

Vegan, dairy-free, refined sugar-free

Ingredients

Dry ingredients

1 cup self-raising wholemeal flour (or flour of choice)

1 scoop chocolate protein powder

1 teaspoon baking powder

2 tablespoons sweetener of choice (Sabrina uses Stevia)

1 tablespoon cacao powder

¼ teaspoon of salt

Wet ingredients

1 tablespoon olive oil/melted coconut oil

1½ cups plant based milk

Method

Preheat your oven to 200°C (400°F).

In a large bowl, combine all the dry ingredients and mix well.

Add the wet ingredients into the dry mixture and stir well with a wooden spoon until a thick batter forms. If your batter is looking too dry, add more milk a little at a time.

Spray a muffin tin with oil and scoop your mixture into 6 muffin holes. Don't over-fill them as they will rise slightly.

Put the tray into the oven and bake for 15 minutes.

After 15 minutes, poke the centre of a muffin with a toothpick. If it comes out clean, they're cooked. If the toothpick comes out with batter on it, pop the muffins back into the over and check every couple of minutes until cooked through. The muffins will feel a bit soft when you first remove them from the oven, but they'll firm up once cooled.

Let muffins cool in the tray for 10 minutes before removing them, then place on a cooling rack to cool completely.

Makes 6 muffins

Vegan Garlic Scrolls with Tomato, Spinach, Olives & Feta

Jessica Thomson @mindfullyjessica

Would you believe that Perth-based recipe developer Jess Thomson was in the kitchen making pizza scrolls from the age of 11? And while this recipe is a healthified, plant-based version of the scrolls she made when she was young, baking them is still a process she finds incredibly cathartic.

'This dish is so nostalgic for me,' Jess says. 'I remember going to my Nana's house and smelling freshly baked bread and wanting to replicate that for myself.'

'People might think baking bread is difficult, but it's really just a series of simple steps. I would tell people to take time making it, slow down and enjoy the entire process; the smell of the dough, feeling it as you knead it. That's what cooking is all about.'

Jess says you can be creative and add your own flavours to these scrolls, but this combo is her all-time favourite.

Vegan, dairy-free

Ingredients

Dough

250 millilitres (8 fl oz) warm water

½ teaspoons sugar

1 teaspoons yeast

360 grams (12½ oz) flour (plus more to knead with)

1 teaspoons sea salt

2 tablespoon olive oil

Filling

2 cloves of garlic

Method

In a small bowl, add the warm water and sugar and mix to dissolve. Add the yeast, stir and put aside for 5-10 minutes.

Add the flour and salt to a large mixing bowl. After around 5-10 mins add the yeast mixture and the olive oil to the flour. Mix well to combine and then place on a floured surface and knead for a few minutes. Lightly form into a ball of dough.

Place the kneaded dough in a lightly oiled bowl and flip the ball of dough around so it is covered in oil. Let the dough sit in a warm place for around 1 hour or until doubled in size.

Transfer the dough onto a floured surface or a piece of baking paper. Using a rolling pin, roll the dough into a roughly 25x30 rectangle.

1 tablespoons vegan butter, softened

1 teaspoon mixed herbs

4 olives, chopped

2 tablespoons red capsicum, finely diced

½ a tomato, finely chopped

½ cup spinach, shredded

¾ cup dairy-free shredded cheese

Mix the the butter, garlic and mixed herbs together in a small bowl, then spread evenly over the dough. Place the olives, capsicum, tomato, spinach and cheese evenly on top of the dough, leaving a 5cm (2") space border.

Roll the longest side of the dough up towards the other side of the dough, to form a log.

Preheat the oven to 200°C (400°F).

Slice your dough log into 3-4 cm (1-2") thick slices. Arrange the slices onto a baking tray lined with baking paper. Allow them to rise for another 30 minutes and then bake in the oven for around 20 minutes or until golden.

Makes 8-10 scrolls

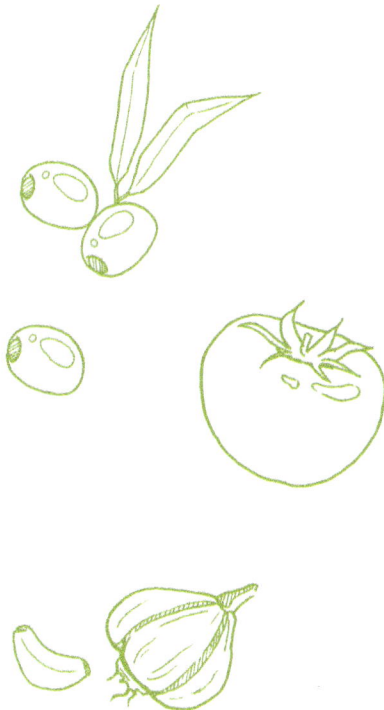

Vegan Garlic Scrolls
with Tomato, Spinach,
Olives & Feta - Pg. 182

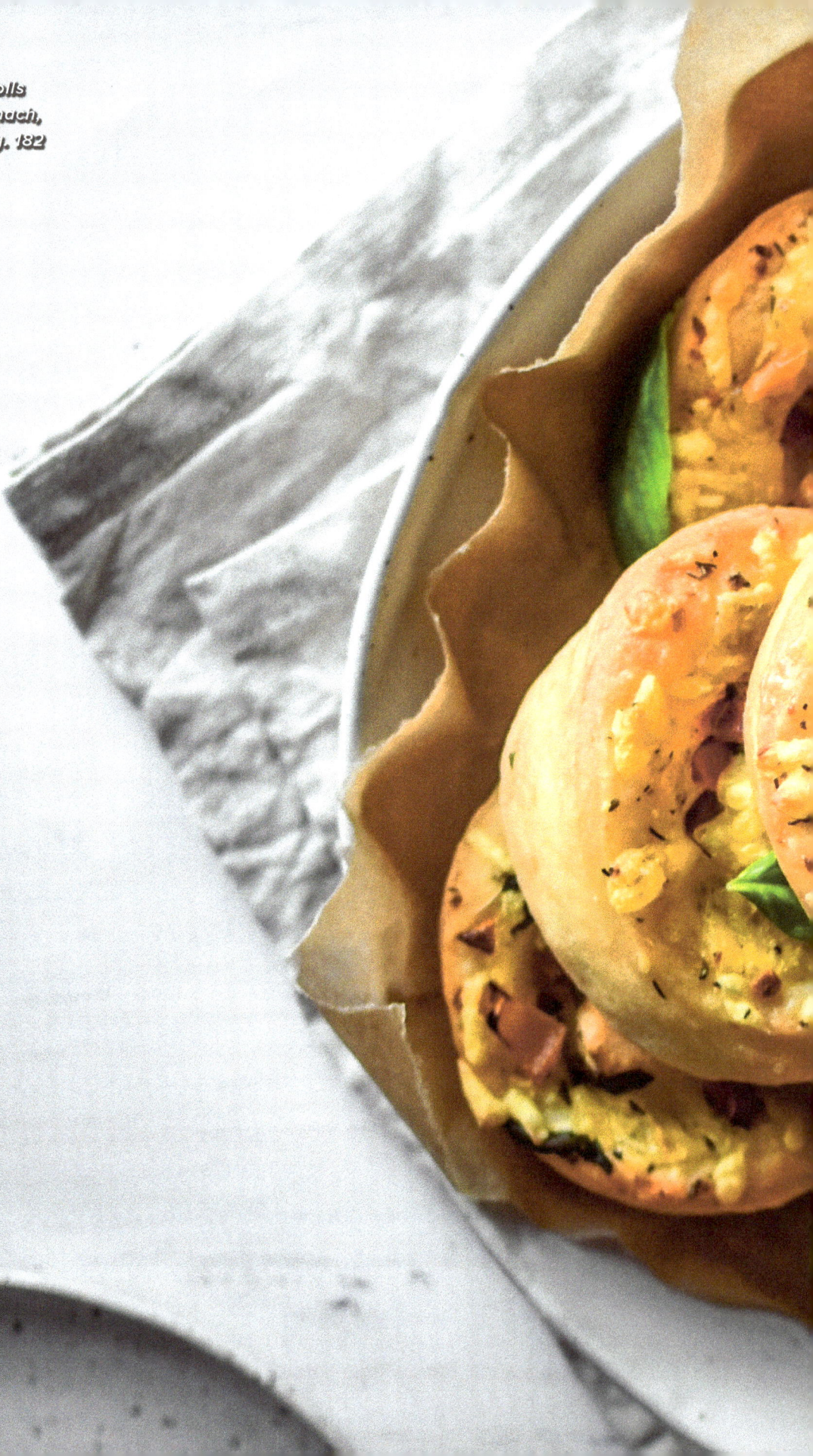

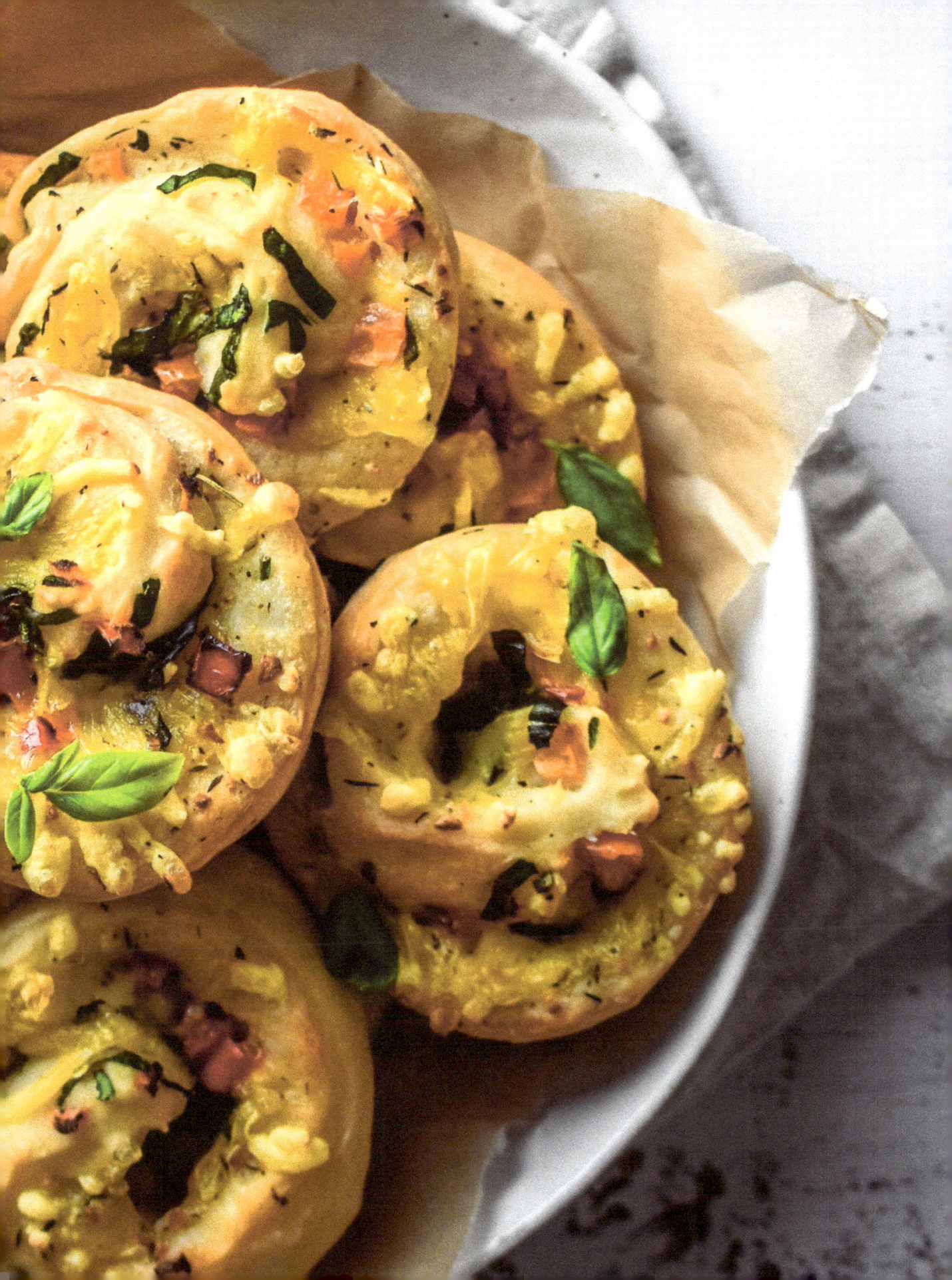

Mini Vegan Quiches

Michelle Chen @run2food

Raised with Chinese parents who didn't enjoy cooking Western food, passionate foodie Michelle Chen was forced to learn to cook for herself when she became vegan. One place she always tuned to for inspiration was popular cooking program Master Chef, which always sparked her creativity.

'I saw an episode where contestants had to make a quiche, so I wanted to try and replicate a vegan version of this, which was quite a challenge as they're typically made with eggs, milk and butter,' she says.

Containing chickpea flour, this is a great high-protein savoury snack that's ideal for vegans or those who can't eat eggs and dairy. Feel free to add whatever vegetables, herbs and vegan cheese into the mix.

Vegan, gluten-free, dairy-free, refined sugar-free

Ingredients

2 cups of chickpea (besan) flour

2 ¼ cups of water

2 tablespoons nutritional yeast

1 teaspoon dried parsley

2 cloves of garlic, minced

1 small carrot, finely diced

½ onion, diced

½ zucchini, diced

½ cup of corn kernels (cooked)

1 teaspoon sea salt

Method

Preheat your oven to 160°C fan-forced (325°F). Line your muffin tins or spray them with oil.

In a large mixing bowl, combine the chickpea flour, water, nutritional yeast, parsley and 1 clove of minced garlic. Mix well and set aside.

Add a dash of oil to a pan on medium heat and sauté the remaining garlic with the carrot, onion and zucchini until soft and cooked through. Season with salt to taste.

Add the cooked veggies and corn kernels to the chickpea flour batter and fold the mixture together until the vegetables are well combined.

Divide the batter evenly among the muffin tins and fill until almost level to the top. Place muffin tin into the oven and bake for about 15 minutes.

Turn up the heat to 180°C (350°F) and bake for another 5 minutes until the tops of the quiches are beautifully golden.

Remove from oven and cool before removing the muffins from the tin.

you may choose to add in whatever you like into the batter i.e. different variations of veggies, vegan ham or vegan cheese etc.

Makes 16 mini quiches

Beetroot Hummus

Gabrielle O'Dea @nourishtheday

There was a general consensus among us that hummus is life. For this reason, it was difficult choosing just one hummus recipe to include in this book, but the pretty radiant pink of this beetroot hummus by Gabrielle O'Dea sold us.

'I really want to encourage people to include more legumes in their diets,' explains the Adelaide-based dietitian. 'They have such a wealth of important nutrients, like protein, zinc, and fibre, but I think a lot of people aren't quite sure how to cook with them. Hummus is a simple, delicious stepping stone to eating more.'

'You can eat this snack anyway you want. With crackers, spread on sandwiches, served on a cheese board - but I often just stand at my fridge and dig straight in with some fresh veggie sticks,' Gabby laughs.

Vegan, gluten-free, dairy-free, refined sugar-free

Ingredients

½ large beetroot, grated (about 1 cup)

1 x 400 gram (14 oz) tin chickpeas (or 1¼ cups cooked), drained

3 tablespoons extra virgin olive oil

1 clove garlic

Juice of 2 limes or 1 lemon

1 heaped tablespoon tahini

Salt and pepper

Cumin and fresh mint, to serve

Method

Place all the ingredients in a blender and blend until you reach your desired consistency. Blend for longer if you like a smoother hummus, or less if you like it to be a little chunkier.

Season to taste with salt and pepper. This is lovely finished off with a garnish of fresh chopped mint and a sprinkle of ground cumin.

Makes 2 cups

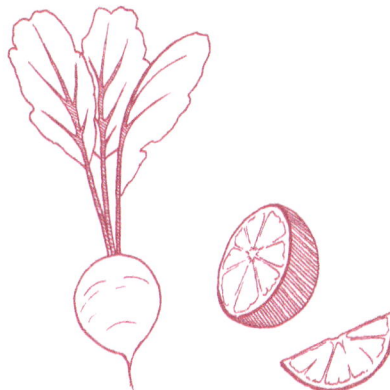

*Beetroot Hummus
- Pg. 187*

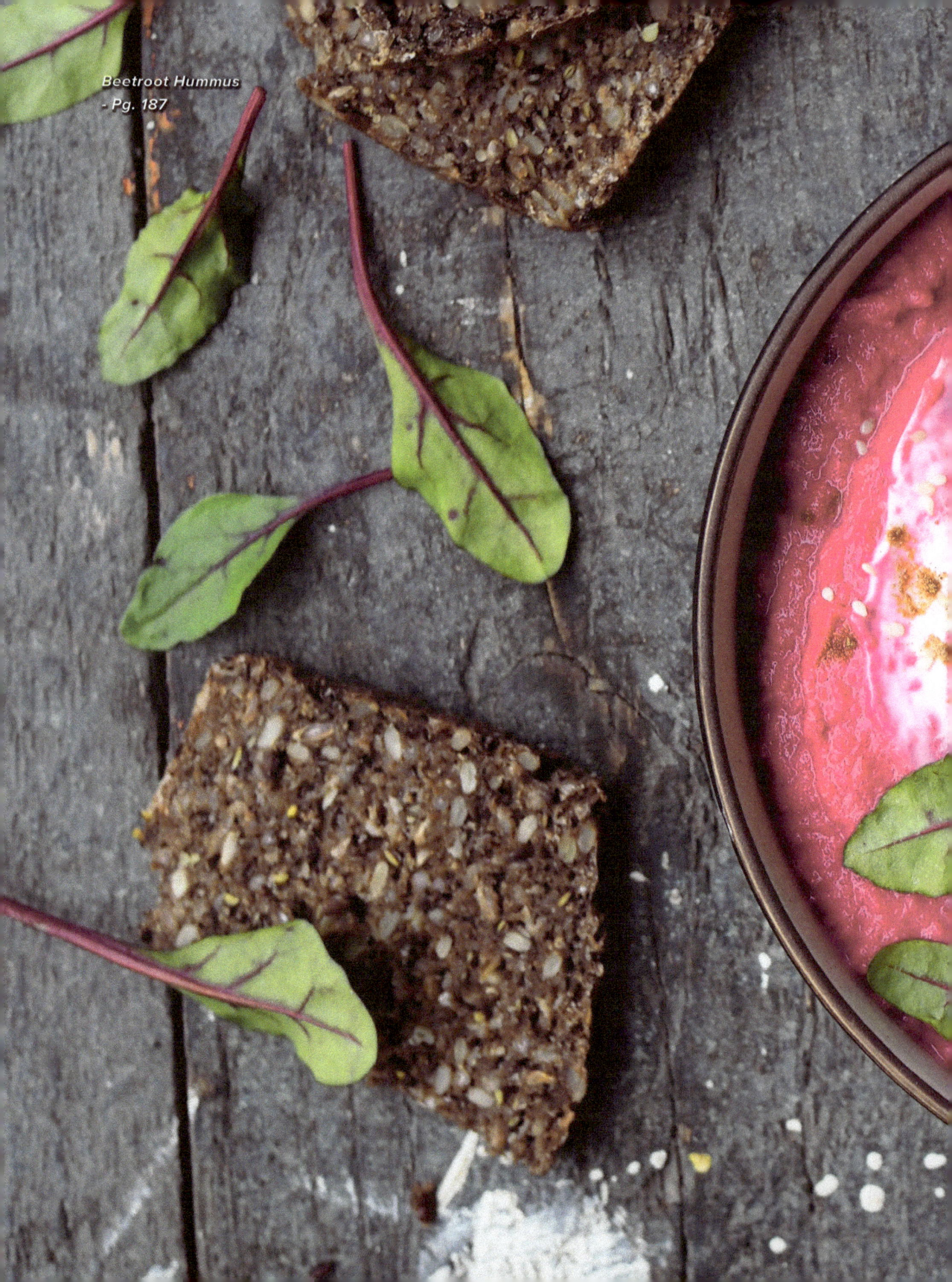

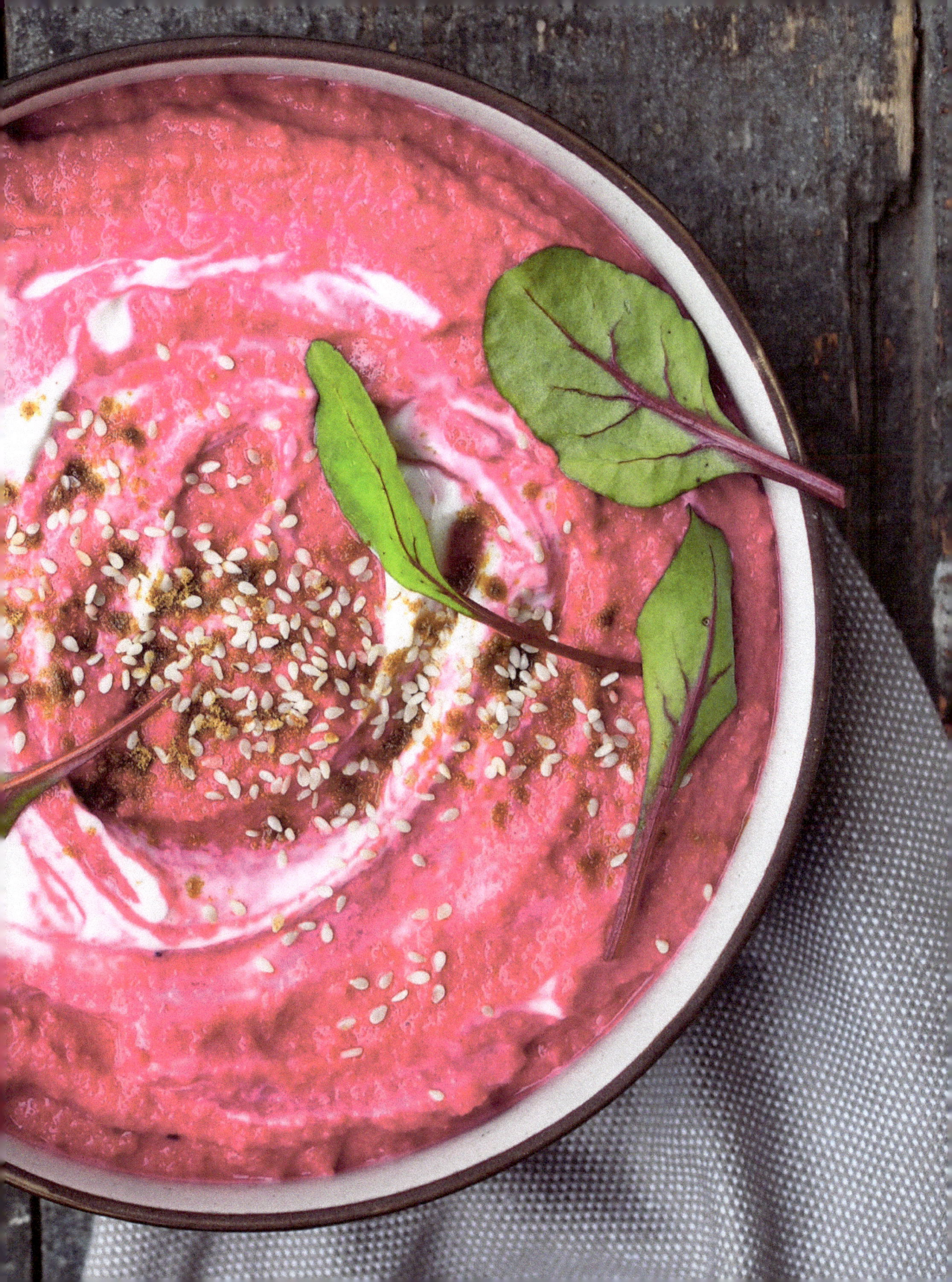

Ally Sheehan on Why it's Cool to be (Self) Kind

Ally Sheehan @agirlnamedally

Though 'Self-Love' may be a buzzword right now, we can't emphasise enough the importance of showing yourself kindness and compassion. For so many years, women in particular, have been made to feel as though we must be constantly selfless, always giving and putting the needs of others before our own. More often than not, this leaves us feeling exhausted, depleted and, perhaps worst of all, completely ignorant to what it is that our bodies and minds really need. Often, anything less than this self-effacing behaviour is seen as "selfish", as if in some way by not giving 100% of ourselves to others, we're being self-centered or greedy.

We want you to challenge this notion, instead thinking of self-respect and compassion as a way that you can better your lived experience and the world in which you live.

'Once you learn to speak to yourself from this place of kindness, you can open up your heart, mind and soul to all of your potential,' says YouTuber, content creator and councillor, Ally Sheehan.

'It's so important to see that when you come from a place of self-love, you can really achieve anything because you don't have negative thoughts or self-doubt holding you back. You can't reach your full potential when you're stifling yourself, and unfortunately this is something a lot of women are doing, because that's how society positions us to feel,' she explains.

Ally grew up in Melbourne and developed a passion for nutrition and wellness at a young age, having been raised in a health-conscious family. As her dedication to wellness progressed, so too did her influence as a blogger, and she found many young girls turning to her for advice and assistance regarding their negative relationships with food. What Ally noticed was an enormous lack of self-worth and self-compassion occurring amongst this group of women, who were feeling an increasing pressure to be 'perfect' - always healthy, happy, fit, smart and kind to others. In striving to reach these unattainable goals, many were manipulating food and exercise, as they felt they weren't "deserving" of food and adequate nourishment.

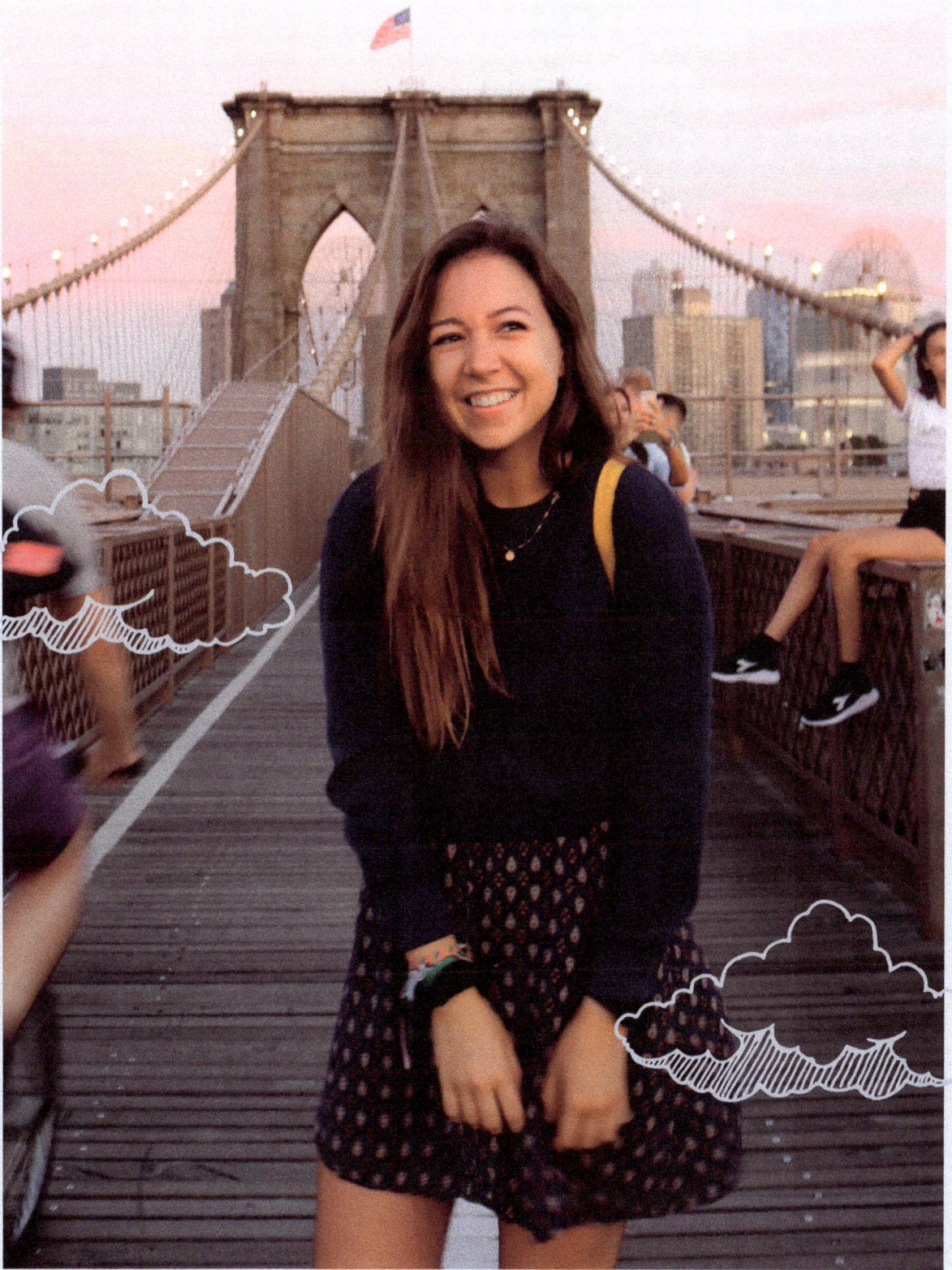

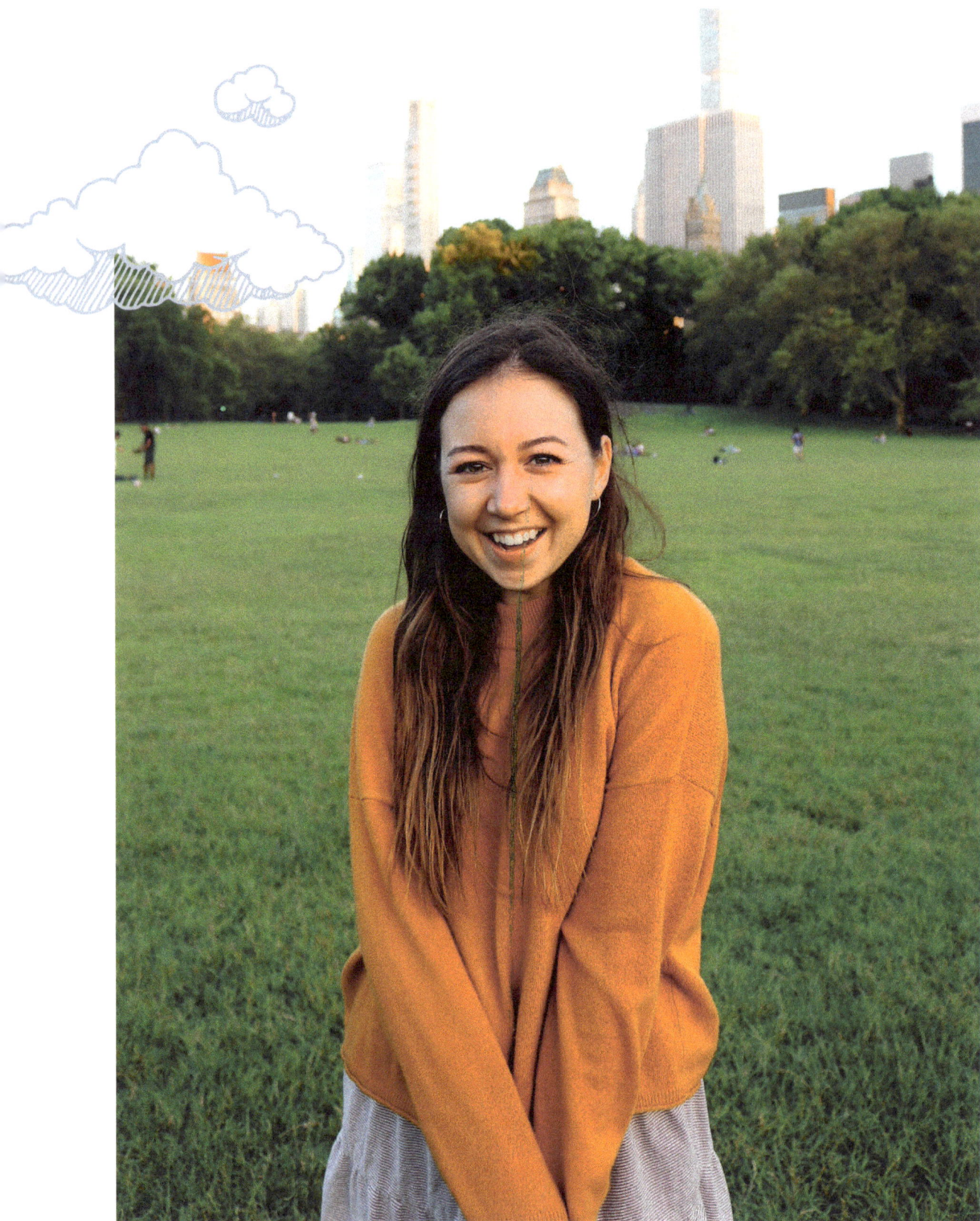

'I started to see the flip-side of nutrition,' Ally says. 'There was a whole other world where young women had exceptionally damaging relationships with food that was seeing them restrict and under-nourish themselves because they didn't feel worthy of proper nutrition.'

'Our society and the media talk about food as though it's something we need to "earn", as if you need to be some kind of perfect human in order to deserve eating. That's not the case; if you are human, you deserve to eat. And you deserve to eat freely without fear or judgement.'

'I want to help inspire women to take care of themselves, be kind to themselves and live in a way where they don't have to be constantly wondering whether they're worthy or deserving.'

Ally has since gone on to complete a degree in Psychology at the University of Melbourne, which has led her to become a councillor to young women and boys both in Australia and America.

Recognising & Asking for Help

According to Ally, self-love and compassion starts with recognising when you need help - and then asking for it. This is something she struggled to do for years, keeping her from being diagnosed with depression long after it had begun. Much like the notion that women need to earn the right to eat, so too are we made to feel as though asking for help is something we just shouldn't do. As if it's indulgent or self-centered to assert when we're not coping emotionally.

'I didn't want to reach out because I was in denial, I didn't think I was "allowed" to be depressed, because it wasn't who I was or who I thought people wanted me to be,' explains Ally. I was always supposed to be the happy one. Being positive was so intrinsically tied to who I was.' This very much fits into the external pressure we receive to appear to be coping, happy and abiding

to a certain stereotype laid out by society. If you feel like you can't reach out to family or friends without looking selfish or for fear of being labelled an attention seeker, know you're not alone.

Thankfully, Ally believes it is slowly becoming more accepted to talk about mental health difficulties you may be experiencing. What's important to remember, she adds, is that no one should be unkind to themselves for feeling a certain way. Just as anyone can break their leg, anyone too can feel sadness, anxiety or struggle to cope when life gets hard.

'I would say to anyone experiencing any level of fear, sadness, depression or anxiety that even if it doesn't feel serious, you deserve help,' she says. 'Reach out for assistance because people will want to help. You deserve their support and you deserve to be happy.'

Food & Self-Love

The manipulation of food and exercise seems to be an increasing way in which women of all ages cope with a sense of low self-worth and general dissatisfaction. Food in itself is a symbol of life. It's a tool by which we can nurture ourselves and show ourselves kindness. Just the very act of feeding yourself shows that you believe you are deserving of energy, growth and possessing a strong life force. But for so many of us, it's difficult to even contemplate deserving these wonderful things.

A good place to start when it comes to improving your self-compassion and kindness then, is to begin healing this relationship with food. Rather than looking at food as something that needs to be deserved, think about it as fuel you're giving yourself in order to be the very best version of yourself. After all, a car can't function without servicing and good quality petrol and your body is just the same.

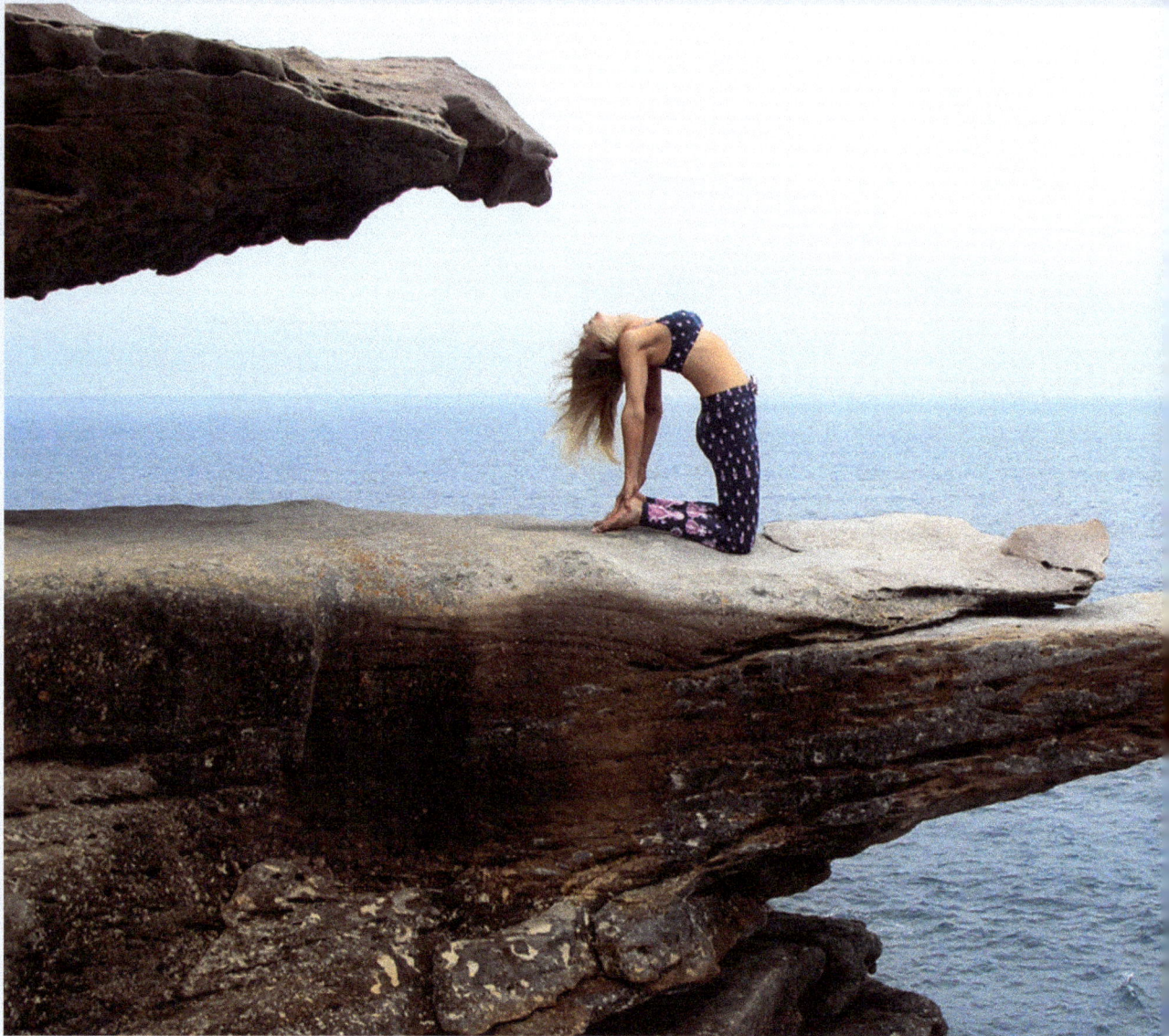

Ally suggests that if you find you're judging yourself for eating certain foods, or even for just enjoying food, try and talk to yourself as you would to a friend. 'We would never say some of the nasty things we say about ourselves to a close friend,' she says. 'You need to start treating yourself as though you are your own best friend.

This can be hard at first and you'll likely find that these negative comments often pop into your head without you even realising, but it's important to stop yourself and change the thought to something positive. It's this act of changing the thought that

actively begins to form new pathways in your brain that will, overtime, help you think more kindly towards yourself.'

What Ally refers to here is called manifestation; it's the act of making a thought or perception become real. Ally says this played a crucial role in her being able to practice self-compassion.

'A lot of young women came to me and would say that they wanted to be happier with who they were, but none of them were actually trying to change the negative thoughts they were having about

Photographer: Louisa Seton

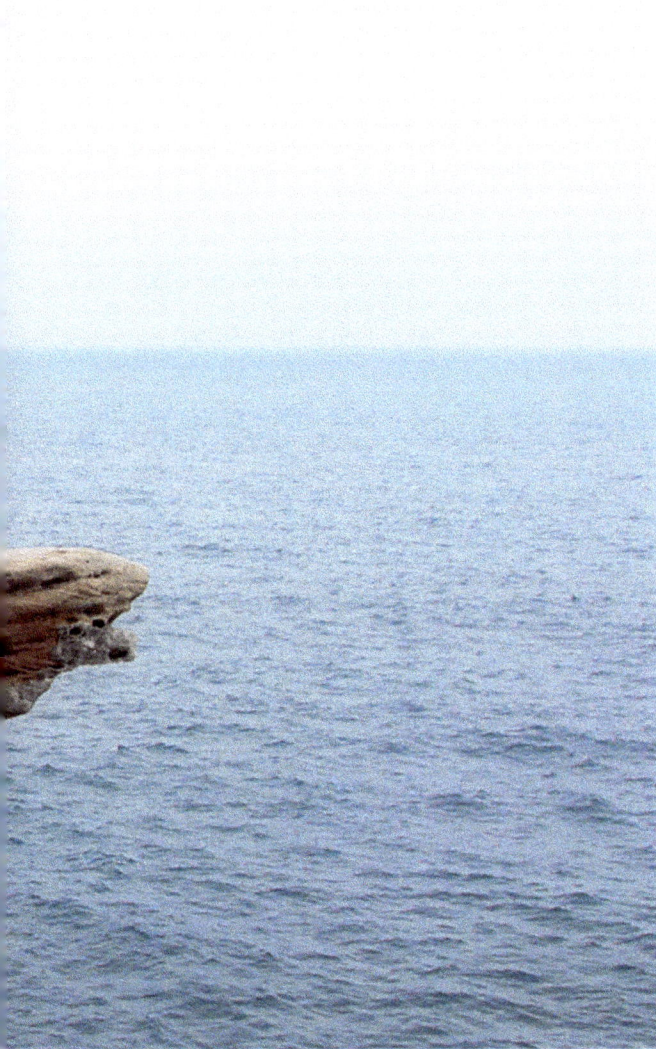

that's normal, but your constant thoughts of self-dissatisfaction are unlikely to remain. It sounds a little unbelievable, but there's a huge body of science behind this. When you do anything new, your neurons (the brain cells that transfer neurotransmitters for communication) form new connections with other neurons. This means that if for some reason one path can't be accessed (like when you block a negative thought), there are other paths that can be taken (the paths to positive thoughts). It also means that as you continue to use your positive thinking path, you continue to strengthen it.

Be Mindful on Social Media

Given the time we spend on social media, it's really important to be aware of the impact it can have on your mental health and wellbeing. And while we hope that you're able to recognise those accounts you may be following which aren't so helpful, we know it sometimes isn't so easy.

'There's definitely a way social media can be incredibly positive, but it really all does come down to who you follow,' says Ally. 'When you think about the content you consume, you really are what you eat. If you surround yourself with accounts and images that don't make you feel good, or that you're constantly comparing yourself to, then these are the messages you'll always carry around in your head. They become your world and your reality.'

What so many people don't realise is the incredible amount of editing, lighting, make-up and time that goes into creating some of these photos. The representation of life on social media is skewed, and this is something that's always so important to remember. The more you obsess about looking and being like someone else, the further you move away from self-acceptance and self-kindness. Instead of identifying your own beautiful qualities, you're demonising yourself for not having someone else's. But you will never be that person, just as that person looking back at you from your Instagram feed will never be you.

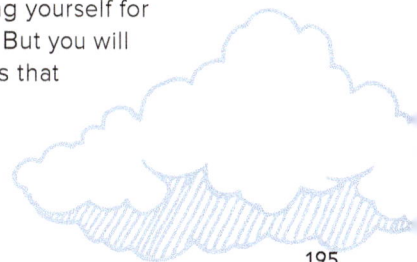

themselves. Instead, they were getting more angry and frustrated with themselves that they seemingly couldn't change the way they were thinking,' she says.

This is when, as Ally says, you need to "fake it till you make it". The idea being that if you change a thought - for example, "I don't like myself" to "I feel good about the person I am" - enough times, your brain will naturally begin to rewire itself to the point where those negative thoughts are no longer constantly present. Sure, you might still feel a bit down on yourself from time to time,

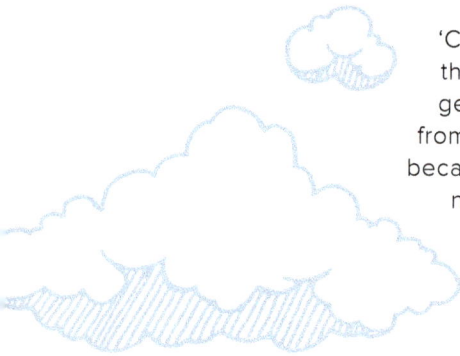

'Comparison is the thief of joy,' Ally says. 'It gets you further away from self-acceptance, because, in reality, you'll never be someone else and you'll never look like someone else. Because you weren't meant to! You were born the way you are for a reason, and there's a time in your life where you just need to come to peace with that.'

If self-kindness and compassion seems impossibly out of reach, don't worry, you're not alone. And reaching this place can feel like a really daunting challenge. But there are small changes you can start incorporating into your life which will help you move towards this place and away from negative self talk.

Here are some practical tips from Ally to help you start living a life that promotes self-compassion. She recommends aiming to incorporate one of these small acts of kindness into each day. It may feel uncomfortable at first, but eventually it will become natural.

1. The Only Good Detox is a Social Media Detox

Go through your social media accounts and ask yourself whether the photos you look at make you feel good about yourself. You may follow some accounts under the guise of 'fitspo', but if you find yourself making comparisons to the images in a way that makes you feel negatively about yourself, then unfollow them.

It can also be helpful just to give yourself a few hours of time away from your social accounts each day. Scheduling some time in your day to do this is a good idea, so that you can hold yourself accountable.

2. Spend Time with Loved Ones

Spending time with those who make you feel positive and supported will have an enormous impact on your overall mental health. If you surround yourself with kind and caring people who treat you well, you begin to see that this is the way you deserve to be treated.

Try to spend quality, face-to-face time with these important people in your life. We so often default to simply texting or messaging someone, but that doesn't stimulate the same kind of positive emotions as physical human interaction.

3. Eat Foods that Make you Feel Happy

We've become so consumed by what macro nutrients our food contains or what 'diet' we should follow, but food was never meant for that purpose. 'Food is for energy - it's the fuel that is our lifesource and is something to be celebrated, not manipulated', says Ally 'One of the best and simplest acts of self-kindness is allowing yourself to eat something you really, really want to without judgement and guilt.'

Try to see eating as a normal bodily function, just like breathing or blinking. You would never try to stop yourself from doing those things, so why do the same when you're hungry? Becoming hungry is your body's natural signal and is something we shouldn't try to ignore or repress. Listen to your body and give it what it's asking for.

4. Journal Your Thoughts

Journaling for just a few minutes each day is a fantastic way to get in touch with your own thoughts, to give them the space and time they deserve away from the stimuli of the outside world. Ally says she found writing in a journal as a way to better understand her feelings and issues that she was having trouble voicing to loved ones. Getting them down on paper first allowed her to clarify them and look at them with a more objective view.

5. Mindful Movement

Movement is a great way to give yourself a boost of endorphins when you're feeling low, but it always needs to come from a place of self-love and shouldn't be used as a form of punishment, Ally says.

Do something that you find joyful and makes your body and mind feel good. This could be walking your dog, doing a yoga class, playing a game of netball with your friends or taking a dance lesson.

Try to leave any step-counting or calorie tracking devices at home. While they can be helpful in specific circumstances, for most people this level of data analysis isn't necessary and can create even more judgemental thoughts about yourself.

6. Get Back to Nature

Have you ever felt inexplicably better about yourself and the world when you immerse yourself in nature? Well, there's actually some science to back up this phenomenon.

Back in 1984 a dude called Edward O. Wilson published his 'biophilia hypothesis' (also called BET), which suggests that humans possess an innate tendency to seek connections with nature and other forms of life.

Essentially, as humans we feel happy and healthy spending time in nature because of the genetic wiring of our brains. Neural pathways formed long ago (we're talking before dial-up modems were even a thing) that told our ancestors that being in nature - close to food, water and shelter - was 'safe'. These environments put the human brain into a state of calm, allowing it to rest and recover, rather than worry about staying alive.

While our stresses are very different to those of our distant ancestors (think paying your phone bill on time rather than running away from a raging wildebeest) similar rules apply. So if you're feeling stressed, overwhelmed or have lots of negative self-talk going on in your head, try to spend some time outside. 'You don't have to go for a hike up a mountain, a simple walk through your local park or sitting in your garden will do', Ally says. 'Inhale the fresh air and picture all the negative self-talk and judgement flowing out of you as you exhale.'

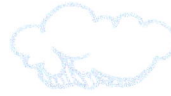

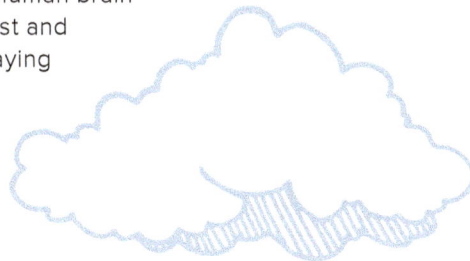

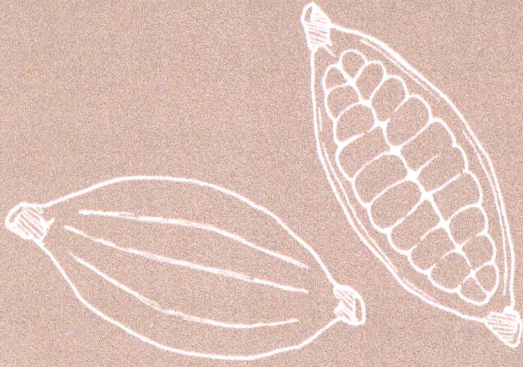

Desserts

This collection of recipes is here to show you that all foods can and should be included in a healthy, balanced diet. Many of these recipes will substitute white flour for wholemeal, raw sugar for agave and butter with mashed banana, so you're still getting a delicious sweet treat with the bonus of added nutrients.

That doesn't mean you always need to choose these healthier alternatives, but opting for these recipes over commercial choices will mean you get to make your raw vegan caramel slice and eat more of it too. And in our opinion, that can only be a good thing.

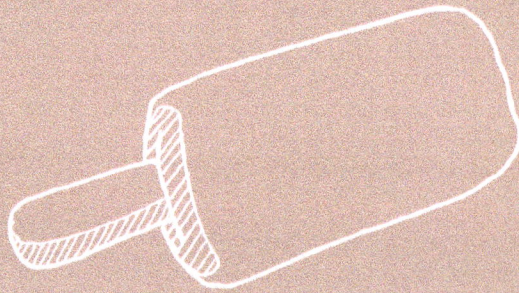

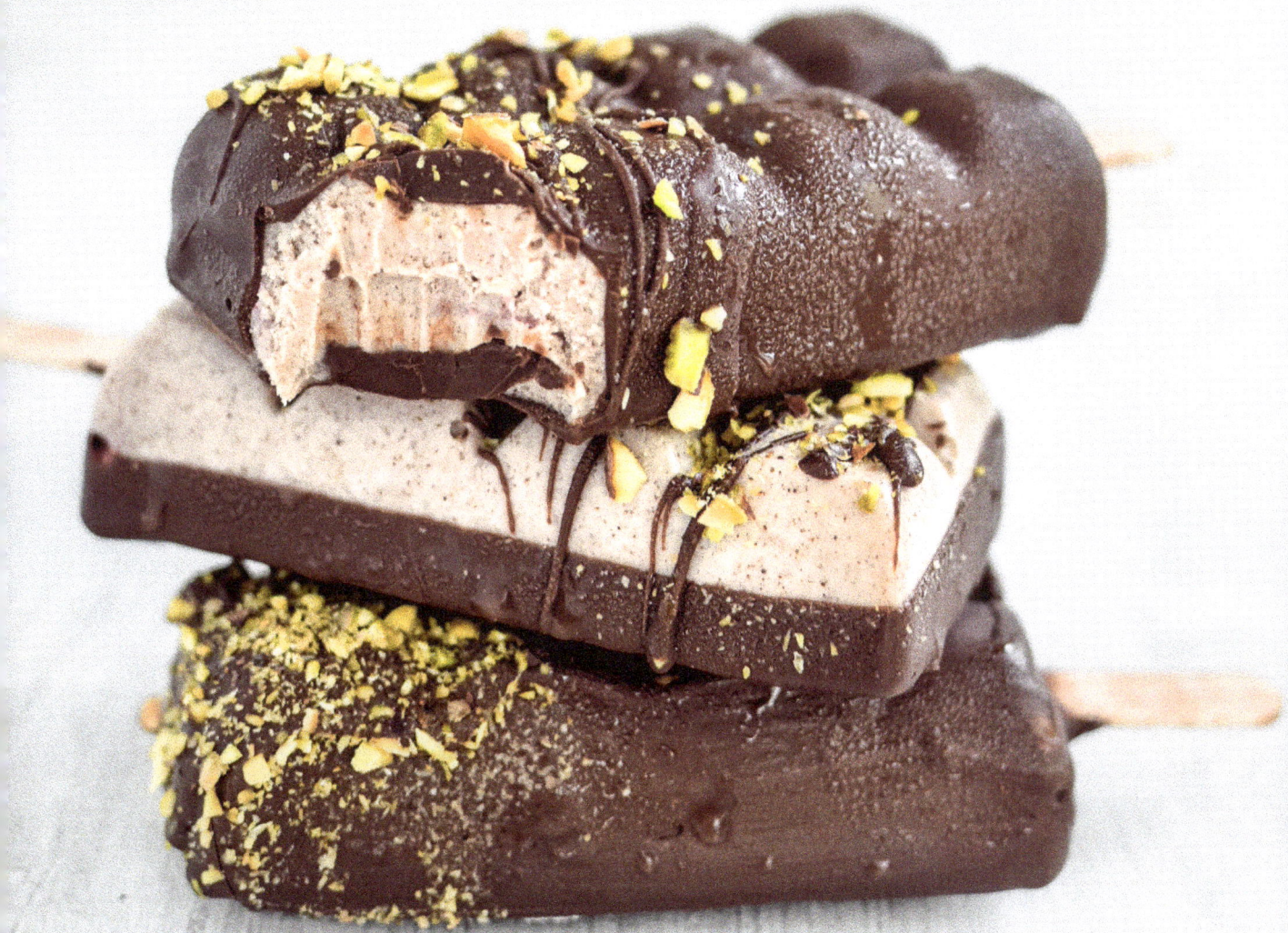

Pecan Caramel Tarts with Chocolate Sauce

Talida Voinea @hazel_and_cacao

Don't be intimidated by these incredibly pretty tarts. All you need is a high-powered blender and you'll be able to whip these up to impress your friends and family. But they're not just good looking, says Talida, the health food enthusiast behind the Hazel and Cacao blog, they're also incredibly rich in nutrients.

'The reason I love raw desserts is because you can pack so much nourishment into them,' she says. 'When you're dealing with hormonal imbalances like I was, nuts and seeds are your go to because they have the vitamins, minerals, protein and fat that you need to build up your hormone levels again.'

Vegan, dairy-free, refined sugar-free

Ingredients

For the base

1 cup rolled oats

½ cup pecans

½ cup cashews

2 tablespoons maple syrup

2 tablespoons sunflower oil

½ teaspoon cinnamon

¼ teaspoon ground ginger

Pinch of salt

For the filling

½ cup pecan butter

1 cup pitted dates

½ cup soy or almond milk

Pinch of salt

For the chocolate sauce

2 tablespoons cacao powder

2 tablespoons maple syrup

2 tablespoons melted coconut oil

Drop of vanilla extract

Method

Preheat the oven to 180°C (350°F).

For the base, process all the ingredients in a food processor until sticky.

Evenly press the mixture into the base and sides of 4 lightly greased tart pans and place in the oven to bake for 15 minutes.

For the filling, start by making the pecan butter. Roast the pecans for 10 minutes on a lined baking tray in the oven at 180°C. Whizz them in a food processor until they turn into a butter. This can take quite a few minutes, so be patient and trust the process!

Add pitted dates and almond milk to the pecan butter and blend until you achieve a thick and smooth consistency. Spoon out caramel over the cooked tart bases and spread evenly.

For the chocolate sauce combine all ingredients in a bowl and mix until smooth. Pour over the caramel layer of the tart.

Serves 4

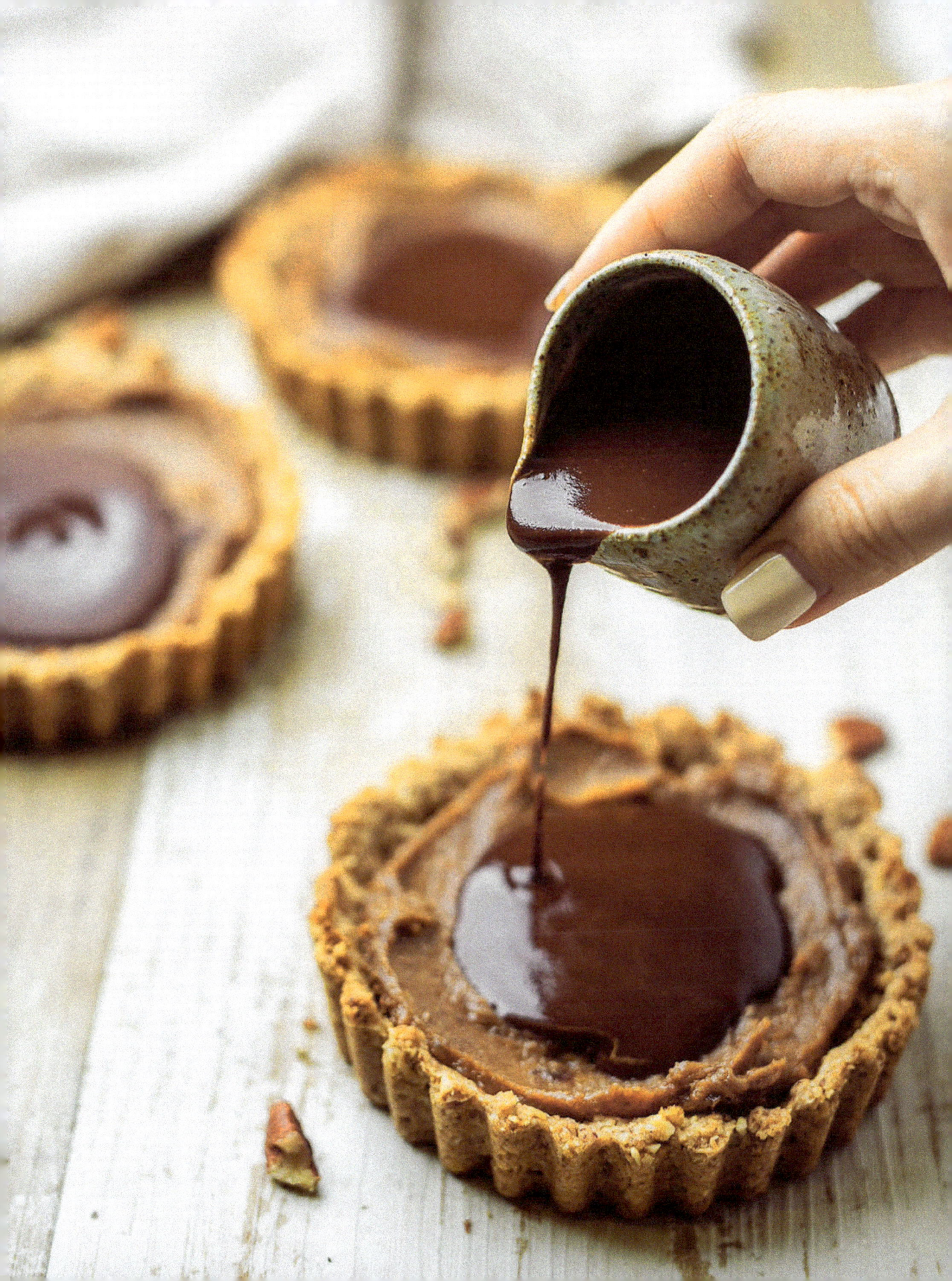

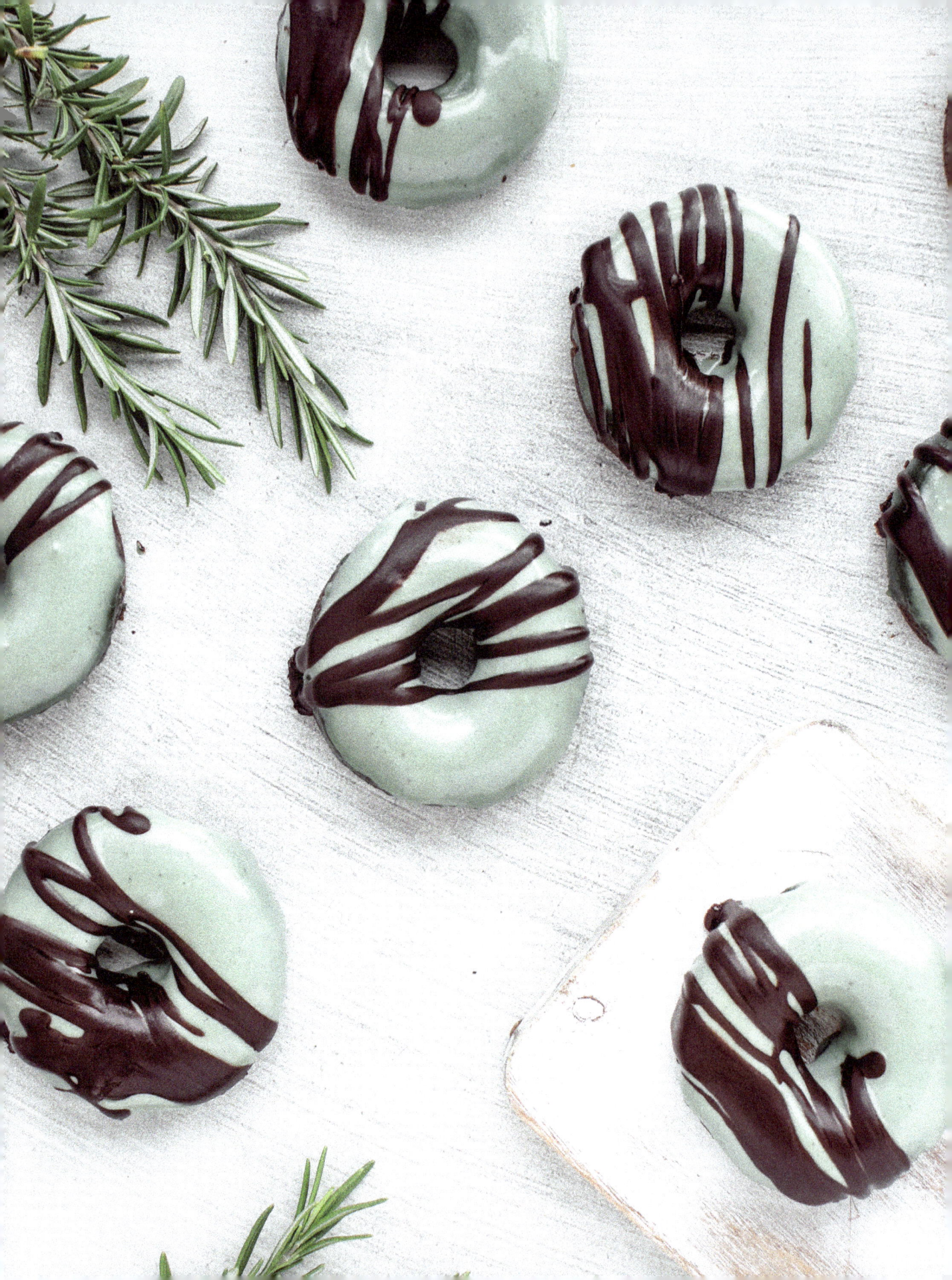

Chocolate Mint Donuts with Cashew Glaze

Zoe Lyons @wildblend

Confession time, guys. Recipe developer and food photographer Zoe Raissakis has never actually had a conventional fried donut. But somehow, despite this, her nutritious adaptation of the cult classic is moorish and delicious.

'I don't think I'm a donut lover, but healthy donuts are fun,' laughs Zoe. 'I love the shape, playfulness and I like to experiment with different glazes, flavours and colours.'

'I've always been passionate about food and became obsessed with styling food at a very young age. Whenever my mum hosted a dinner party she'd have me help with dessert and I'd spend hours creating and decorating.'

Vegan, gluten-free, dairy-free, refined sugar-free

Ingredients

For the donuts

¾ cup gluten-free oats

¾ cup almonds

12 Medjool dates, pitted

¼ food-grade peppermint essence

½ teaspoon vanilla bean essence

4 tablespoons cacao powder

Pinch of teaspoon sea salt

2 tablespoons plant-based protein powder (optional)

For the mint glaze

½ cup coconut cream

¾ cup soaked cashew nuts (soaked in filtered water for 3-4 hours)

2 tablespoon coconut oil

¼ cup maple syrup

¼ teaspoon food-grade peppermint essence

⅛ teaspoon vanilla powder

⅛ teaspoon liquid chlorophyll (or spirulina powder, optional for colour)

Method

To make the donuts, add the oats and almonds to a food processor and process into flour.

Add the cacao, protein powder and salt to the food processor and blend for a second so they're evenly mixed. Add the dates, vanilla, and peppermint essence and blend until you get a moist, thick dough that holds its shape.

Press the dough into a donut mould and place in the freezer until solid, around 1-2 hours.

To make the mint glaze, blend all ingredients (except the chlorophyll) in a high-speed blender until smooth. Slowly add the chlorophyll (if using) to the mixture until you get the green colour you want. Place the glaze in the fridge for at least 20 minutes to thicken before you dip the donuts.

Once solid, remove your donuts from the freezer and drizzle or cover with the mint glaze. Decorate as you please and store the donuts in an airtight container in the fridge or freezer.

Makes 14 donuts

Vegan Brioche Cinnamon Scrolls

Kitch Catterall @soybabie_

Growing up in England meant it was often dark and cold by the time Kitch Catterall got home from school. And while most of us might have plonked down on the couch to watch cartoons for the afternoon, Kitch headed straight for the kitchen.

'I used to get home from school and I would go straight to the kitchen and put some yeast in a bowl to start it rising for whatever creation I was going to cook,' she says. 'Growing up in a cold climate always made me crave comfort food, so I just wanted to bake all the time!'

Now living in Melbourne, the vegan food blogger still find something wonderfully therapeutic about dedicated her Sundays to baking a batch of these fluffy cinnamon scrolls. While she admits they're a little time consuming, one bite into these scrumptious, fluffy buns and you'll know they were well worth the effort.

Vegan, dairy-free

Ingredients

2 tablespoons yeast

60 millilitres (2 fl oz) warm water

3 tablespoons sugar + 1 extra teaspoon (to activate yeast)

1 cup vegan butter

1 cup soy milk (or other plant-based milk)

2 cups flour

Nuttelex, to grease

Cinnamon

Coconut sugar

Method

Start off by activating the yeast. To do this, combine the yeast, warm water and 1 teaspoon of the sugar in a bowl and leave to sit until the mixture becomes foamy and bubbly.

In a pan, melt the vegan butter with soy milk and the rest of sugar until combined. Don't let it bubble or boil, just melt the ingredients together until warm.

Remove from the stove and add one cup of flour and stir together. This creates a roux. Place your roux in a large bowl and let it sit for a few minutes to cool.

Add your bubbly yeast mixture and remaining flour into the large bowl with the roux and mix well to combine. You may need to add a bit more flour if the mixture if it's too sticky. You want the dough to be soft and bouncy.

Once all ingredients are combined, microwave a tea towel for 30 seconds and place over the bowl. Leave this to sit for an hour and go do something fun in the meantime!

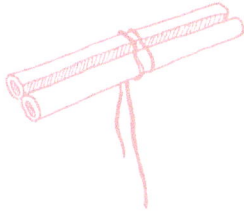

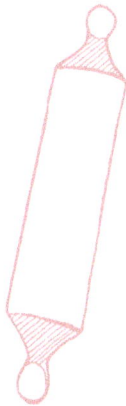

After an hour the dough should have risen and almost doubled in size. Remove dough from the bowl and knead for about 10 minutes.

Place the kneaded dough back in the bowl and allow it to stand for another hour, to let it expand again. Sometimes the dough doesn't expand however, which could be due to the temperature of your home. If this is the case, Kitch suggests placing the bowl over a pan of hot water and covering it with a towel to help achieve a light fluffy dough.

Preheat the oven to 180°C (350°F). Remove the dough from the bowl and place onto a floured surface. Roll out with a rolling pin until you have a large rectangle about 2-3 centimetres thick.

Rub nuttelex onto the side of the dough facing upwards. Liberally sprinkle with cinnamon and coconut sugar.

Begin rolling the dough horizontally in on itself to form a long dough roll. Gently rub nuttelex over the top of the dough.

With a knife, cut slices of the dough log into your desired width. Kitch finds thicker slices of dough work best and turn out more like the store bought varieties.

Place your scrolls onto an oiled or lined baking tray and leave again to sit and expand - there's a lot of this, but this is how you'll get fluffy scrolls!

Once the scrolls have increased in size, use spray oil to spray the tops of each then sprinkle over extra coconut sugar and cinnamon.

Place in the oven and bake for 20 minutes or until slightly golden.

Makes 6 scrolls

Vegan Brioche
Cinnamon Scrolls
- Pg. 204

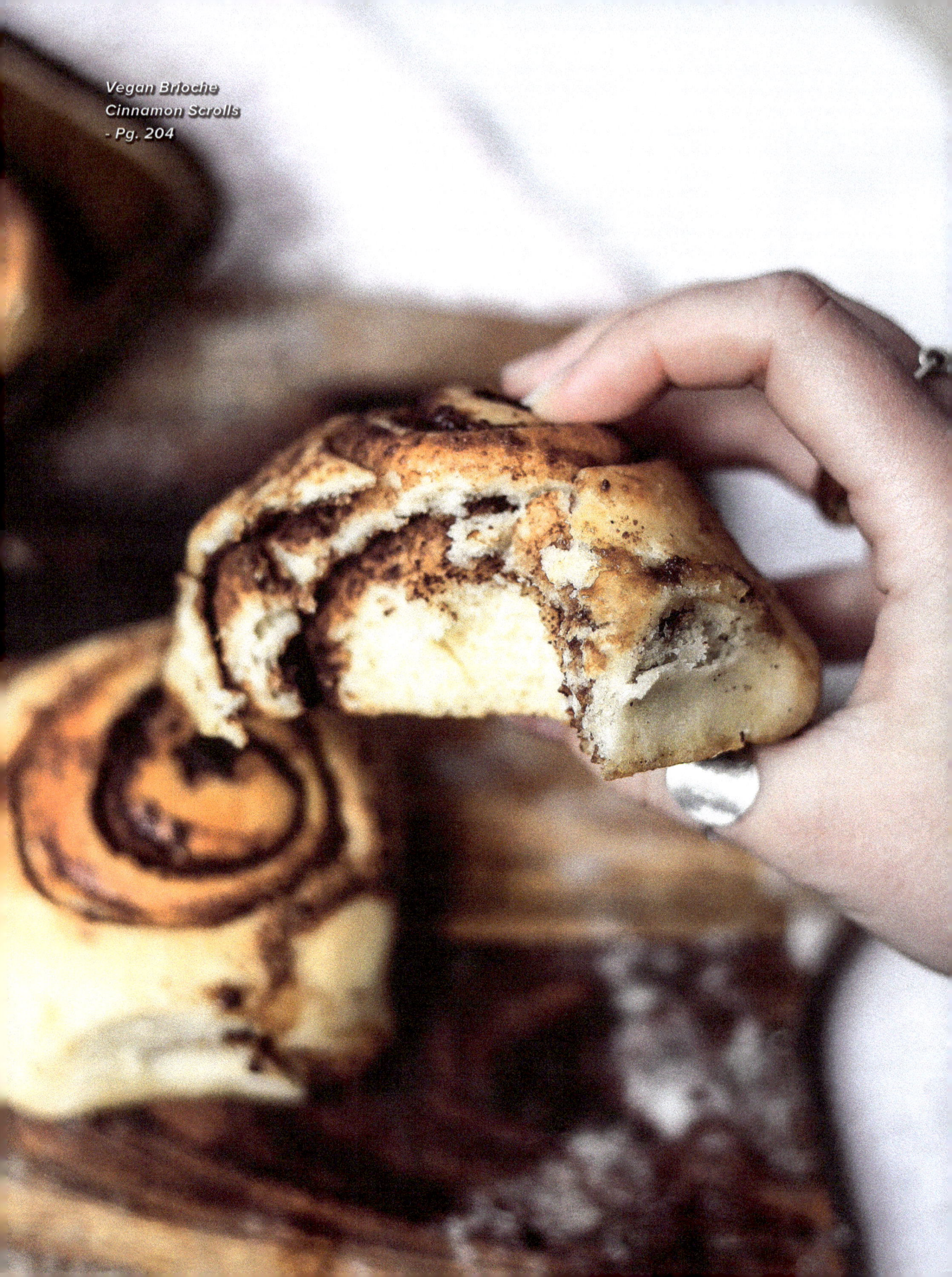

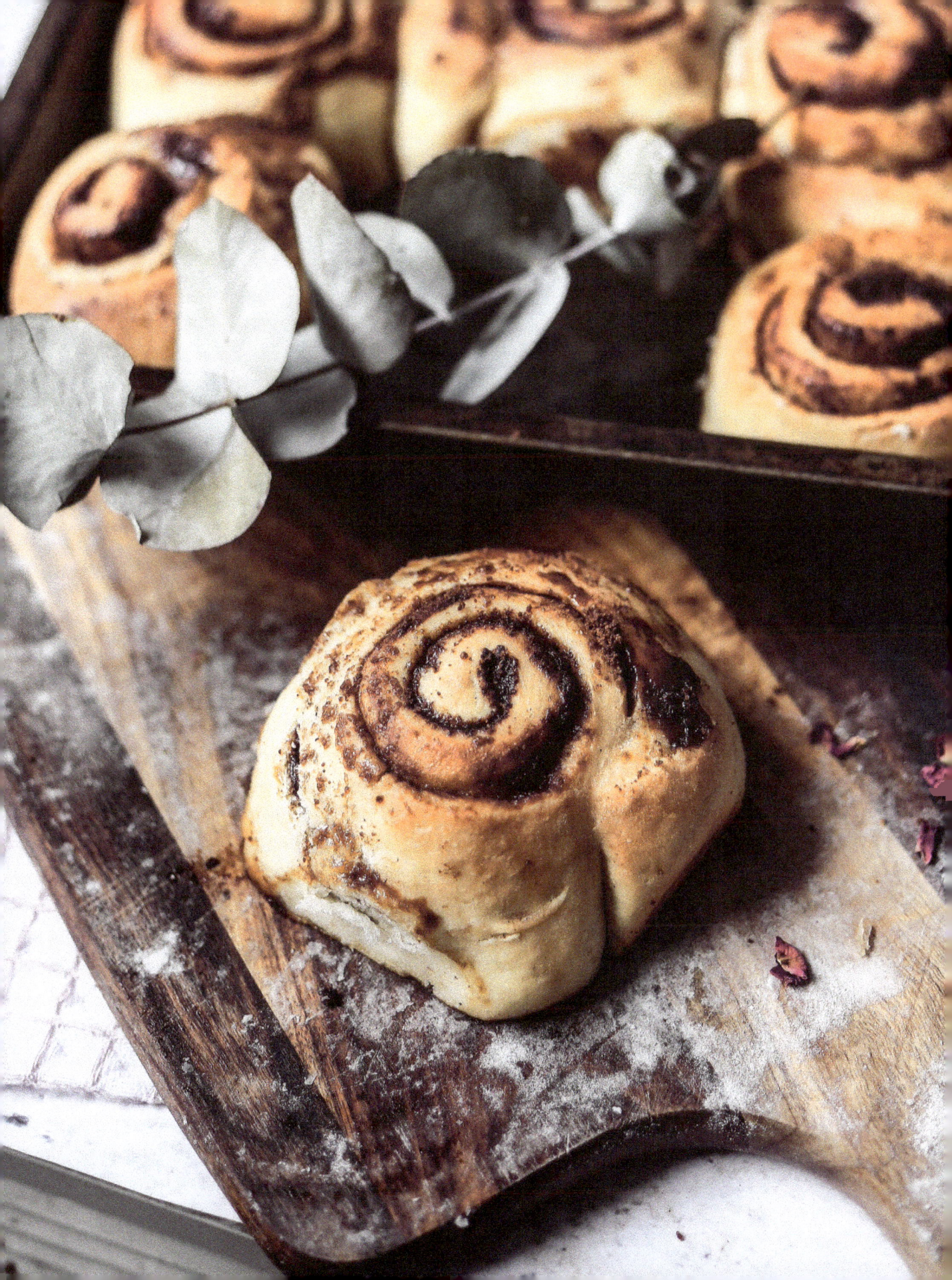

Vegan Lemon Slice

Lauren Mariano @lm_nutrition

When she was in high school Lauren Mariano would often walk past the bakery on her way home from school and pick up a piece of lemon slice as an afternoon snack. Now an accredited practising dietitian and personal trainer, Lauren had reimagined a more nutritious version of her favourite after school treat.

'I love being able to recreate sweets and desserts that contain more nutrients and less added sugar than the traditional versions,' explains Lauren. 'The combination of the toasty coconut with fresh, zingy lemon in this recipe is delicious - what's not to love!'

Vegan, dairy-free, gluten-free option, refined sugar-free

Ingredients

For the crust

¼ cup desiccated coconut

1 cup oats

1 cup almonds

½ teaspoon salt

½ cup medjool dates

2 tablespoons maple syrup

4 tablespoons coconut oil, melted

Method

First, do some prep. Soak raw cashews in boiling water for 30-60 minutes and preheat your oven to 180°C (350°F). Line 25cm x 25cm (10" x 10") tray with baking paper.

Blend coconut, oats, almonds and salt in a processor until a meal-like consistency.

Add the dates and process until the mixture begins to clump together. Add the coconut oil and maple syrup and process again for 30-60 seconds.

Transfer mixture to a lined baking tray and spread evenly. Place baking paper on top and use glass to press the mixture into the try firmly.

Place the crust into the oven and bake for 15 minutes. Increase heat to 200°C (400°F) and bake for a further 5 minutes, or until it starts to become golden brown. Remove from the oven and reduce oven temperature to 180°C (350°F).

For the filling

1 cup raw cashews

1 cup coconut cream

2 tablespoon plain flour

Juice and zest of 3 medium lemons

¼ cup maple syrup

50 grams (1½ oz) dark chocolate (optional for topping)

Drain the cashews and add to a food processor with coconut cream, flour, lemon juice, lemon zest, and maple syrup. Blend until you reach a creamy, smooth consistency.

Pour the filling over the baked crust. Place the slice back in the oven and bake for 25 minutes. You'll know when it's cooked perfectly, as the top will be quite firm.

Once cooked, remove from the oven and let the slice rest for 10 minutes, then refrigerate for 2-4 hours.

Melt the dark chocolate (if using) and drizzle over the slice. Cut into 16 squares and serve.

Makes 16 small squares

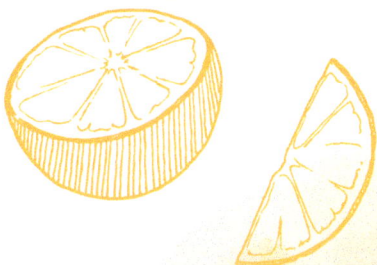

Substitutes

You can substitute the normal flour for 2 tablespoons of gluten-free oats or flour to make this slice gluten-free.

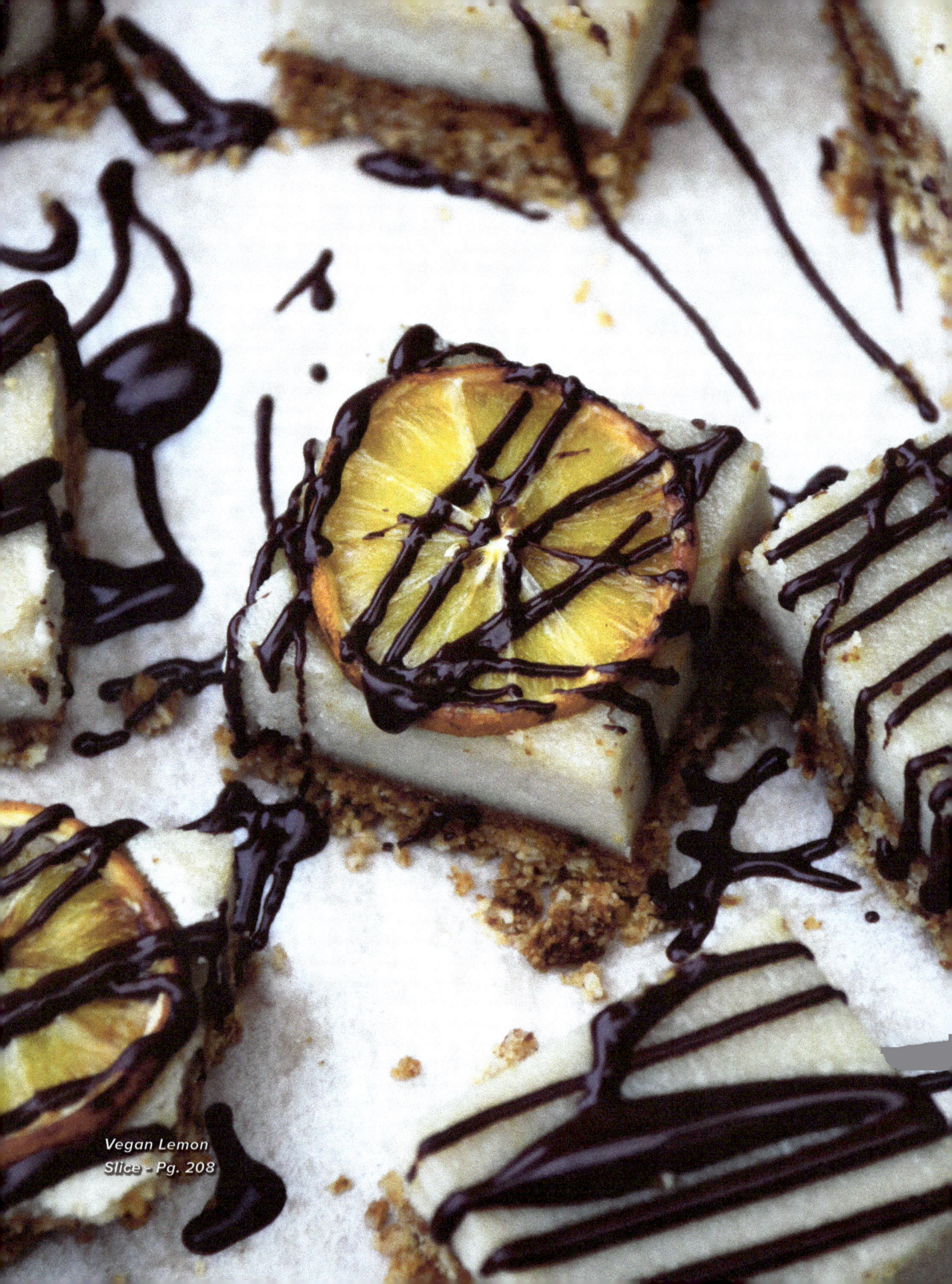

Vegan Lemon Slice - Pg. 208

Raw Mars Bar Slice

Jessica Thomson @mindfullyjessica

'This is one of my favourite recipes ever,' says vegan recipe developer, Jessica Thomson. 'I just love the combination of caramel and chocolate.'

Yas Queen!

When Jess was creating her eBook, *7 Slices of Heaven*, she asked her Instagram followers what recipe they'd like her to include. Unsurprisingly, a plant-based Mars Bar was the resounding winner, and so this dreamy dessert came to life.

The creamy caramel made with peanut butter coupled with a layer of decadent chocolate makes this slice a rich treat that will satisfy any sweet tooth and impress anyone who eats it.

Vegan, gluten-free, dairy-free, refined sugar-free

Ingredients

Base

¾ cup almonds

¾ cup pitted medjool dates

½ tablespoon cashew butter

½ tablespoon cacao powder

Pinch of salt

Nougat layer

⅔ cup cashew butter

¼ cup rice malt syrup

1 tablespoon coconut oil, melted

1 teaspoon cacao powder

Caramel

⅓ cup rice malt syrup

1 tablespoon peanut butter

Pinch of sea salt

100 grams (3½ oz) raw chocolate, melted

Method

In a food processor, add the almonds and process into fine pieces. Add the remaining base ingredients and process until a sticky mixture is achieved. Press into base of a lined cake tin, or silicone loaf tin.

Combine all the ingredients for the nougat layer in a bowl and mix until completely combined.

Spread the nougat layer over the base. Pop into the freezer to firm up a little, before you get ready to add the next layer.

Mix together the caramel ingredients in a bowl until well combined. Spread over the top of the nougat layer and place in the freezer to firm up for at least an hour. This will make it easier to slice!

After the hour, remove from the freezer and slice into bars. Return to the freezer to firm up again.

Meanwhile, melt the chocolate over a double boiler. Remove your slice from the freezer and dip the surface of each Mars Bar into the chocolate to coat completely. Return the slices to the tray and place back in the freezer to set completely - around 2 hours.

These are best kept in the freezer and left out for a moment or two to soften before enjoying.

Serves 9

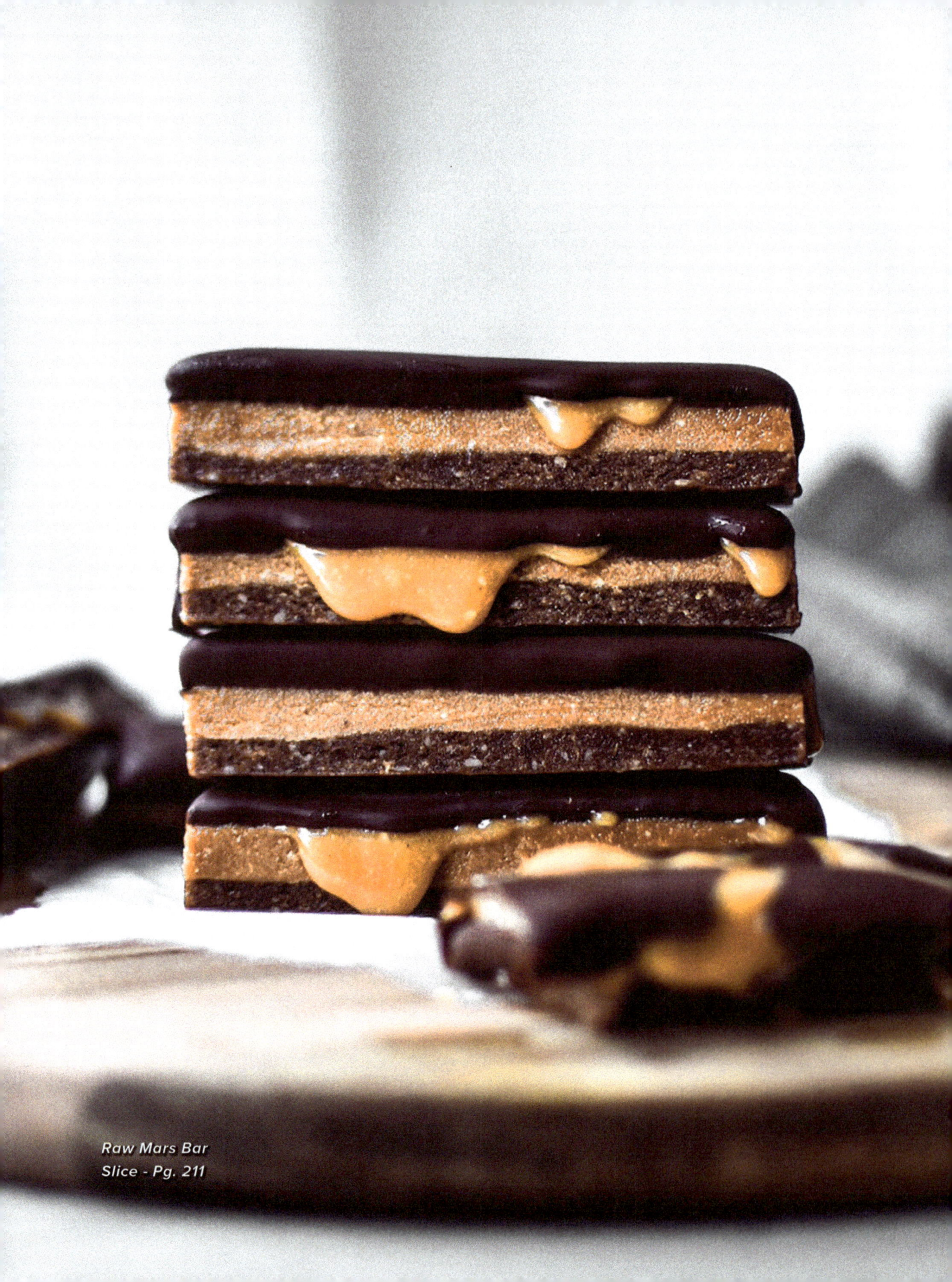

Raw Mars Bar
Slice - Pg. 211

Healthier Twix Bars

Jess Lirosi @jess_mycleantreats

An obsession with nutella in her early twenties drove Melbourne-based recipe developer Jess Lirosi in search of a more nutritious way to satisfy her insatiable sweet tooth. Her inspiration was sparked when she stumbled across a few vegan desserts online and the rest, they say, is sweet, sweet history.

This healthier Twix bar's ingredients might be far away from the processed store-bought version, but with its crumbly biscuit and gooey caramel it tastes just as good.

'I never want my desserts to taste "healthy"', laughs Jess. 'I want them to taste like the real deal. I love proving to people that you can create something that tastes rich and decadent while using more nutrient dense ingredients.'

Vegan, gluten-free option, dairy-free, refined sugar-free

Ingredients

For the biscuit base

1 cup flour of choice

½ teaspoon baking powder

Pinch of salt

¼ cup coconut oil, melted

¼ cup rice malt syrup

Dash of almond milk

Dash of vanilla extract

For the caramel

⅓ cup rice malt syrup

⅓ cup almond butter

⅓ cup coconut oil

Pinch of salt

Coating

200 grams (7 oz) 70% dark chocolate

1 tablespoon coconut oil

Method

Preheat your oven to 190°C (375°F) and line a baking tray with baking paper.

For the biscuit base, add all the dry ingredients to a large bowl and stir to combine.

In a separate bowl, combine the coconut oil, rice malt syrup, almond milk and vanilla extract and mix well. Make a well in the centre of the dry ingredients and pour in the wet mixture, folding it through until a biscuit-like dough forms.

Roll out the biscuit base with a rolling pin until it's around 1.5cm (½") thick. Cut out a thin, Twix-sized rectangle and repeat until all the dough has been used.

Carefully transfer the rectangles of dough onto your baking tray and place in the oven for 10 minutes, or until cooked through and slightly browned. Remove from the oven and allow to cool.

To make the caramel, combine all the caramel ingredients in a medium bowl and chill in the fridge for 10 minutes.

Continued over page.

Once the biscuit bars have cooled, add a tablespoon of caramel over each bar and mould with your fingers until it covers the entire bar, including all the edges.

Once each bar is covered in the caramel, place in the freezer for 20-30 minutes.

Meanwhile, microwave the chocolate with coconut oil in a heatproof bowl until melted. Dip each bar in chocolate using a fork until the bar is completely covered in chocolate.

Place the chocolate coated bars on a tray lined with baking paper. Repeat until each bar is coated in chocolate.

Place the tray back in the freezer for 1-2 hours, or until completely set.

You can store these in the fridge for up to 5 days, or the freezer for up to a month.

Makes 24

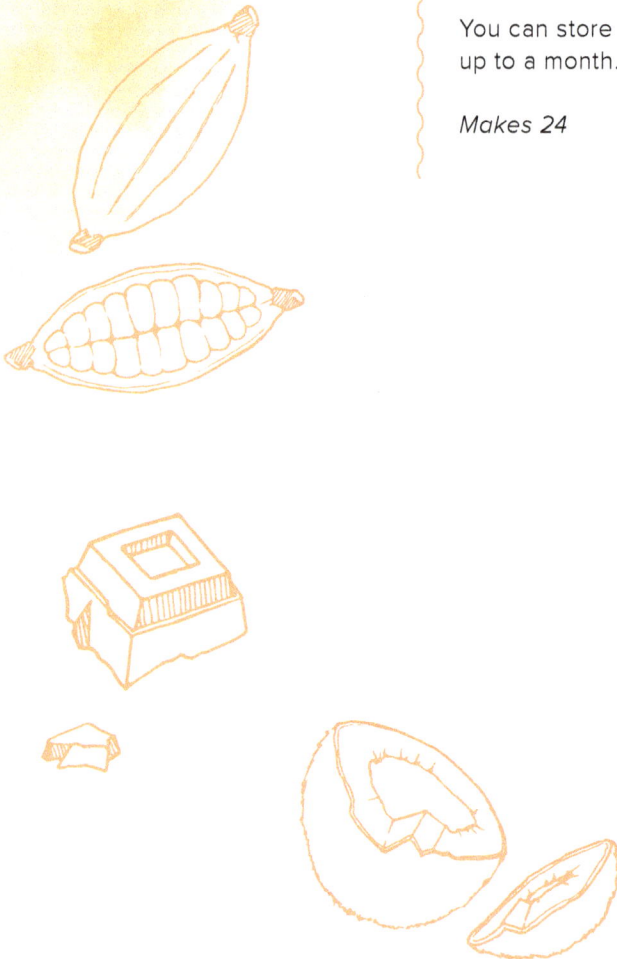

Rocky Road

Courtenay Perks @wholeremedy

Health coach and vegan recipe developer Courtenay Perks' daughters may look angelic, but point them at a plate of her healthier rocky road and chaos will ensue.

'My kids nick my rocky road straight off the bench and run around the house with chocolate all over themselves,' laughs the mother of four. Despite the mess, these delicious treats are something Courtenay still loves to make her family, especially around Christmas time.

Filled with nuts and fruit, there is something wonderfully festive about this chocolatey treat, though we're not suggesting you can only make it at Christmas. Filled with healthy fats and antioxidants, this is a recipe you should enjoy all year round!

Vegan, gluten-free, dairy-free, refined sugar-free

Ingredients

For the chocolate

¾ cup coconut oil, melted

¾ cup raw cacao powder

¾ cup pure maple syrup

For the rocky road

½ cup almond butter (can substitute for nut butter of choice)

¼ cup raw hazelnuts

¼ cup raw almonds

¼ cup raw pistachios

¼ cup goji berries

¼ cup glacé cherries

¼ cup sulphur-free dried apricots

¼ cup toasted coconut flakes

Pinch of Himalayan sea salt

Method

Line a square baking tin with baking paper that's been lightly greased with coconut oil.

Make the chocolate sauce by whisking all the chocolate ingredients in a saucepan over a very low heat until well combined. Remove from heat.

Mix all the rocky road ingredients (except salt) into the saucepan and mix well to ensure all the chunks are coated with your chocolate.

Transfer the mixture to your lines baking tin and level out by banging the tin on your kitchen bench a couple of times. The mixture should be roughly mixed with gooey clumps of almond butter throughout.

Scatter a few extra ingredients over the top of the rocky road for decoration and colour, and sprinkle over the Himalayan sea salt.

Place in the freezer to harden for at least an hour or overnight. Remove from the freezer, carefully remove from the tin and slice with a hot sharp knife into square portions. Store in the fridge.

Sulphur is a naturally occurring chemical compound that is commonly used as a preservative in dried fruit. While considered safe for consumption, Courtenay recommends sourcing sulphur-free dried fruit for her recipe, as some people can be sensitive to it.

Mocha Caramel Slice

Leah Boston @simplyleahboston

This dessert is the love child of recipe developer Leah Boston's two favourite things: mocha donut holes and caramel slice. Because who wouldn't want to add caramel to a mocha donut, amiright?!

This recipe combines the rich notes of cacao and earthy tones of coffee with sweet, carmel-ey dates, which will make you a crowd favourite with your friends.

'These bars are definitely extra,' Leah laughs 'They're perfect for those over-the-top sweet cravings you sometimes just can't kill, or your best friend's birthday celebration.'

Chances are, you'll end up being everyone's best friend after rocking up to a party with a tray of these decadent treats.

Vegan, gluten-free, dairy-free, refined sugar-free

Ingredients

For the mocha base

½ cup gluten-free oats

¼ cup raw cacao

¾ cup raw almonds

⅓ cup unsulfured apricots

¼ cup coconut butter, melted

2 tablespoons maple syrup

3 tablespoons coconut milk

1 teaspoon vanilla bean powder

½ teaspoon cinnamon

Pinch of Himalayan sea salt

For the caramel

20 medjool dates, pitted and soaked

2 tablespoons coconut cream

Method

For the base, line a 9cm x 5cm (3.5" x 2") loaf pan with baking paper.

Add the oats, cacao and almonds to a food processor and pulse until combined.

Add apricots, coconut butter, maple syrup, coconut milk, vanilla, cinnamon and salt to food processor along with the oat mixture and pulse until a dough is created. Don't over blend here, the dough should hold its shape but still be a but chunky.

Remove the mixture from the blender and press evenly into the lined loaf pan. Place in the fridge while you make date caramel and chocolate layer.

Add all the ingredients for the caramel into your food processor and blend until a smooth paste forms. Be patient and continue to blend until it reaches a really smooth consistency. If your dates won't break down, you can add 1-2 tablespoons of warm water, but be careful to not add too much or your mixture will become too thin.

Spread your caramel on top of your mocha base and return to the fridge to set.

1 tablespoon almond butter

1 teaspoon vanilla bean powder

1 teaspoon cinnamon

For the chocolate layer

1 bar dark vegan chocolate (Leah recommends Eating Evolved or Loving Earth brands)

Break up your chocolate into chunks and place in a double boiler over medium heat. Stir continuously until chocolate is fully melted. Alternatively, you can place your chocolate in a heat-proof bowl and microwave in 30-second bursts, stirring in between until it's melted.

Allow the chocolate to cool for about 10 min before pouring over the caramel layer.

Place loan tin back in fridge or freezer to set for at least 2 hours.

Once completely set, slice and store in the fridge for up to a week, or in the freezer for 2 months.

Makes 9-12

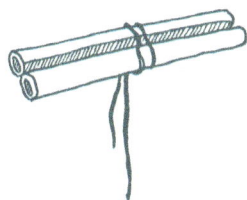

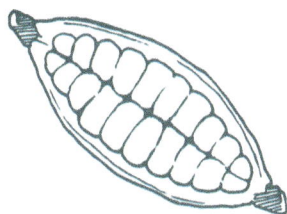

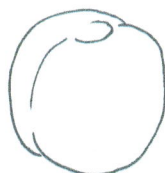

Jammy Blackberry Slice

Lauren Mariano @lm_nutrition

With an Italian background, dietitian Lauren Mariano grew up around food, cooking fresh pasta and minestrone with her Nonna on weekends. This saw cooking become a creative outlet, allowing her to experiment with ingredients and recipes to devise healthier versions of the dishes she grew up eating.

'This dish just popped into my head one day after I made some berry chia jam,' says Lauren. 'My Italian family is very sceptical about vegan food, so when they tasted this and loved it, I knew I was on to a good thing.'

Rather than being packed with added sugar, Lauren's homemade jam uses berries to add natural sweetness, antioxidants and vitamin C, which is great for immunity and skin health.

Don't feel like you have to stick to blackberries. Use whatever berries you have on hand, either fresh or frozen that have been thawed.

Vegan, gluten-free, dairy-free, refined sugar-free

Ingredients

For the base

½ cup of fresh dates

1 cup of almonds

¼ cup of coconut

1 tablespoon coconut oil, melted

For the blackberry jam layer

1½ cups of fresh blackberries

3 tablespoons chia seeds

1 tablespoon coconut oil, melted

Melted dark chocolate, to serve (optional)

Method

Mash the blackberries until pureed with a few little chunks. Stir through the chia seeds and melted coconut oil. Let sit for 15 minutes.

Blend all base ingredients in a food processor. Press the base mixture into a small pan, top with blackberry jam layer and drizzle with chocolate.

Place slice in the freezer for an hour and serve.

Makes 8 slices

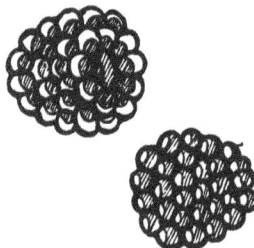

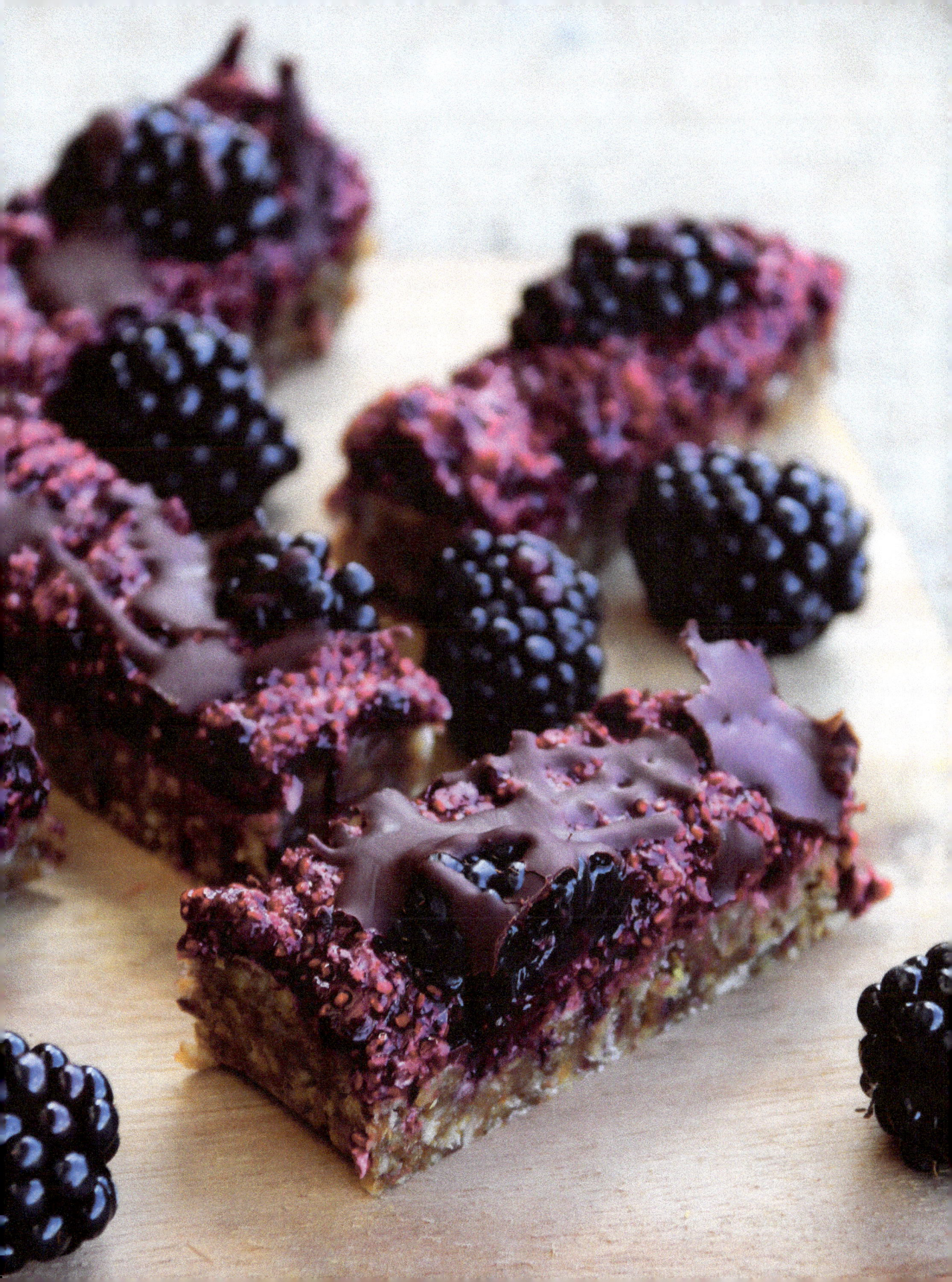

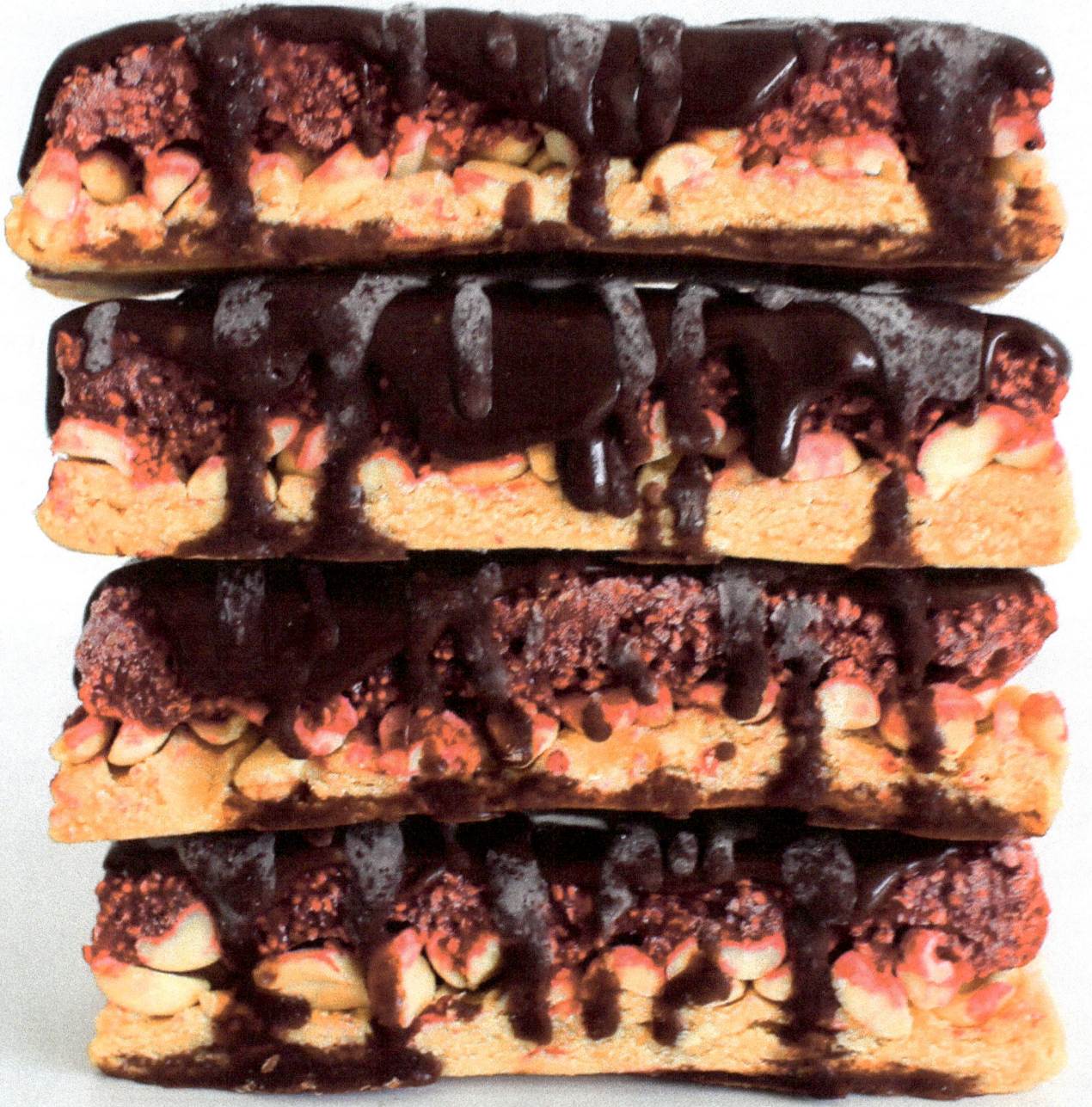

Raw Peanut Butter Jelly Bars

Cassidy Bates @healthiielife

She may be a little ray of sunshine now, but when she was younger Gold Coast vegan recipe creator Cassidy Bates had a dark secret. She hated peanut butter.

But don't worry, she's finally come around and has since joined our peanut butter cult, redeeming herself with these incredibly moorish peanut butter and jelly bars.

Making your own jam might seem like a nuisance, but this recipe is quick, simple and contains none of the added sugars that you find in store-bought versions. Chia seeds are a high-fibre addition to the jam and are what give it a thick, jelly-like consistency.

Vegan, gluten-free, dairy-free, refined sugar-free

Ingredients

For the base

1 cup peanut butter

½ cup rice malt syrup

½ cup coconut flour

¼ cup coconut oil

½ cup peanuts

For the jelly layer

1 cup of frozen or fresh raspberries

¼ cup chia seeds

For the chocolate layer

⅓ cup cocoa powder

¼ cup rice malt syrup

2 tablespoons coconut oil, melted

Method

To make the base, mix all the base ingredients (except peanuts) together until well combined.

Press the mixture evenly into a baking tray and sprinkle the peanuts on top. Press the nuts lightly into the base and set this in the freezer while you make the next layer.

To make the jelly layer, microwave the berries in a small bowl for 30-60 seconds. Add the chia seeds to the bowl and mash together with a fork until well combined.

Pour the jam mixture over your base layer and set back into the freezer for 2-4 hours.

For the chocolate layer, combine all the ingredients in a bowl and mix well.

Once your base and jam layer has been in the freezer for at least two hours, cut into rectangular bars.

Pour the chocolate over the top of each bar and set them back into the freezer for the chocolate to harden.

Makes 6 bars

Chai, Carrot And Olive Oil Cake

Olivia Kaplan @livinbondi

When she was younger, you could find Olivia Kaplan making jewellery, origami, knitting or sewing. Fast forward many years, and the Sydney-based nutritionist's creativity has manifested in another way: cooking. One of the things she loves most about this creative outlet is recreating favourite recipes from her childhood. First up was the humble carrot cake, which has received a modern tasty twist.

'Olive oil is one of my favourite ingredients - my inner Italian Nonna thinks olive oil will cure the world,' Olivia laughs. 'I've used it in this recipe in place of the usual butter or coconut oil. It's distinctive flavour compliments desserts and here it offers subtle savoury and nutty undertones to this cake.'

Vegetarian, gluten-free, dairy-free, refined sugar-free

Ingredients

200 grams (2 cups/7 oz) almond meal

1 tablespoon monk fruit sweetener

2 teaspoons baking powder

5 eggs

⅔ cup extra virgin olive oil

3 medium carrots, grated (about 280-300 grams (10 oz-11 oz)

1 cup walnuts, roughly chopped, plus extra to serve

1 teaspoon cinnamon, ground

1 teaspoon ginger, ground

2 teaspoons mixed spice

1 cup coconut yoghurt, or regular yoghurt, to serve

Fresh figs, to serve

Method

Preheat the oven to 180°C (350°F) and line a 20cm (10") baking tin with baking paper.

In a medium bowl combine almond meal, monk fruit and baking powder.

In another bowl, whisk eggs then stir in the olive oil. Gently fold in the grated carrot followed by the almond meal mixture. Stir in the walnuts.

Spread mixture into the lined baking tin and place in the oven for 40-50 minutes or until a skewer inserted comes out clean. Leave to cool in the tin before turning out.

To serve, spread over coconut yoghurt, place fresh figs on top and sprinkle over extra cinnamon.

Serves 10

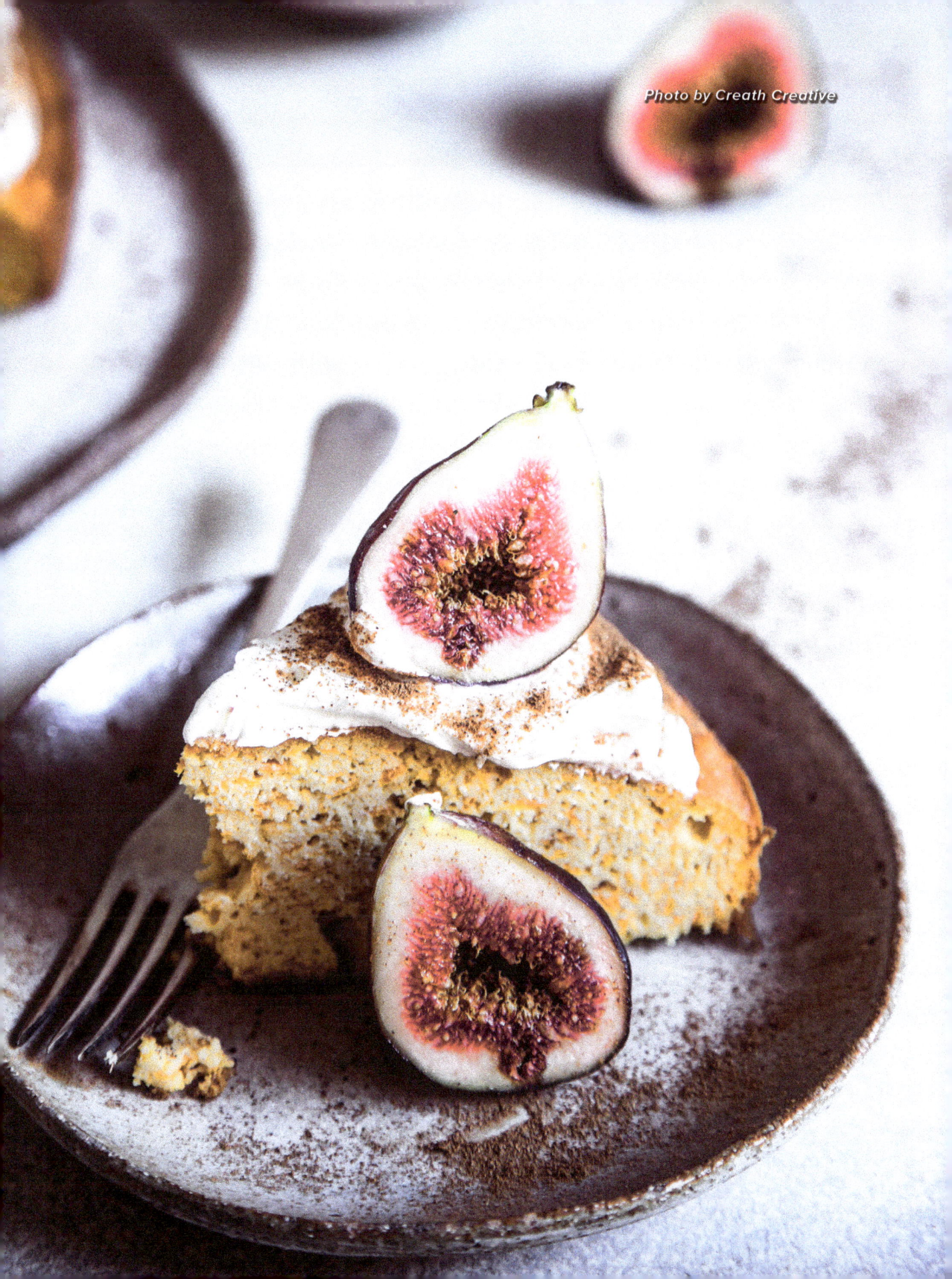

The Best Raw Vegan Carrot Cake

Gabriella O'Dea @nourishtheday

'I want to see our focus on nutrition turn towards giving our bodies the nutrients we need to thrive, instead of just calories and weight loss,' explains Adelaide-based dietitian Gabrielle O'Dea.

Based on this ethos, Gabby has created a nourishing take on the classic carrot cake, which allows you to enjoy a sweet treat while also giving yourself a good dose of healthy fats from the addition of nuts, and vitamin C from the fresh carrot.

Gabby recommends playing around with this recipe, adding in chopped dried figs, walnuts or candied ginger to make it your own. You can even skip making the frosting and roll them into balls for grab-and-go bliss balls.

Vegan, gluten-free, dairy-free, refined sugar-free

Ingredients

For the cake

1½ cups walnuts

¾ cup almonds

¾ cup shredded coconut

1 cup Medjool dates, pitted (around 10-11 dates)

1¾ cup grated carrot (about 2 medium)

2 teaspoons cinnamon

¼ teaspoons ground ginger

1 teaspoons vanilla extract

Pinch of salt

¼ cup sultanas (feel free to sub for other dried fruit)

Extra walnuts, to decorate

Method

You will need a decent quality food processor or high-speed blender for this recipe.

For the frosting, soak the cashews in boiling water for 30 minutes or more. Get this going while you make the rest of the cake.

Place the walnuts, almonds and coconut in a food processor or high-speed blender. Blend briefly on medium until broken up, crumbly and fine. Don't over-blend into a paste. Tip this into a large mixing bowl.

Add the dates to the processor or blender, dropping them in one by one with the motor running. This should form a paste-like consistency, but a few lumps are ok.

Add half the grated carrot and pulse briefly to break down a bit more and release a little juice.

Scoop this mix into your bowl with the ground nuts.

For the frosting

1¼ ups raw cashews

⅓ cup coconut cream (Gabby recommends Ayam brand)

Juice of 1 lime or ½ lemon

Finely grated zest of one lime/lemon

3-4 tablespoons maple syrup

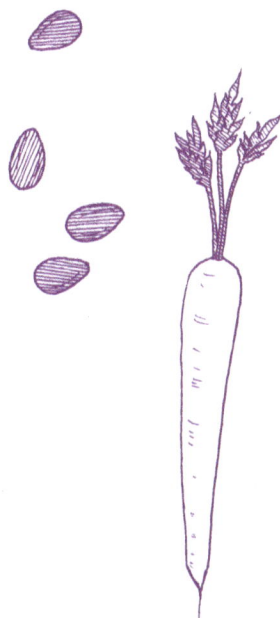

Add the remaining half of the carrot, spices, salt, vanilla and sultanas to the bowl and mix until well combined, mashing the carrot/date paste into the mix to form a dough. If it's looking a bit sticky, add extra almond meal or coconut flour. If it's very crumbly and not sticking together much, place half the mix back in the food processor and pulse a few times to release more of the natural carrot juices, then mix back into the rest of the mixture.

Press the dough into a small cake pan or loaf tin lined with baking paper. Place in the freezer to chill while you make the frosting.

To make the frosting, drain the cashews. Wash out your processor bowl and add the drained cashews along with juice and zest of the lemon/lime and maple syrup. Scoop the thick cream from the top of the coconut cream can (don't shake it first!) and add this to the blender.

Blend this all up until smooth and creamy. Taste and if it needs more sweetness, add more maple syrup, if it needs more tartness, add some more lime juice.

Remove the cake from the freezer and spread the frosting over the cake. Sprinkle with some extra walnuts and place back in the freezer for a few hours until set.

Remove from the freezer 30 minutes before serving. If you like slightly softer icing it can also be stored in the fridge.

Makes 1 small cake

Substitutes

If you don't have medjool dates you can substitute 1 cup of dried dates which have been soaked in boiling water for 10 minutes and drained.

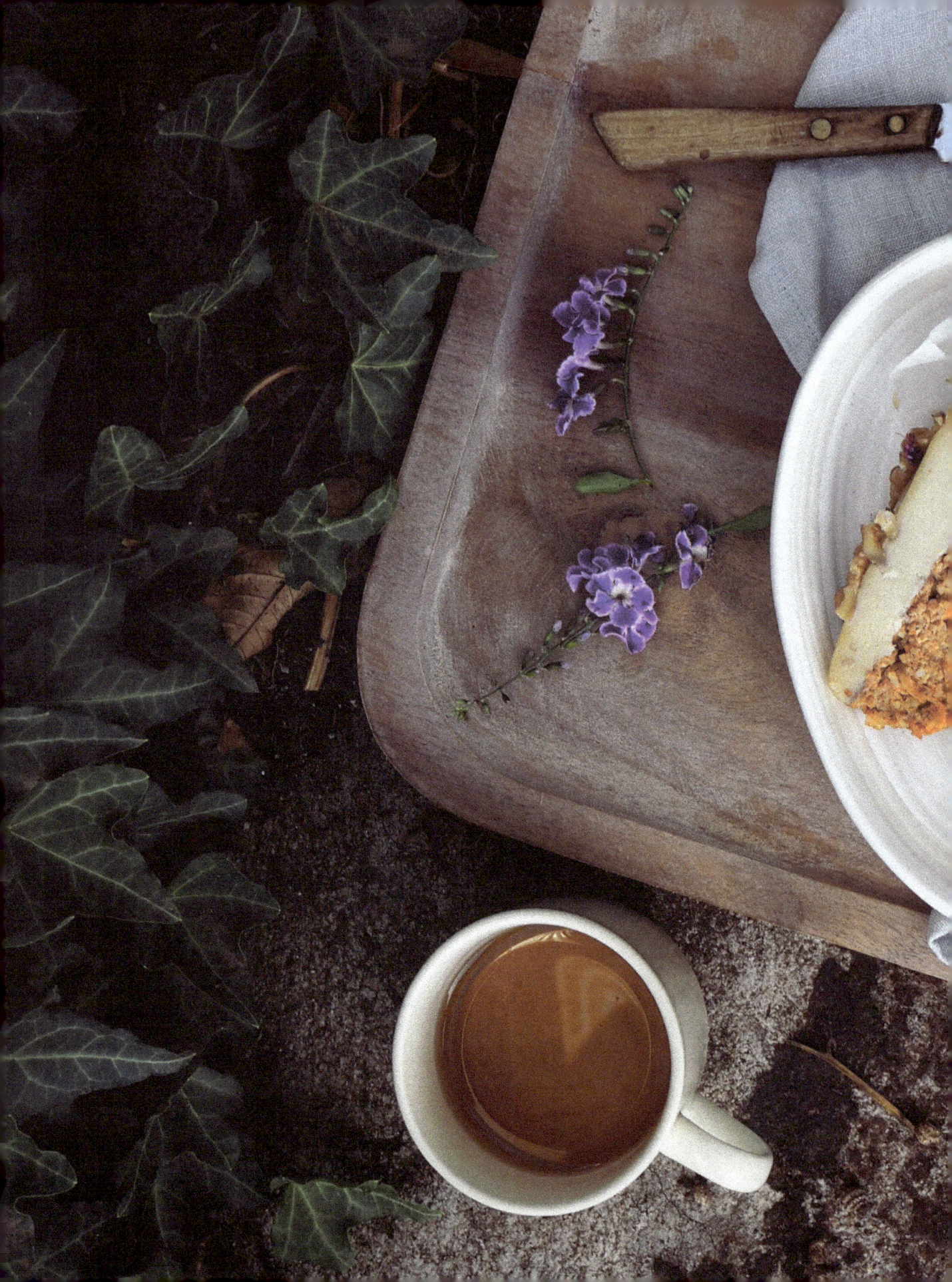

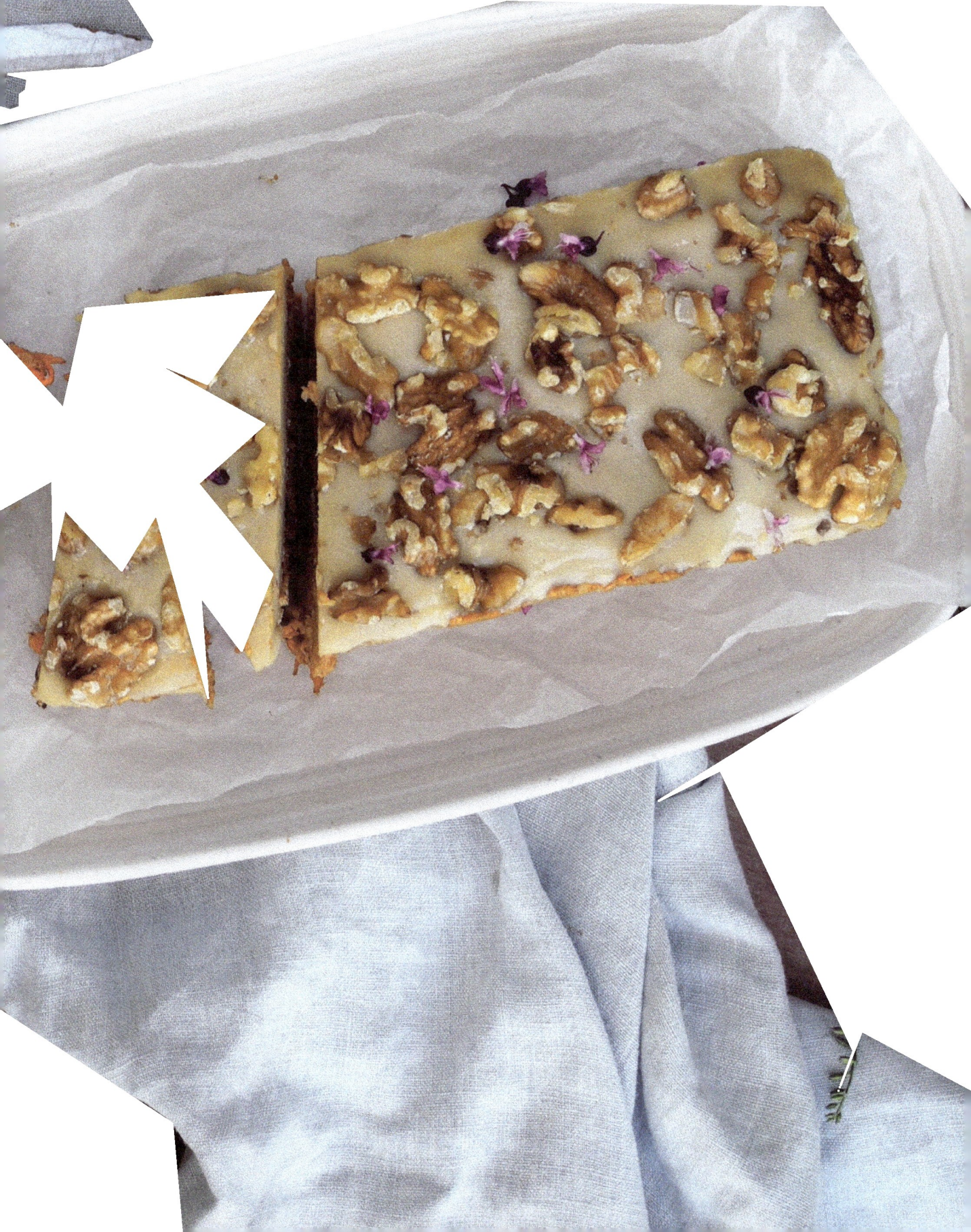

Baked Vanilla Cheesecake

Talida Voinea @hazel_and_cacao

During her pregnancy, health food blogger Talida Voinea found herself completely averse to the taste of coconut. After reaching out to her community, she found many women had experienced a similar thing, spurring her on to experiment in the kitchen.

The result was this cheesecake that, instead of using coconut, achieves a creamy, cheesecake-like consistency using cashews.

'I took up the challenge of making a cheesecake that people could enjoy even if they don't like coconut,' Talida says. 'And while this doesn't necessarily taste like a traditional cheesecake, it's incredibly delicious and much more nutrient dense!'

Vegan, gluten-free option, dairy-free, refined sugar-free

Ingredients

For the crust

1 cup oats (can sub for gluten-free if)

3 cups blanched almond meal

4 tablespoons grapeseed or sunflower oil

Pinch salt

4 tablespoons maple syrup

For the filling

1 cup cashews (soaked for 3-4 hours)

1 packet good quality organic silken tofu

6 tablespoons maple syrup

1 tablespoon nutritional yeast

1 tablespoon vanilla extract

1 teaspoon tahini

Fresh raspberries and pomegranate seeds, to serve

Method

Preheat your oven to 180°C (350°F).

For the crust, mix all the ingredients in a bowl with a spoon until slightly sticky and moist.

Press the mixture evenly on the base and sides of a lightly greased cake tin. Try to go as high up the sides as you can, as this will hold in the filling of the cake.

For the filling, add all the ingredients to a blender and blend until smooth.

Pour the filling over the base and bake for around 30- 40 minutes. Check whether the cake is cooked by shaking it from time to time. Remove from the oven once the filling had set and has a jelly-like consistency.

Allow the cake to cool completely, then decorate with raspberries and pomegranate seeds.

Serves 8-10

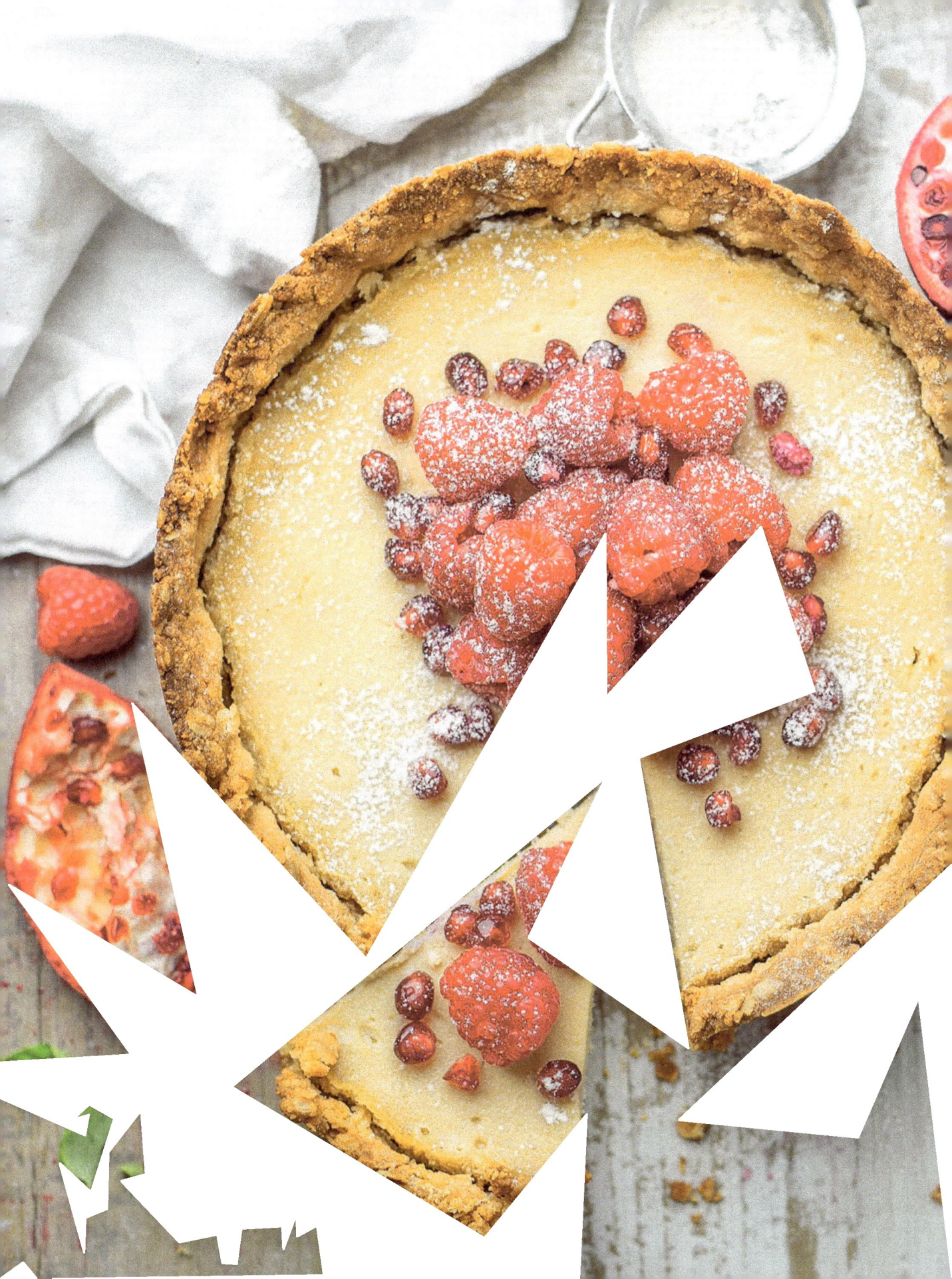

Brownie Base Raspberry Cheesecake

Zoe Lyons @wildblend

This brownie-bottom raspberry cheesecake combines two crowd favourites: gooey brownie and creamy cheesecake.

'Baked cheesecake was my mum's go-to dessert and a family favourite,' says Queensland recipe creator Zoe Lyons. 'And ever since I made my first dairy-free, cashew-based cheesecake, I was in love. I still think it's one of the most satisfying vegan treats.'

Zoe creates three different colours for her cheesecake, which she admits is a bit more work, but gives a lovely marbled pattern. This cake takes a little bit of love, but it's the perfect dessert to show someone how much they mean to you.

Vegan, gluten-free, dairy-free

Ingredients

For the brownie

½ cup non-dairy butter, melted

½ cup granulated sugar of choice

2 flax eggs (see note)

1 teaspoon vanilla extract

¾ teaspoon baking powder

¼ teaspoon sea salt

½ cup raw cocoa powder

¾ cup almond flour

For the cheesecake

2 cup raw cashews, soaked

⅓ cup coconut cream

2 tablespoons coconut oil

2 tablespoons maple syrup

½ teaspoon vanilla essence

Method

For the brownie base, preheat oven to 180°C (350°F) and line a 20cm (8") round baking tin with baking paper.

Prepare flax eggs in a small bowl and let rest for 5 minutes. Once flax eggs are ready, add all brownie ingredients to a large mixing bowl and whisk to combine until a smooth batter forms.

Pour batter into lined baking dish and bake on the middle rack for 25 minutes, or until toothpick comes out clean. The centre of the cake should feel firm and slightly springy to the touch.

Remove brownie base from oven and leave to cool completely before you add the cheesecake layer. Don't remove from baking dish.

For the cheesecake, combine all cheesecake ingredients (except frozen raspberries and pitaya powder) in a high-speed blender and process until smooth and creamy.

Divide mixture into three bowls and add different amounts of pitaya powder to each bowl. Whisk to combine. This is how you will create the marble effect. Feel free to skip this stage if you wish and simply combine all the cheesecake ingredients with the pitaya powder in the one bowl.

2 teaspoons pitaya powder

⅓ cup frozen raspberries

For the raspberry jelly

2 cups of fresh or frozen raspberries

1 teaspoon agar agar (or gelatine)

1 teaspoon maple syrup

1 teaspoon fresh lemon juice

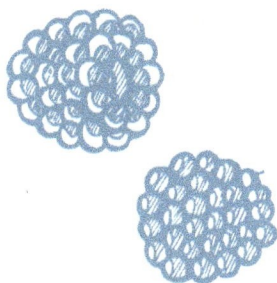

Pour cheesecake mixture on top of the brownie base. Alternate between different shades of pink (if using) for marble effect.

Stir in frozen raspberries and smooth top with a silicone spatula.

Cover and place in freezer for 4-6 hours or overnight.

For the raspberry jelly, heat the frozen raspberries, maple syrup and lemon juice in a small pot over medium heat until raspberries start to break down.

Once broken down, add agar to the pot, stir well and let soak for approximately 10 minutes. Then gently bring to the boil and let simmer for 5 minutes, stirring constantly. Set aside and allow to cool.

Once your cheesecake is fully frozen, pour the cooled raspberry jelly on top. It should set almost immediately.

Once the jelly is fully set, remove from the pan and serve.

Serves 8-10

To make your flax eggs, simply combine 2 tablespoons of flaxseed meal with 6 tablespoons water in a bowl and leave to soak for 5 minutes.

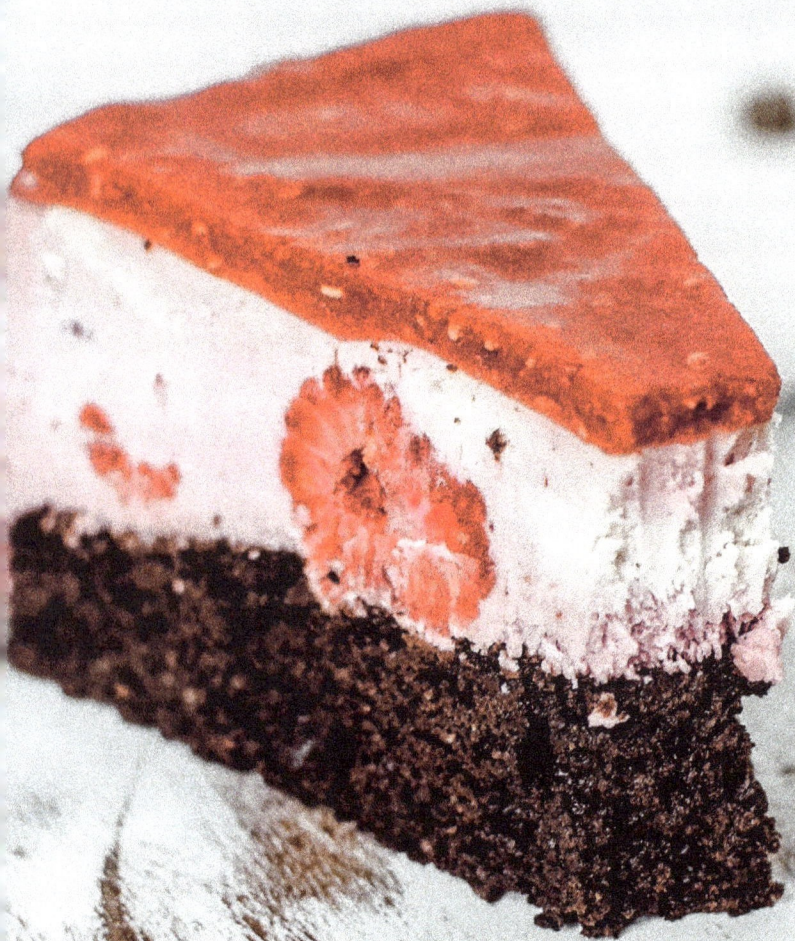

Brownie Base Raspberry
Cheesecake - Page 230

Lemon, Blueberry and Date Cake

Jessica Lirosi @jess_mycleantreats

Scroll through the Instagram of self-confessed Dessert Queen Jess Lirosi and you'll be greeted with an abundance of chocolate, nutella and caramel-flavoured treats. This zesty, elegant cake might diverge from her usual recipes, but we guarantee it's just as delicious.

'This cake isn't super indulgent or rich,' Jess says. 'The flavours are subtle and a little more sophisticated, so it's perfect for a beautiful high tea with friends.'

'I've always loved the ceremony of high tea. Sometimes we take food so seriously, and afternoon tea is an experience that gives you the chance to relax and enjoy the act of eating with friends and family.'

You heard the woman, get baking and stick your little pinky out!

Dairy-free

Ingredients

2 cups wholemeal flour

1 teaspoon cinnamon

Pinch of salt

2 teaspoon baking powder

½ cup rice malt syrup

½ cup coconut oil, melted

2 teaspoon lemon zest

¼ cup lemon juice

1 teaspoon vanilla essence

2 eggs

1 cup almond milk

1½ cup frozen blueberries, plus extra for serving

14 dates, finely chopped

Method

Preheat your oven to 160°C (325°F) and line a circular cake tin with baking paper.

In a large bowl combine the flour, salt, baking powder and cinnamon.

In a separate bowl, mix coconut oil, rice malt syrup, vanilla, lemon zest and lemon juice. Add one egg at a time and beat through mixture. Pour in milk and stir until well combined.

Make a well in the centre of the dry mixture and pour in the liquid ingredients, mixing until combined. Add the dates and blueberries and fold lightly until they are evenly distributed throughout the mixture batter. Transfer mixture to your lined cake tin.

Place the cake in the oven for 40 minutes, or until cooked through. Leave it to cool in the tin and then turn out onto a serving dish to serve. Top with extra blueberries.

Serves 8-10

Vegan Raspberry Jam Magnums

Zoe Lyons @wildblend

Austrian-born recipe developer Zoe Lyons believes that the 'wilder' we live the better - that being in sync with nature and connecting to our food is important for living a long and healthy life. This mantra is captured within this better-for-you, homemade version of a childhood favourite that contains none of the additives or preservatives of the original.

'Cooking from scratch is paramount. It keeps you from eating processed foods, which generally contain ingredients you'd never use at home, and I really just love the process,' she says.

'Our bodies are wild and our food should be the same! I'm a nature child and Wildblend represents this strong connection to anything untamed and natural.'

Vegan, gluten-free, dairy-free, refined sugar-free

Ingredients

For the cream filling

1 cup cashews, soaked

2 tablespoon maple syrup

⅓ cup pecan butter

⅓ cup coconut milk

For the jam

1 cup frozen raspberries

1 tablespoon maple syrup

1 tablespoon chia seeds

For the chocolate coating

1 cup dairy-free chocolate chips

2 tablespoons coconut oil

Method

For the cream filling, add all ingredients to a high-speed blender and process on high until smooth and creamy.

Fill your ice cream moulds half way (about 1 ½ tablespoons of cream in each mold) and placed them in the freezer while you make the jam.

For the jam, add frozen raspberries and maple syrup to a small saucepan and heat over medium heat until the raspberries start to break down. Add the chia seeds, stir until well until combined and turn off the heat. Set aside for 15 minutes or until cooled.

Once jam is completely cooled, add around 1 tablespoon of jam on top of the cream filling in each mould.

Once each ice cream mold has jam, place back in the freezer to set and cool down. Once set, top the jam layer with another 1 ½ tablespoons of the remaining cream and spread evenly with a spatula.

Set in freezer for 4 hours or overnight.

For the chocolate coating, melt chocolate chips with coconut oil in a double boiler.

De-mould your mangums and dip them in the chocolate. Drizzle with crushed pistachios or your favourite nuts and place back in the freezer until the chocolate is set.

Makes 4 magnums

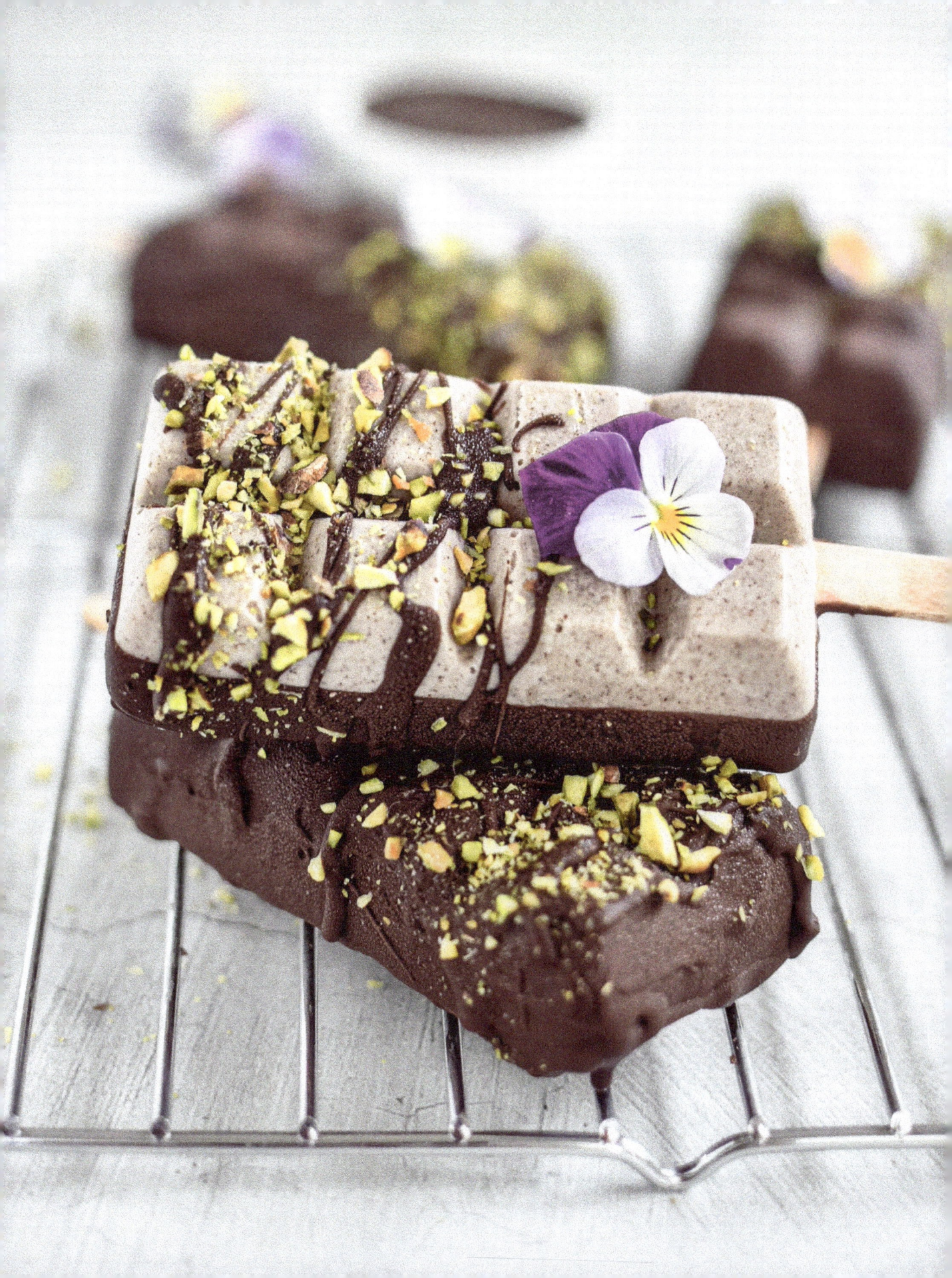

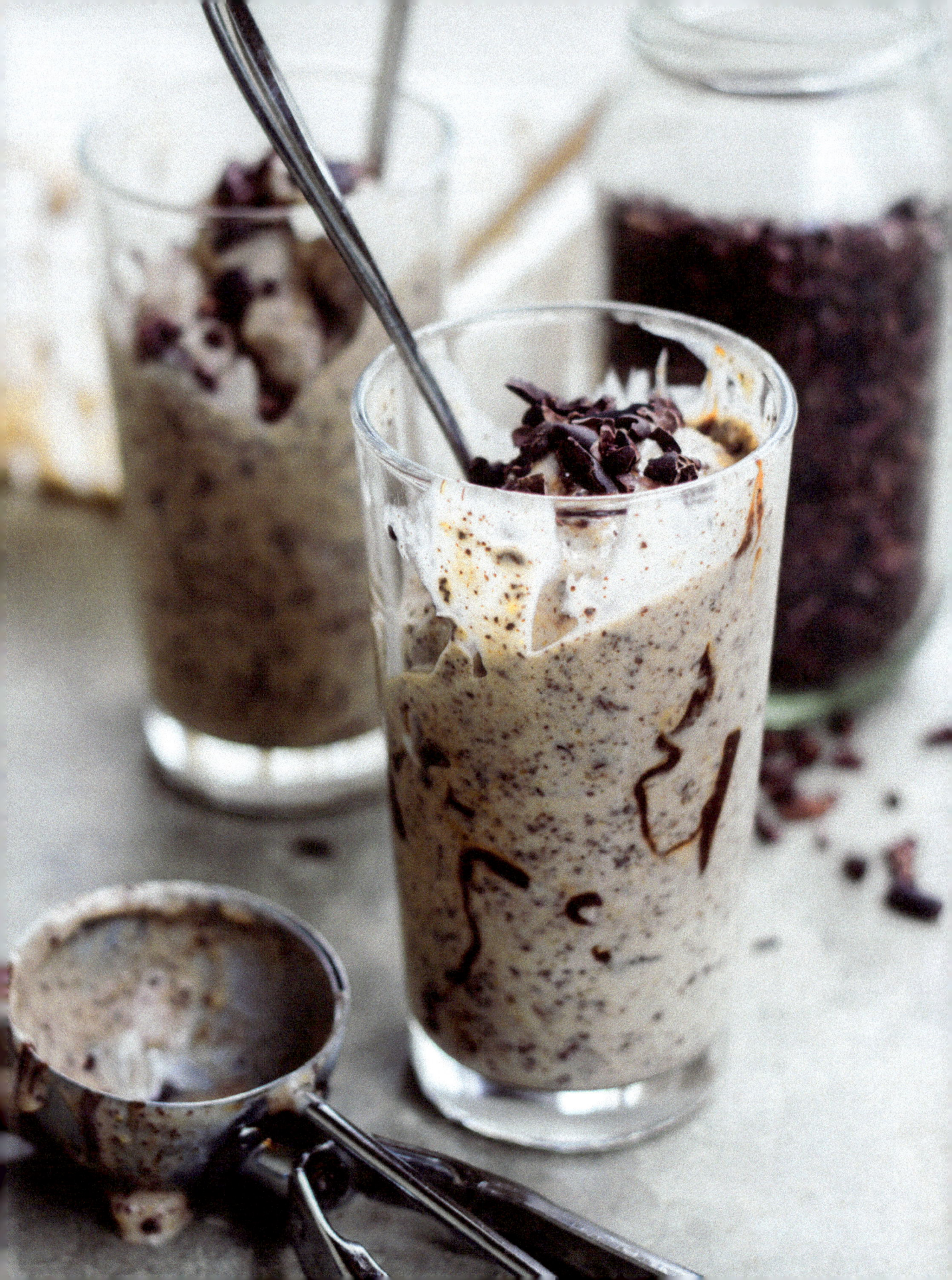

Peanut Butter Chocolate Chip Nice Cream

Phoebe Conway @Pheebsfoods

Chocolate, peanut butter and bananas. Has there ever been a more holy trinity of flavours? If there is, we're yet to discover it!

This dessert is a far cry from the ice cream covered in sprinkles that Phoebe Conway remembers from her childhood, but it satisfies her sweet tooth just as much.

After studying nutrition, Phoebe discovered her passion for creating healthier alternatives to her favourite foods, so naturally ice cream was on the list. She threw three of her favourite flavours into a blender and the result was one delicious frozen dessert.

Vegan option, vegetarian, gluten-free, refined sugar-free

Ingredients

4 frozen bananas

2 tablespoons peanut butter

1 tablespoon honey or maple syrup

1 teaspoon vanilla extract

½ cup milk kefir

1 dash of coconut milk

100 grams (3½ oz) dark chocolate

Method

Place the bananas, peanut butter, honey, vanilla, kefir and a dash of coconut milk into a high powered blender or food processor

Blend the mixture until thick and creamy, scraping down the sides of the processor as necessary and add a small amount of additional coconut milk if needed.

Roughly chop the dark chocolate and add it to the blender. Give it a pulse just to incorporate it, you don't want to break it up too much!

Spoon the mixture into a tub or bowl and place into the freezer to set until it's a bit firmer, around 30 minutes. You can skip this stage if you wish and serve immediately. Serve with extra peanut butter and melted chocolate drizzled on top.

Serves 2

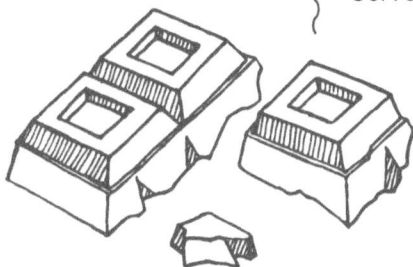

Metric Conversions

Approximate Equivalents - Weight	
Metric	**Imperial**
15 grams	½ ounce
30 grams	1 ounce
60 grams	2 ounces
90 grams	3 ounces
125 grams	4 ounces
155 grams	5 ounces
185 grams	6 ounces
220 grams	7 ounces
250 grams	8 ounces
280 grams	9 ounces
315 grams	10 ounces
345 grams	11 ounces
475 grams	12 ounces
410 grams	13 ounces
440 grams	14 ounces
470 grams	15 ounces
500 grams	16 ounces

Approximate Equivalents - Liquid Measures

Metric	Imperial
30 millilitres	1 fluid ounce
60 millilitres	2 fluid ounces
100 millilitres	3 fluid ounces
125 millilitres	4 fluid ounces
150 millilitres	5 fluid ounces
190 millilitres	6 fluid ounces
250 millilitres	8 fluid ounces
300 millilitres	10 fluid ounces
500 millilitres	16 fluid ounces
600 millilitres	20 fluid ounces
1000 millilitres	1¾ pints

Approximate Equivalents - Temperature

Metric	Imperial
120°C (Celcius)	250°F (Fahrenheit)
150°C (Celcius)	300°F (Fahrenheit)
160°C (Celcius)	325°F (Fahrenheit)
180°C (Celcius)	350°F (Fahrenheit)
190°C (Celcius)	375°F (Fahrenheit)
200°C (Celcius)	400°F (Fahrenheit)
220°C (Celcius)	425°F (Fahrenheit)
240°C (Celcius)	475°F (Fahrenheit)

Contributors

Aliza Strock

Ally Sheehan

Ami Shoesmith

Cassidy Bates

Chloe Munro

Courtenay Perks

Gabrielle O'Dea

Hannah Singleton

Jessica Lirosi

Jennifer Murrant

Jessica Thomson

Kat Nguyen-Thai

Kitch Catterall

Laura Ford

Lauren Mariano

Leah Boston

Leanne Ward

Liz Miu

Melanie Lionello

Michelle Chen

Nadia Felsche

Olivia Kaplan

Phoebe Conway

Sabrina Lu

Sally O'Neil

Sami Bloom

Sarah Bell

Sarah Cooper

Sarah Holloway

Sasha Back

Stephanie Geddes

Talida Voinea

Tarni Deutsher

Tully Humphrey

Zoe Lyons

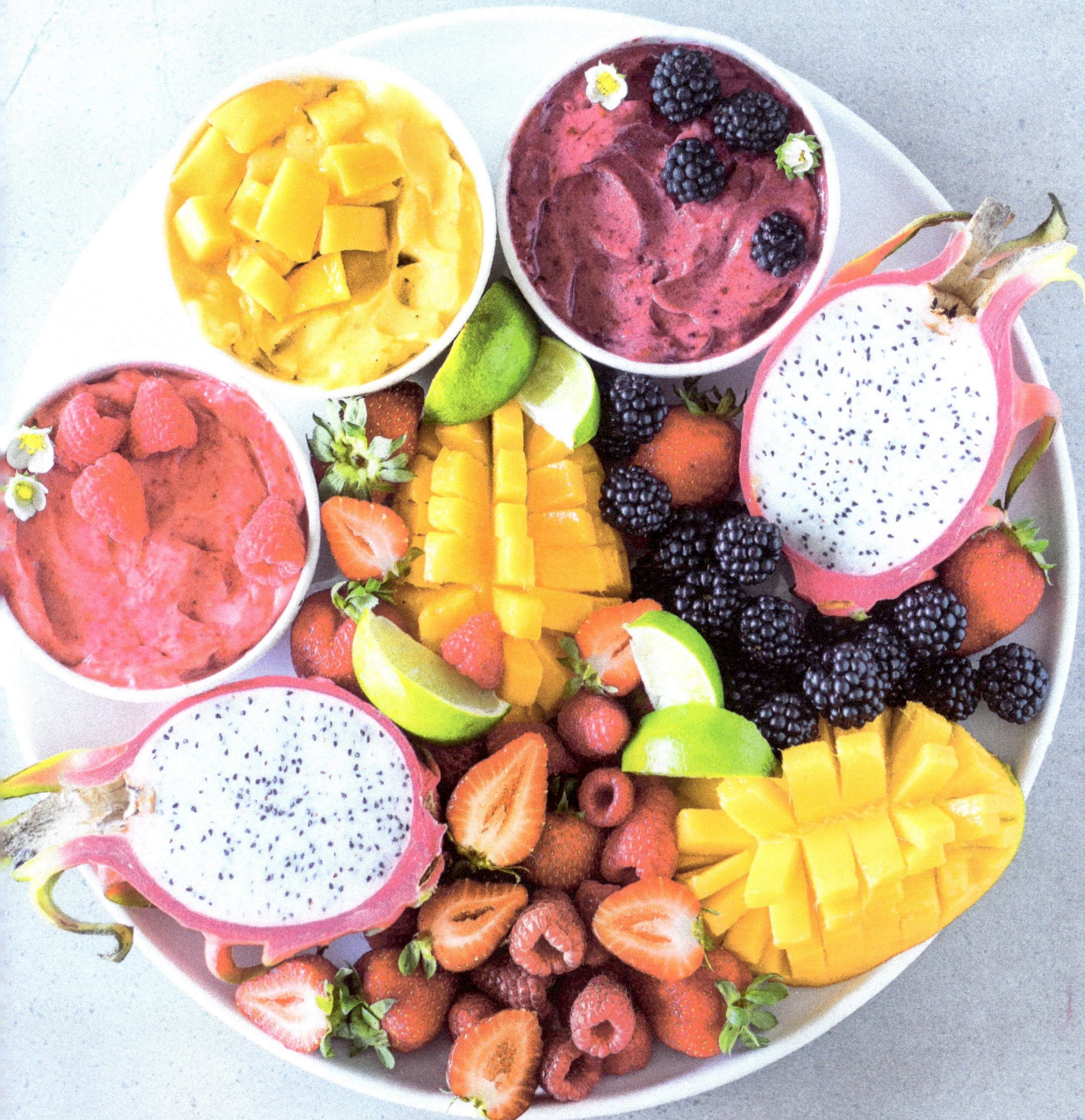

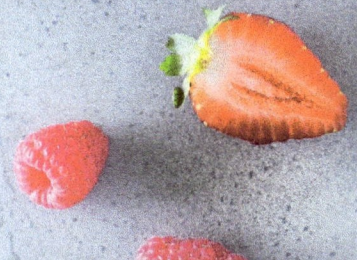

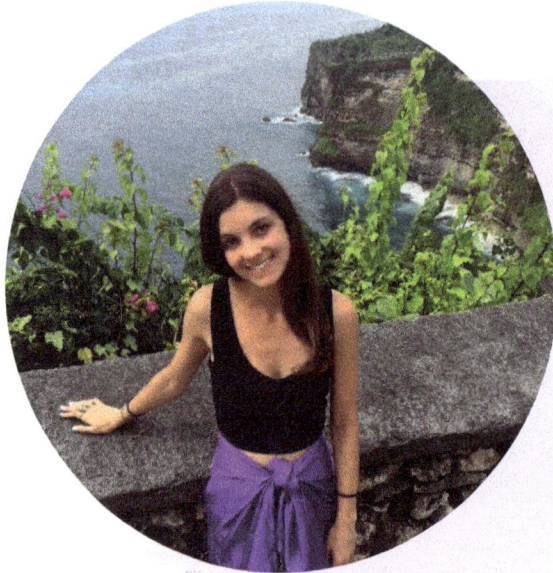

About the Author

Born and raised in Melbourne, Amelia Mills is a former journalist who began her career writing for cultural authorities, including Broadsheet and Mamamia. After writing for a newspaper in regional NSW focusing on the areas of mental health, culture, education and multiculturalism, she returned home to begin her career as a marketer and content creator.

Her passion for health, wellness and cooking, coupled with her dedication to writing and interest in mental health, has resulted in her first book, Recipes for Life. After years of struggling with her relationship with food, Amelia sought to create a resource that helps people view food, not as the enemy, but as a vehicle for self-love and compassion. With recipes collected from like-minded Australian women in the health and wellness industry.

Recipes For Life

Copyright © 2019 by Amelia Mills

All recipes and corresponding photography has been provided by contributors.
Cover photo by Creath Creative
ISBN: 9780648708704 (paperback)

Instagram: @recipesforlifecookbook
Website: www.recipesforlifecookbook.com

www.ingramcontent.com/pod-product-compliance
Lightning Source LLC
Chambersburg PA
CBHW051558030426
42334CB00031B/3256